Psychology Revivals

Parent–Baby Attachment in Premature Infants

Originally published in 1983, in the two decades prior to publication, specialised neonatal units for the treatment of sick or preterm babies had been set up in most major neonatal centres. In the early years these units did little to prevent separation of parents and babies and evidence accumulated of the ill effects of this situation. In addition, we had gradually become aware of the difficulties of building a relationship with a sick or immature baby even under more ideal circumstances.

This book, in a series of authoritative review chapters, sets out to describe the process by which social relationships develop after birth and the ways in which this process may be distorted by separation, the condition of the baby or by the process of medical treatment. Experienced practitioners describe practical steps which may be taken to support parents and foster their relationship with their babies in treatment situations. The final section of the book examines the organisation of neonatal care in a number of widely different settings and indicates that diverse approaches may be successful in achieving the same ends.

Parent–Baby Attachment in Premature Infants

Edited by
J.A. Davis, M.P.M. Richards
and N.R.C. Roberton

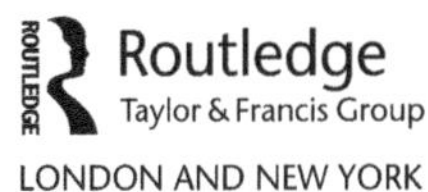

LONDON AND NEW YORK

First published in 1983
by Croom Helm Ltd

This edition first published in 2015 by Routledge
27 Church Road, Hove BN3 2FA

and by Routledge
711 Third Avenue, New York, NY 10017

Routledge is an imprint of the Taylor & Francis Group, an informa business

Publisher's Note
The publisher has gone to great lengths to ensure the quality of this reprint but points out that some imperfections in the original copies may be apparent.

Disclaimer
The publisher has made every effort to trace copyright holders and welcomes correspondence from those they have been unable to contact.

A Library of Congress record exists under ISBN: 031259657X

ISBN: 978-1-138-81228-4 (hbk)
ISBN: 978-1-315-74889-4 (ebk)
ISBN: 978-1-138-81229-1 (pbk)

PARENT-BABY ATTACHMENT IN PREMATURE INFANTS

EDITED BY DAVIS
RICHARDS & ROBERTON

CROOM HELM London & Canberra
ST. MARTIN'S PRESS New York

Croom Helm Ltd, Provident House, Burrell Row,
Beckenham, Kent BR3 1AT

Croom Helm Australia, PO Box 391, Manuka,
Act 2603, Australia

British Library Cataloguing in Publication Data

Parent-baby attachment in premature infants.
1. Mother and child 2. Infants
I. Davis, J.A. II. Richards, M.P.M.
III. Roberton, N.R.C.
155.4'222 BF723.2

ISBN 0-7099-0817-2

 For information, write:
St. Martin's Press, Inc., 175 Fifth Avenue, New York, NY 10010
Printed in Great Britain
First published in the United States of America in 1983

Library of Congress Cataloging in Publication Data
Main entry under title:

Parent-baby attachment in premature infants.

Includes bibliographical references and index.
1. Infants (Premature) – Family relationships.
2. Parent and child. 3. Neonatal intensive care –
Psychological aspects. I. Davis, John A., 1923-
II. Richards, M.P.M. (Martin P.M.)
III. Roberton, N.R.C. [DNLM: 1. Infant, Premature.
2. Intensive care units, Neonatal. 3. Parent-child
relations. 4. Object attachment. WS 105.5.F2 P2269]
RJ250.P37 1984 618.92'011'019 83-40171
ISBN 0-312-59657-X (St. Martin's Press)

CONTENTS

PREFACE

In 1978 the monograph *Separation and Special Care Baby Units*[1] drew attention to the fact that many aspects of neonatal unit care then current were open to question. In particular the widespread beliefs that such units could do no harm, causing no hazards or problems for the babies in them or their parents, and that admitting a large proportion of all newborn babies to them was largely responsible for the fall in neonatal mortality and morbidity over the preceding decade, were scrutinised and found wanting.

In the subsequent years, considerable modification in the practices of perinatal care has reduced the number of babies admitted into neonatal units and improved the lot of parents of newborn babies for whom neonatal intensive care is indicated, not to say life-saving. Yet, many problems remain; too many babies are *still* admitted to neonatal units throughout the world. In many of the units facilities for the parents to visit and the understanding of parental problems leave a lot to be desired.

This book has been conceived in an attempt to provide a practical manual for those trying to improve these aspects of care for low birthweight and sick babies. The first section provides the background information about the development of neonatal care, and its subsequent problems, and also about parent-baby attachment. We have then tried to provide two practical 'cook book' sections, the first on how specific problems are handled by professionals experienced in neonatal care, and the second comprising descriptions of how a number of different neonatal units are run. We hope that, by building up on these models, all readers will be able to provide a steadily improving service not only for the sick, low birthweight infant who must always be their major preoccupation, but also for his parents, who in the past have been neglected to a greater or lesser extent.

Reference

1. Brimblecombe, F. S. W., Richards, M. P. M., and Roberton, N. R. C. (1978). *Separation and Special Care Baby Units*. London, Spastics International Medical Publications/Heinemann Medical Books.

CONTRIBUTORS

Harry Bard, MD, Professor of Pediatrics and Director of Perinatology, Hôpital Sainte-Justine, 3175 Chemin Ste-Catherine, Montreal, Quebec, Canada H3T 1C5.

J. D. Baum, MA, MSc, MD, FRCP, DCH, Clinical Reader and Honorary Consultant in Paediatrics, John Radcliffe Hospital, Headington, Oxford OX3 9DU, UK.

Helen Bender, BA, Dip ICP (London), Principal Child Psychotherapist, Department of Child Psychiatry, The London Hospital, London E1, UK.

Jean Boxall, MA, SRN, SCM, Neonatal Unit, Royal Devon and Exeter Hospital (Heavitree), Exeter, Devon, UK.

F. S. W. Brimblecombe, CBE, MD, FRCP, Honorary Professor of Child Health, University of Exeter, and Honorary Consultant Paediatrician, Royal Devon and Exeter Hospital, Exeter, Devon, UK.

L. Joseph Butterfield, MD, The Family Care Program, The St Luke's Hospital/The Children's Hospital Perinatal Program, Department of Perinatology, The Children's Hospital, Denver, Colorado, USA.

Perry M. Butterfield, MA, The Family Care Program, The St Luke's Hospital/The Children's Hospital Perinatal Program, Department of Perinatology, The Children's Hospital, Denver, Colorado, USA.

D. M. Campbell, BScN, MA, PhD, Division of Community Health Science, Faculty of Medicine, University of Calgary, Calgary, Alberta, Canada.

D. P. Davies, BSc, MD, FRCP, DCH, DObst, Professor of Paediatrics, University of Hong Kong; former Senior Lecturer, University of Leicester Medical School and Neonatal Unit, Leicester Royal Infirmary Maternity Hospital, Leicester, UK.

John A. Davis, MA, MB, MSc, FRCP, Professor, University Department of Paediatrics, Addenbrooke's Hospital, Hills Road, Cambridge, CB2 2QQ, UK.

C. M. de Cates, BSc, MB, MRCP, Neonatal Unit, Maternity Hospital, Mill Road, Cambridge, UK.

Peter de Chateau, MD, Associate Professor, Head of Neonatal Division, Karolinska Hospital, Karolinska Institute, Box 60500, S-104 10 Stockholm, Sweden.

F. M. Derbyshire, SRN, SCM, RSCN, Nursing Officer, Neonatal Unit,

Leicester Royal Infirmary Maternity Hospital, Leicester, UK.

Chloe Fisher, SRN, SCM, MTD, Nursing Officer, Community Midwives, University Department of Paediatrics, John Radcliffe Hospital, Headington, Oxford OX3 9DU, UK.

Gillian C. Forrest, MB, BS, MRCPsych. MRCGP, Consultant Child Psychiatrist, The Park Hospital for Children, Oxford, UK.

G. M. Gandy, MD, DCH, Neonatal Unit, Cambridge Maternity Hospital, Cambridge,UK.

Donald H. Garrow, BM, FRCP, Consultant Paediatrician, High Wycombe and Amersham General Hospitals, Bucks., UK.

Edward Goldson, MD, The Family Care Program, The St Luke's Hospital/The Children's Hospital Perinatal Program, Department of Perinatology, The Children's Hospital, Denver, Colorado, USA.

Joanna T. Hawthorne Amick, MA, PhD, 5802 S. Blackstone Avenue, Chicago, Illinois 60637, USA; formerly of The Child Care and Development Group, University of Cambridge, UK.

Nicola C. S. Jaques, MSc, BPhil, Department of Social Administration and Social Work, University of Exeter, Exeter, UK.

R. A. K. Jones, MD, MRCP, Senior Registrar in Pediatrics, Norfolk and Norwich Hospital, Norwich, UK.

John Kennel, MD, Department of Pediatrics, Case Western Reserve University, Cleveland, Ohio 44106, USA.

Marshall Klaus, MD, Department of Pediatrics/Human Development, Michigan State University, East Lansing, Michigan 48824, USA.

Sheldon B. Korones, MD, Professor of Pediatrics, University of Tennessee, Center for the Health Sciences, and Director of Newborn Center, E. H. Crump Women's Hospital and Perinatal Center, Memphis, Tennessee, USA.

Francine Lefebvre. MD, Assistant Professor of Paediatrics, University of Montreal, in charge of Neonatal Follow-up Clinic, Hôpital Sainte-Justine, 3175 Chemin Ste-Catherine, Montreal, Quebec, Canada H3T 1C5.

Martin P. M. Richards, MA, PhD, Child Care and Development Group, University of Cambridge, Free School Lane, Cambridge, UK.

N. R. Clifford Roberton, MA, MB, FRCP, Consultant Paediatrician, Addenbrooke's Hospital, Hills Road, Cambridge CB2 2QQ, UK.

Roberta Siegel, MSW, Family Care Program, The St Luke's Hospital/ The Children's Hospital Perinatal Program, Department of Perinatology, The Children's Hospital, Denver, Colorado, USA.

Alison Swan-Parente, BA, Dip ICP (London), Psychotherapist, The Women's Therapy Centre, London, UK.

Contributors

Jorge Torres Pereyra, MD, Assistant Professor of Paediatrics, Catholic University of Chile, Santiago, Chile.

Samuel Wayburne, MB, BCh, FRCP, DCH, Department of Paediatrics, Baragwanath Hospital and the University of the Witwatersrand, Johannesburg, Republic of South Africa.

Chris Whitby, SRN, SCM, Nursing Officer, Neonatal Unit, Cambridge Maternity Hospital, Cambridge, UK.

Part One

THEORETICAL BACKGROUND

1 PARENT-CHILD RELATIONSHIPS: SOME GENERAL CONSIDERATIONS

Martin P. M. Richards

Introduction

The aim of this book is to improve the services that are designed to care for pre-term and other sick babies and their families. In particular, we focus on the relationship of parent[1] and child, its potential vulnerability and the ways in which it may be fostered and supported. Our concern is both with the elimination of medical practices and hospital routines that may distort or inhibit the initial phases of parental relationships and with the development of procedures that may positively encourage their growth and provide good experiences for mother, father and other family members. To have any chance of success, a programme designed to support parenthood must be based on a clear understanding of the nature of relationships between parents and children, their growth and development and the factors that may damage or enhance them. To claim that we have such a full understanding would be overoptimistic, if not a little arrogant. But I believe that some of the broad principles are reasonably clear and it will be these that I shall describe in this chapter.

In the past decade the discussion of parent-child relationships in the neonatal period has been dominated by the concept of 'Bonding'. This notion was originally proposed by the American paediatricians Marshall Klaus and John Kennell[2]. From their observations of the unsatisfactory mother-infant relationships that they saw after a period of separation caused by the admission of the baby to a neonatal unit or simply unnecessary limitation of mother-infant contact through maternity hospital routines, they suggested that there may be a sensitive period in which a mother is especially ready to form a good relationship with her baby. If separation keeps the two apart during this time, which they hypothesised lasts a day or so, they thought a permanently damaged relationship might ensue. This dramatic proposal became accepted very widely, though uncritically, and has done much to focus attention on some of the undesirable aspects of hospital rountines for parents and children. While the idea that a mother's relationship to her baby might be particularly sensitive to separation at birth was not a new one (see

Chapter 2), it had not been stated in quite such stark terms in recent times.

The wide acceptance of the idea of bonding also reflected a growing questioning from both parents and some professionals about the ways in which hospital care seemed to disrupt patients' social relationships. Already there were examples where such questioning had led to improvements in practice; for instance, the acceptance of fathers in the delivery room, the provision for parents to stay with their sick children in hospital, the encouragement of breast feeding and a general relaxation of rigid routines in lying-in wards. Given these changes, it was not surprising that attention was turned to neonatal units (NNUs) and the separation of parents and children that they might bring about. The idea of bonding provided a convenient rallying point for those who wished to improve things for parents and their infants in NNUs. It is unlikely to be an accident that the interest in bonding arose at a time when this form of neonatal care was developing very rapidly and an increasing proportion of babies were being admitted to these units[3] (see also Chapter 2).

However, the notion of bonding has not been without its critics.[4-8] As a way of organising the discussion in this chapter I shall first deal with some of the objections to it. Though I believe that the evidence for the existence of a process of bonding is unsatisfactory, there is no reason to assume that separation of parent and child at birth is of no consequence. The concept was simply one attempt to unify a series of observations about the effects of the neonatal separation of mother and child. In putting it forward Klaus and Kennell provided a great stimulus for further research as well as opening up the discussion about the needs of parents and their babies in neonatal units. More recent research may have shown the concept to be over-simple, but it has also demonstrated the vulnerability of social relations in the neonatal period to interference. It is this broader view of growing parent-infant relationships that will form the subject of the final part of the chapter.

Some Criticisms of the Concept of Bonding

As originally proposed by Klaus and Kennell[2], the support for the concept of bonding came partly by analogy with the behaviour of certain animals. They described observations on sheep and goats which were interpreted as evidence for a brief sensitive period in which a mother learnt the specific characteristics of her kid or lamb. If separation occurred during this sensitive period, the offspring might be permanently rejected.[9]

The main problem about using the analogy between the behaviour of sheep and goats and our own species is that parental behaviour is organised in a quite different way in each case and any similarity is likely to be quite coincidental. Sheep and goats live in herds and their young move around with the group almost immediately they are born. Breeding takes place at a specific season. This means that at certain times of the year there are likely to be a large number of lactating females and of young in the herd. Selection seems to favour a system whereby a mother suckles only her own young. While young are apparently ready to approach any mother, the mothers are selective and only allow their own offspring to feed from them. In order for them to achieve this selectivity they must be able to recognise their own young from birth, hence the need for a system of rapid learning of the individual characteristics and for rejecting 'alien' young.

Our own species organises social life and reproduction in quite a different way. As most human generations were passsed in hunting and gathering, it is in that kind of society that our reproductive patterns developed. The evidence suggests that hunter-gatherer groups were small and that births were widely spaced – perhaps by four years if we take the example of surviving hunter-gatherers like the !Kung San.[10] Thus at any time there are unlikely to be more than a couple of newborns in the group so that questions of confusion in identification do not arise, especially as our offspring take many months to develop independent mobility. Furthermore, human fetuses are large and relatively difficult to deliver, so that childbirth was probably the major cause of adult female mortality. If a mother died but the infant survived it would be most maladaptive if the offspring were rejected by other adults.[11] Short of a maternal death, a mother might be unable to cope with her baby for some time after delivery; again it would not be advantageous for her to reject her baby permanently after this kind of experience.

It is difficult to think of a plausible reason why our species might have developed a brief sensitive period for the formation of parental relationships. All speculation seems to run in the opposite direction and to suggest that the optimal system would be one in which a mother (or other adult) would build the social relationship at a time and pace which could vary with the particular circumstances. Indeed, the great variety of social arrangements for birth and the neonatal period that may be found around the world is a testament to the adaptability of human behaviour.

The second general point of criticism of the 'bonding' concept concerns the process by which a sensitive period – supposing one existed – was produced and then brought to an end. We have no independent evidence that there is such a period and we cannot observe or measure it directly. It is simply a concept postulated to account for the observations made in some of the studies of the consequences of early separation. There are many psychological phenomena that lack any kind of satisfactory explanation. But the bonding concept simply describes a state of affairs – that relationships appear to be inhibited if separation occurs – and it provides no account of why this should be or how such a process occurs. It also, of course, fails to account for cases where good parental relationships arise despite separation after birth and those, for instance, that may form between infants and step or adoptive parents.

Another difficulty with the bonding concept is that it ignores the general human concern for the meaning and interpretation of events and the point that individuals may react to the same external event in widely differing ways. In this sense universal laws may only be found at a level of generality that makes them of little practical utility. Separation at birth may well influence a parent in a number of ways depending on the circumstances and the way in which these are seen by those involved. Consider two hypothetical mothers: the first has just given birth to a healthy baby; her labour was relatively easy, the mother had prepared herself well; and, as she had planned, she was able to avoid all drugs except some gas and oxygen. Immediately the cord was cut, her baby was removed for bathing, weighing, etc., because this was the policy of the hospital. Despite the mother's protests and those of her husband who was with her, they were unable to see or hold the baby for 40 minutes until they were all reunited in the post-natal ward. Even then her husband was only allowed to stay for a few minutes as it was now late evening and it was felt he would disturb the other patients if he remained in the ward. During the pregnancy this couple had read widely about childbirth and talked to other couples. They were familiar with the concept of bonding and one of the reasons why they felt it was important to avoid drugs in labour was that they believed that these might blunt the mother's feelings and make it difficult for her to bond to the baby.

Our second mother had a rather different view of childbirth and medical care. She was only too happy to let the doctors and midwives take over and manage the delivery. Her labour was induced and accelerated and she was given Pethidine but despite the oxytocin she had a rather long labour. She also had an epidural anaesthetic and the baby was eventually born by forceps. Beyond a little bruising from the manner of the delivery, the baby was in good shape. But this hospital had a rule that 'forceps babies' should go to the special care unit for a period of observation. As with the previous mother, the birth occurred in the evening and the mother was very sleepy and rather confused after the delivery. She was content to sleep it off having been told that she would see her baby before breakfast. This mother did not hold her baby for eight hours after delivery.

Would we expect 'separation' to influence these two mothers in similar ways? It is clear that we must consider the experience of separation as it is perceived by each parent. We need a theory that can embody both the general assumptions of the society in which they live and the individual's particular beliefs. In our own society the issue of control seems to be central for many parents and the extent to which a mother feels in charge at her delivery may be of vital importance (see below).

Here we might note that the use of the word bonding seems to have originated with Winnicott[12]. But when he referred to the growth of the relationships between mother and baby with this term he clearly had something rather different in mind than the way the term has come to be used in recent writing on early separation. Winnicott saw the process as quintessential to humans, involving complex and changing feelings on both sides, in contrast to the static and rather mechanical view that seems to be behind some of the recent work.

The final general point I shall raise about the bonding concept is that it incorporates the idea that a single event – separation – can have long-term or even permanent effects on the mother-child relationship and the development of the child.

Human (and other) evolution is about means and not ends. The developmental process is one that is well 'buffered' against the changes and chance of our fleeting world so that children growing up in varied circumstances and situations all have a reasonable chance of reaching a satisfactory adulthood. This implies that the developmental process can be self-correcting. The model used by the great developmental biologist C. H. Waddington[13] to illustrate this process was a three-dimensional map of the Alps. The developmental organism was likened to a marble rolling down a valley. Periodically the marble will encounter some irregularity in the floor of the valley which makes it run up the side for a short distance. But, unless it hits a major obstacle which knocks it hard enough to go right over the dividing ridge into the neighbouring valley, the marble will pass down the valley until it reaches its mouth. The case of an obstacle sufficiently large to push it over into the next valley can be likened to major developmental catastrophies that have such a drastic effect on the system that self-correction can never be complete. Examples here would include the major genetic abnormalities which set the developmental process off down a new (and wrong) valley, like Down's Syndrome or massive brain damage that produces permanent spasticity.

The important point in this view of development is that there are great powers of recovery from a single disruptive event. Permanent disability is usually the result of both damaging events and a poor environment that does not facilitate recovery. It is interesting that we have a strong tendency to overestimate the extent to which single untoward events have permanent effects and to believe that development is an inevitable and unchangeable process.[14] Several examples can be cited of what is usually seen as 'unexpected' powers of recovery from early insult.

Ten years ago it was considered that germinal layer and intraventricular haemorrhage in low birthweight babies was generally fatal and that any survivors would have serious neurological handicaps. However, the use of computerised tomography[15] and ultrasound[16] for examination of the heads of these babies has shown that such bleeds are relatively common. In many cases they do not seem to produce symptoms in the neonatal period and they may be associated with normal development on follow-up.[17,18] Similar evidence of developmental plasticity comes from registers of children with cerebral palsy. A study in Western Australia found a significant number of children who showed a change from one cerebral palsy diagnostic category to another or from a cerebral palsy syndrome to a non-cerebral palsy syndrome in the first five years of life.[19] This kind of indeterminancy can be found throughout development, including its behavioural aspects[20] and there is no reason why it should not apply to social relationships. Therefore, it is inherently unlikely that an event like early separation will have persistent effects on children and/or their relationships with their parents and we would expect to encounter processes that bring about recovery.

However, one caveat is in order here: there are examples of a kind of negative feedback loop that can be set up between parent and child which can have the effect of maintaining or exaggerating what would otherwise be a brief and temporary disturbance in development. Obstetric drugs provide an example here. Narcotics given to a mother tend to make her baby sleepy and unresponsive at feeds for several days after birth. These 'dopey' babies get a lot of stimulation from their mothers during feeds trying to get and keep them awake. Interestingly enough, some weeks after birth when the baby's behaviour has returned to normal their mothers are still stuck in this pattern of extra stimulation and are behaving as if their babies are still unresponsive.[21] As far as we know, in this example, the continuing response of the mother to an infant behaviour pattern that has dropped out has no effect on the infant's behaviour. But, in theory, one can construct models where such a feedback loop would maintain and amplify the effects of a single short-acting disruptive event.

A corollary of what I have said about buffers should be that prediction over time of development should only be possible in rather broad terms. Only when events of sufficient magnitude to override the buffering system have occurred is it likely that there will be permanent changes in development that are in some way predictable. So, for instance, we can predict the developmental pattern of a child with Down's Syndrome in so far as there is a typical pattern for Down's children in general. Given the variability within a group of Down's children this may not be saying a lot beyond the fact that the syndrome persists and is recognisable throughout development and into adulthood.

Within a group of 'normal' children, consistency of individual differences is not strong. Over the first year, for example, though there are correlations in the pattern of mother-infant interaction, these are quite modest and seem to be the result of combination of mothers adopting particular styles of interaction and of the individual characteristics of the children.[20]

Much discussion of bonding implies that parent-infant relations can be reduced to this dimension: the presence or degree of bonding. At worst bonding is discussed as if it was a state of grace into which mother and infant may have passed – and woe betide those whom God has not smiled on. In fact, if you examine the various aspects of what goes on between a parent and children – the amount of smiling, mutual looking, physical proximity and so on – the striking finding is that these do not all co-vary in the way the discussion of bonding would suggest. Positive aspects of the relationship, say smiling and physical closeness, do not necessarily go together. One couple may smile at each other a lot but not be particularly close physically while in another both measures may be high.[22] This demonstrates the complexity of social relationships and the fact that they cannot be easily reduced to a single dimension.

The proposal of the concept of bonding has proved to be a great stimulus to research and over the last decade there has been a large body of studies that have attempted to assess the effects of early separation of mother and infant on their subsequent relationship and the infant's development. Such studies have involved both full-term and pre-term babies. This work has been reviewed many times in recent years[2,4-8,23-25] and new studies continue to appear[26-30]. This research is of varied quality in terms of design and methodology[31,32], uses very varied measures of the quality of mother-infant relations, defines separation and/or extra contact in a number of ways and involves widely differing populations. Not surprisingly the conclusions it reaches are rather inconsistent. Many studies, but by no means all, do show differences between separated and non-separated pairs of mothers and babies. Such differences are generally small – both groups would fall into what most people would see as a normal, non-pathological group – and tend to disappear within a matter of weeks or months of birth. Where differences are found they are generally in the direction that the optimal outcome in terms of a close mother-infant relationship or a more satisfied and positive maternal attitude is found in the non-separated or extra-contact group. But, as in most things, there are exceptions to this. For instance, an English study[24] which compared mothers in NNUs with more and less open visiting found that mothers who had experienced more separation described themselves as being more attached to their infants and more responsive to their crying. If then, within the imperfections and variations of the research, one might tentatively infer that early separation does, in general, have slight negative effects on maternal relations, how could these be explained? I have already outlined some rather substantial theoretical objections to the concept of bonding but this discussion does not, of course, provide any explanation of separation effects that may be found. In the next section I shall outline a few of the broad characteristics of parent-child relationships and in each case I think it will be clear that separation is likely to have an inhibitory (if any) effect on the aspects I describe.

A final note is required here about breast feeding. In contrast to other aspects of mother-child relationships, separation appears to have a much more consistent effect on lactation. Both the chance of a mother establishing lactation and its duration, if established, are reduced by separation, unless a mother takes special steps to stimulate her milk production. The breast requires frequent stimulation to set up the production of milk and separation of mother and infant normally removes this stimulation.[33-34] If such stimulation is absent in the postpartum period it may be possible to establish a lactation after an interval, especially in multiparous women. Breast feeding may foster the growth of mother-infant relations and so be particularly important with pre-term infants.[35]

Some Aspects of Parent-child Relationships

Becoming a Parent

Though the last decade has seen a period of very active research on parent-child relationships, surprisingly little attention has been paid to the psychological process of becoming a parent and to the social institution of parenthood. Parents do not appear *de novo* the day their child arrives, but are people who have gone through a long period of anticipation and preparation for this event. Here I am not referring to active processes of learning about parenthood by attending classes and reading that some go through, but the more or less universal and fundamental evolution that occurs as part of everyday life for those who are going to have a child. It has many aspects related to such things as employment, attitudes towards and from relatives and friends as well as psychological adjustments.[36] Most women are employed outside the home when they conceive their first child and will leave this work towards the end of pregnancy, perhaps not to return for several years. Employment may be an important source of friendships, social support and self-confidence and its loss can mean that some women face the birth of their child with a considerable sense of deprivation.[37] Psychoanalytic work has stressed the psychological changes in a parent's, especially a woman's, position towards her own mother and father and the fact that entering parenthood represents a completion of the generational cycle.[38,39] Recently more attention has been paid to the effects of these psychological and social processes in fathers.[40,41]

From the point of view of a pre-term delivery one proposition in this work seems of particular importance: that the processes of pregnancy, ideally at least, create a state in which a mother is psychologically prepared for the relationship with her newborn. Various writers express this in different ways. Winnicott, for instance, described the state of a new mother as 'primary maternal preoccupation'.[12] This he says 'gradually develops and becomes a state of heightened sensitivity during and especially towards the end of pregnancy' and 'the mother who develops this state . . . provides a setting for the infant's constitution to begin to make itself evident, for the developmental tendencies to start to unfold, and for the infant to experience spontaneous movement and become the owner of the sensations that are appropriate to this early phase of life . . . only if a mother is sensitized in this way I am describing can she feel herself into her infant's place, and so meet the infant's needs'. A pre-term birth will not only cut short any process of preparation for parenthood (psychological or indeed socially – perhaps the baby's room has not been painted) but any separation after the birth will delay the development of the parental relationship. The latter part of pregnancy may also be a time when an infant develops capacities needed for the evolution of social relationships after birth and these may be immature in the pre-term baby (see next section below). But matters may be more subtle than this because the timing of delivery and the social and psychological processes of pregnancy are linked. Pre-term birth is more common among those who are very young,[42] unsupported, or living under stress[43,44]. In these situations those who are at least ready for delivery in psychological terms may well have fewest resources to cope.[45] A pre-term birth may be seen by the mother as a failure to nurture the fetus adequately and so the birth in this situation becomes a source of guilt[46] and it may be very hard for the mother to bring herself to face her baby.[47] The crisis of a pre-term birth may make the mother feel depressed or she may be mourning for a lost baby: perhaps one of a twin pair who has died or simply for the healthy full-term baby that was expected and has been replaced by a sick 'prem'. Both depression and mourning may inihibit a mother's capacity to feel close to her baby (see Chapter 14).

A common preoccupation during pregnancy is that the baby will be malformed or damaged in some way. If a baby is born prematurely and taken away to a neonatal unit before the parents have had a chance to examine him or her properly these fears may grow until they become certain that there is a serious malformation. This is perhaps one reason why a photograph of the baby and even a brief time with the baby at birth can be so important for parents in this situation. It is not clear why this preoccupation with malformation is so common. Perhaps it relates to the way in which the management of pregnancy has been taken over by medicine so that more general anxieties about becoming a parent tend to be expressed in specific medical terms (see[48]). Often there is little opportunity or encouragement for parents to discuss any aspect of pregnancy and parenthood beyond the physiological.

Parent-child Interaction

We now have abundant evidence of the mutual dependence of the behaviour of parent and child. What the parent does, influences the behaviour of the child and what the child does, influences the parent, all operating within a particular social and psychological climate. Mutual interaction may be seen on a minute-to-minute basis as in the way a mother's talking to her infant is organised around the temporal pattern of bursts of sucking and pauses as the infant feeds.[49] It has been suggested that such turn-taking and interdependence represents the origin of dialogue and so it is quite fundamental in the emergence of social relations.[50]

At the other end of the time scale a parent's view of a child is moulded and shaped by the ease or difficulty of coping with a particular child. Babies who cry a lot may, for instance, 'turn off' their parents and get less attention. As such patterns emerge gradually they are, in part at least, a response to the characteristics of the baby.[51] Equally, such processes work the other way round so that styles of caretaking influence the development of children.

Pre-term babies, because of their immaturity and because they may be sick, show neither the same degree of organisation in their behaviour nor the same ability to enter into dialogue-like exchanges as full-term babies. One could say that they may be neurologically immature for interaction. This makes them hard for parents 'to read',[52] to understand what they are doing or to feel close to them. As one might expect, behavioural observations demonstrate clear differences between interaction by parents with pre-term and full-term babies and these differences may persist for several months after birth.[53-55] Parents may feel frustrated and unsatisfied with their relationship with their 'prem' and this may be a reason why sleeping and feeding problems are commonly reported.[45]

One feature of neonatal units is that caretaking is usually carried out by a large number of different people who are seldom able to learn individual characteristics of a particular baby so that their interventions tend to bear little or no relation to what the baby is doing.[56,57] Feeding or other caretaking is seldom related to whether or not a baby in an incubator is crying. We do not know whether it matters that some children only begin to experience the mutual interdependence of caretaking after some days, weeks or even months of life.

A common complaint of mothers after a period of neonatal separation is that they do not 'know' their baby. It seems likely that this feeling arises from the mother's inability to experience the usual interdependence of a relationship with a young baby. Almost always this feeling is shortlived but at least on an anecdotal level there are cases where the sense of distance persists throughout childhood. The ex-prem is seen as a kind of changeling who remains aloof from the rest of the family. It is plausible that early separation plays some part in the evolution of these distorted relations. Clearly a prime aim of neonatal care must be to provide a peaceful and calm atmosphere in which parents can get to know their infants. This will involve providing privacy and the avoidance of interruptions or distractions.

Whose Baby?

It is usual for parents to say that they did not feel their baby was theirs until they all got home from hospital. These feelings are particularly often expressed if a baby has been in a neonatal unit.[58] In a sense these parents are being quite realistic because given the way in which most hospitals and neonatal units are organised it is very difficult for mothers to feel in control of what is happening to them or their babies. Leaving aside ethical or legal questions, is this of any psychological consequence? Studies of maternity care suggest it may be. Mothers who receive unwelcome interventions and did not feel fully consulted about what was happening to them not only were less satisfied with their deliveries but were more likely to feel depressed in the post-natal period.[37,59,60] A recurrent finding in the studies of early separation and admission to a neonatal unit is that mothers of pre-term and other sick babies tend to feel less confident about looking after their children when they get home.[58,61,62] Some of this may be a direct response to the medical problems that these babies may have and their real or assumed vulnerability. However, part of the mother's feelings seem to arise from the separation itself.[23] Such an effect is understandable as an admission of a baby to a neonatal unit carries the implicit message that the mother (and father) are incapable of looking after their own child. Of course, in a literal sense this may be true and the baby may need all sorts of specialised medical treatment and nursing. However, it does seem to be very important that parents remain as involved as possible by spending time with their baby and undertaking as much caretaking as they want to and feel able to do. Equally important, they need to be fully informed about the baby's condition. Standards of giving information to parents and providing them with opportunities for discussion are not always high[63] but parents do appreciate such opportunities that are given[58]. It is very difficult to generalise about exactly what parents should be told and what can justifiably be withheld. Do you, for instance, tell parents about an apparently asymptomatic intracranial bleeding? Much will depend on their degree of understanding and their wish to know. A generalisation that is probably correct is that the parent's wish to know is almost always underestimated and that more harm has been done by withholding information than providing it in excess.

I have already referred to the emotional problems a pre-term delivery may create for parents. If a baby is damaged and especially if the damage is likely to have permanent consequences, parents may become very angry and this anger may be vented on medical staff. Unjust and unfair as it will feel, messengers may get blamed for the messages they carry. Providing effective care without usurping the parental role is perhaps the most difficult task that faces a neonatal unit. It is also an area where there is most to learn.

Amongst the babies that pass through a neonatal unit are a number who will have extensive and continuing need for medical care.[64] The kind of relationship which parents can build with medical staff in the neonatal period may have a considerable effect on the quality of care their child will receive later. These issues are taken up in detail in Chapter 7.

For some parents the maternity hospital and neonatal unit may act as models of what should be the form of parent-child relations. Doctors and other medical staff have after all become sources of advice about child care and many of the most widely read advice books for parents are written by paediatricians. Parents may assume that the more rigid routines, where babies are fed four-hourly and otherwise placed out of sight in the nursery, or where visiting in a neonatal unit is confined to set times, represent a considered view of experts of how parental relations are best conducted. Worse still they may try to follow the same regime when they get home. How far this may happen is not clear. But if such an effect does exist it would be fruitful to look at this in a positive way and try to create hospitals that would represent models of good child care practice. But either way there can be no excuse for routines that unnecessarily restrict or interfere in relations between parents and children.

Fathers and Other Family Members

An interesting point that emerges from several follow-up studies of pre-term babies or others who have been in a neonatal unit is that fathers seem more than usually involved in the lives of these children.[45,65,66] There seem to be several reasons for this. A study of visiting in a neonatal unit showed that while some fathers did not visit at all until their wives were free to visit and even then came less often, others saw their children frequently right from the beginning and initially were very involved.[67] There is other evidence[68] that fathers who have contact with their babies neonatally tend to interact more at later ages.

In the neonatal unit some men seem less intimidated by the equipment than their partners and sometimes appear to form a relationship with their child via an interest in the monitoring and life support equipment. In other ways the increased paternal involvement in these babies may represent an extension of a traditional male role as it may stem, at the beginning at least, from a stepping in to manage a crisis. This may lead on to a less typically male participation in child care.

While many good reasons can be given for an increased role for men in the rearing of their children[69] it would hardly seem appropriate to organise neonatal care with the intent of altering the sexual division of labour within families. However, these considerations should alert professionals involved in child care to the fact that roles do seem to be changing in some families and that traditional assumptions may no longer apply. It also means that there is wide individual variation between families so that it may be unwise to take for granted any particular role for either parent. The onus is on the staff of NNUs to find out what parents want and to support them in doing it.

As well as giving more prominence to fathers, recent work on family dynamics tends to see children more within a whole network of social relationships and less in dyads with mother and father. Again this may have implications for the organisation of neonatal care. Not only may siblings be important because their care may limit the times at which parents can visit their new baby,[67] but the siblings themselves may need to visit. There may be other family members or friends who may be potentially of particular importance to the baby. Most neonatal units are not designed to accommodate many visitors and some limits may need to be applied. Also, of course, basic precautions against the introduction of infection need to be maintained. But within these constraints efforts should be made to make the parents as free as possible to bring who they want to visit their child. The social unit we refer to as a family has many and varied forms and we should not let our prejudices, preferences or expectations stand in the way of parents' beliefs and wishes. They, after all, carry the responsibility for rearing their child.

Conclusions

In this chapter I have tried to sketch some aspects of our understanding of parent-child relations particularly with reference to the pre-term baby and the issue of early separation. While there is no doubt that the concept of bonding is over-simple, its popularisation has led to a desirable concern to preserve parent-child relationships in maternity hospitals and neonatal units.

We cannot make hospitals like homes, but we can try to understand the varied needs of families and their newborns and attempt to minimise the ways their fulfilment may be thwarted. Reducing separation to the absolute minimum is the first step, but beyond that we need to look at the less obvious and more subtle ways in which one can improve matters. We need to exercise our imagination more extensively so that we may see the world a little more from the point of view of parents and may retain a sense of the uniqueness of each baby. The successful medical treatment of small and sick babies may be becoming more routine for staff but the arrival of a new child is never routine for parents. There are vivid and very sad accounts of how parents and child may suffer quite unnecessarily when the provision of neonatal care becomes an end in itself.[70] Let us hope that such events will soon be part of history and that NNUs will always place the preservation and enhancing of parenthood as their first priority. Later in this book several attempts to do this will be described. Their variety underlines both the point that solutions will vary with the particular circumstances and that there is no one right answer. We will move forward by imaginative experiment, assessment and resisting any temptation to feel that we have achieved a final and satisfactory solution.

Notes/References

1. To avoid confusion I shall use the term parent when referring to both mothers and fathers. Mother and father will be used when one or other parent is specifically indicated. The care of children, and especially infants, is largely undertaken by mothers and not fathers. Often when I speak of parents this will in practice mean mostly mothers and a few fathers. But to use the term mother on these occasions might carry with it the unfortunate and unintended implication that the care of infants is and should be the exclusive concern of women.

2. Klaus, M. H., and Kennell, J. H. (1976). *Maternal-Infant Bonding*. St Louis, C. V. Mosby.

3. Richards, M. P. M., and Roberton, N. R. C. (1978). Admission and discharge policies for special care units. In *Separation and Special Care Baby Units*, F. S. W. Brimblecombe, M. P. M. Richards and N. R. C. Roberton (eds), Clinics in Developmental Medicine, No. 68. London, SIMP/Heinemann Medical Books.

4. Campbell, S. B. G., and Taylor, P. M. (1980). Bonding and attachment: theoretical issues. In *Parent-Infant Relationships*, P. M. Taylor (ed.). New York, Grune and Stratton.

5. Herbert, M., Sluckin, W. and Sluckin, A. (1982). Mother-to-infant 'bonding'.

J. Child Psychol. Psychiat., *23*, 205.

6. Richards, M. P. M. (1979). Effects on development of medical interventions and the separation of newborns from their parents. In *The First Year of Life*, D. Schafer and J. Dunn (eds). Chichester, Wiley.

7. Richards, M. P. M. (1983). The myth of bonding. In *Progress in Child Health*, J. A. Macfarlane (ed.). Edinburgh, Churchill Livingstone.

8. Ross, G. S. (1980). Parental responses to infants in intensive care: the separation issue reevaluated. *Clins Perinatol.*, *7*, 47.

9. More recent work (Guberwick, D. J., 1981, Mechanism of maternal 'labelling' in goat. *Anim. Behaviour*, *29*, 305-6) suggests a somewhat different interpretation of the observations on goats. It appears that when the mother licks the kid after birth she places a specific 'label' on it. She will reject kids with 'labels' from other mothers. So the sensitive period represents a period in which the kids acquire olfactory labels and mothers reject kids with labels from other mothers. For further discussion of this work see reference 5.

10. Lee, R. B. (1979). *The !Kuang San. Men, Women, and Work in a Foraging Society*. Cambridge, Cambridge University Press.

11. At least, by blood relatives of mother and father who will have genes in common with the infant. The study of what sociobiologists have chosen to call 'altruism' alerts us to the point that we would be unwise to rely on any group selection arguments.

12. Winnicott, D. W. (1958). *Collected Papers*. London, Tavistock.

13. Waddington, C. H. (1975). *The Evolution of an Evolutionist*. Edinburgh, Edinburgh University Press.

14. Sameroff, A. J. (1975). Early influences on development: fact or fancy? *Merrill-Palmer Quart.*, *21*, 267.

15. Krishnamoorthy, K. S., *et al.* (1977). Evaluation of neonatal intracranial haemorrhage by computorised tomography. *Pediatrics*, *59*, 165-72.

16. Pape, K. E., *et al.* (1979). Ultrasound detection of brain damage in preterm infants. *Lancet*, *i*, 1261.

17. Lazzara, A., *et al.* (1978). Intracerebral hemorrhage in high-risk prematures. *Pediat. Res.*, *12*, 553.

18. Papile, L.A., Burstein, J., Burstein, R., and Koffler, H. (1978). Incidence and evolution of subependymal and intra-ventricular hemorrhage: a study of infants with birthweights less than 1000 gm. *J. Pediat.*, *92*, 529.

19. Stanley, F. J. (1982). Using cerebral palsy data in the evaluation of neonatal intensive care: a warning. *Developm. Med. Child Neurol.*, *24*, 93.

20. Dunn, J. F. (1975). Consistency and change in styles of mothering. In *Parent-Infant Interaction*, CIBA Foundation Symposium, Vol. 33. Amsterdam, Elsevier.

21. Dunn, J. F., and Richards, M. P. M. (1977). Observations on the developing relationship between mother and baby in the neonatal period. In *Studies in Mother-Infant Interaction*, Schaffer, M. R. (ed.). London, Academic Press.

22. Gaines, R., Sandground, A., Green, A. H., and Power, E. (1978). Etiological factors in child maltreatment: a multivariate study of abusing, neglecting and normal mothers. *J. Abnorm. Psychol.*, *87*, 531.

23. Richards, M. P. M. (1978). Possible effects of early separation on later development of children – a review. In *Separation and Special Care Baby Units*, F. S. W. Brimblecombe, M. P. M. Richards and N. R. C. Roberton (eds), Clinics in Developmental Medicine, No. 68. London, SIMP/Heinemann Medical Books.

24. McGurk, H. (1980). *Maternal Attachment Behaviour and Infant Development: The Significance of Temporary Separation at Birth*. Unpublished report to DHSS, London.

25. Traube, M. A. (1981). Extra postpartum contact: an assessment of the

intervention and its effects. In *Newborns and Parents*, V. L. Smeriglio (ed.). Hillsdale, N. J., Lawrence Erlbaum.

26. Grossmann, K., Thane, K., and Grossmann, K. E. (1981). Maternal tactual contact of the newborn after various postpartum conditions of mother-infant contact. *Developm. Psychology*, *17*, 158.

27. Rode, S. S., Change, P. N., Fisch, R. O., and Sroufe, L. A. (1981). Attachment patterns of infants separated at birth. *Developm. Psychol.*, *17*, 188.

28. Craig, S., Tyson, J. E., Samson, J., and Lasky, R. E. (1982). The effect of early contact on maternal perception of infant behaviour. *Early Human Developm.*, *6*, 197.

29. O'Connor, S., Vietze, P., Sherrod, K., Sandler, H. and Altemeler, W. (1980). Reduced incidence of parenting inadequacy following rooming-in. *Pediatrics*, *66*, 176.

30. Ali, Z., and Lowry, M. (1981). Early maternal-child contact: effects on later behaviour. *Developm. Med. Child Neurol.*, *23*, 337.

31. Yogman, M. W. (1981). Parent-infant bonding: nature of intervention and inferences from data. In *Newborns and Parents*, V. L. Smeriglio (ed.). Hillsdale, N. J., Lawrence Erlbaum.

32. Bell, R. Q. (1981). Comparability and generalizability of intervention research with mothers and infants in hospitals. In *Newborns and Parents*, V. L. Smeriglio (ed.). Hillsdale, N. J., Lawrence Erlbaum.

33. Salariyn, E. M., Easton, P. M., and Cater, J. I. (1978). Duration of breast feeding after early initiation and frequent feeding. *Lancet*, *ii*, 1141.

34. de Chateau, P., Holmberg, H., Jukobsson, K., and Winberg, J. (1977). A study of factors promoting and inhibiting lactation. *Developm. Med. Child Neurol.*, *19*, 575.

35. Richards, M. P. M. (1982). Breast feeding and the mother-infant relationship. *Acta Paediat. Scand.*, Suppl., *299*, 33-9. Neonatal care of pre-term and sick babies often involves feeding by tube directly into the stomach. This, of course, removes the possibility of the baby sucking. In a recent experiment pre-term babies were given a dummy to suck on while being tube-fed. These infants gained weight faster than controls and were discharged home earlier (Ignatoff, E., and Field, T. (1982). Effects of non-nutritive sucking during tube feeding on the behaviour and clinical course of ICU preterm neonates. In *Infant Behaviour and Development: Perinatal Risk and Newborn Behavior*, L.P. Lipsitt and T.M. Field (eds). Norwood, N. J., Ablex Publishing Corp.). This indicates that we need to think of both the infant and the maternal side of the early feeding interaction. It might be that if infants in intensive care were given more experience of sucking, it would be easier to establish a delayed lactation at a later date.

36. Osofsky, H. J., and Osofsky, J. D. (1980). Normal adaptation to pregnancy and new parenthood. In *Parent-Infant Relationships*, P. M. Taylor (ed.). New York, Grune and Stratton.

37. Oakley, A. (1979). *Becoming a Mother*. Oxford, Martin Robertson.

38. Bibring, G. L. (1959). Some considerations of the psychological processes in pregnancy. *Psychoanal. Study of the Child.*, *14*, 113.

39. Deutch, H. (1947). *The Psychology of Women, Vol. 2, Motherhood*. London, Research Books.

40. Beil, N., and Macquire, J. (eds) (1982). *Psychological Studies of Fathers*. London, Junction Books.

41. Richman, J. (1982). Men's experiences of pregnancy and childbirth. In *The Father Figure*, L. McKee and M. O'Brien (eds). London, Tavistock.

42. Ragozin, A. S., Basham, R. B., Crnic, K. A., Greenberg, M. T., and Robinson, N. M. (1982). Effects of maternal age on parenting role. *Developm. Psychol.*, *18*, 627-34.

43. Oakley, A., Chalmers, I., and Macfarlane, J. A. (1982). Social class, stress and reproduction. In *Disease and the Environment*, A. R. Rees and M. Purcell (eds). Chichester, John Wiley.

44. Nuckolls, K. B., Cassel, J., and Kaplan, B. H. (1972). Psychosocial assets, life crisis and the prognosis of pregnancy. *Amer. J. Epidemiol.*, *95*, 431.

45. Jeffcoate, J. A., Humphrey, M. E., and Lloyd, J. K. (1979). Role perception and response to stress in fathers and mothers following pre-term delivery. *Social Science and Medicine*, *13*, 139.

46. Caplan, G., Mason, E. A., and Kaplan, D. M. (1965). Four studies of crisis in parents of prematures. *Comm. Mental Health*, *1*, 149.

47. Minde, K., Ford, L., Celhoffer, L., and Boukydis, C. (1975). Interactions of mothers and nurses with premature infants. *Canad. Med. Ass. J.*, *113*, 741.

48. Oakley, A. (1984). *The Captured Womb*. Oxford, Martin Robertson, in press.

49. Richards, M. P. M. (1971). Social interaction in the first weeks of human life. *Psychiat., Neurol. Neurochir.*, *74*, 35.

50. Kaye, K. (1977). Toward the original of dialogue. In *Studies in Mother-Infant Interaction*, Schaffer, H. R. (ed.). London, Academic Press.

51. Bernal, J. (1974). Attachment: some problems and possibilities. In *The Integration of a Child into a Social World*, M. P. M. Richards (ed.). London, Cambridge University Press.

52. Goldberg, S. (1979). Premature birth: consequences for the parent-infant relationship. *American Scientist*, *67*, 214.

53. Divitto, B., and Goldberg, S. (1983). Talking and sucking: infant feeding behaviour and parent stimulation in dyad with different medical histories. *Infant Behaviour and Development* (in press).

54. Field, T., Sostek, A., Goldberg, S., and Shuman, H. H. (eds) (1979). *Infants Born at Risk*, Jamaica, N. Y., Spectrum.

55. Friedman, S. L., and Sigman, M. (1981). *Preterm Birth and Psychological Development*. New York, Academic Press.

56. Gottfried, A. W., Wallace-Lande, P., Sherman-Brown, S., King, J., and Coen, C. (1981). Physical and social environment of newborn infants in special care units. *Science*, *214*, 673.

57. Prince, J., Firlej, M., and Harvey, D. (1978). Contact between babies in incubators and their caretakers. In *Separation and Special Care Baby Units*, F. S. W. Brimblecombe, M. P. M. Richards and N. R. C. Roberton (eds), Clinics in Developmental Medicine, No. 68. London, SIMP/Heinemann Medical Books.

58. Hawthorne Amick, J. T. (1981). *The Effects of Different Routines in a Special Care Baby Unit on the Mother-Infant Relationship: An Intervention Study*. Unpublished PhD thesis, University of Cambridge.

59. Oakley, A. (1980). *Women Confined*. Oxford, Martin Robertson.

60. Day, S. (1982). Is obstetric technology depressing? *Radical Science Journal*, *12*, 17.

61. Leifer, A. D., Leiderman, P. H., Barnett, C. R., and Williams, J. A. (1972). Effects if mother-infant separation on maternal attachment behaviour. *Child Developm.*, *43*, 1203.

62. Leiderman, P. H., and Seashore, M. J. (1975). Mother-infant neonatal separation: some delayed consequences. In *Parent-Infant Interaction*, Ciba Foundation Symposium, No. 33 (new series). Amsterdam, Elsevier.

63. Bogdan, R., Brown, M. A., and Foster, S. B. (1982). Be honest but not cruel: staff/parent communication on a neonatal unit. *Human Organisation*, *41*, 6.

64. Hack, M., DeMontericke, D., Merkatz, I. R., Jones, P., and Faronoff, A. A. (1981). Rehospitalization of the very low birthweight infant. *Amer. J. Dis. Child*,

135, 263.

65. Blake, A., Stewart, A., and Turcan, D. (1975). Parents of babies of very low birthweight: long-term follow-up. In *Parent-Infant Interaction*, Ciba Foundation Symposium, No. 33. Amsterdam, Elsevier.

66. Benfield, D. G., Leib, S. A., and Reuter, J. (1976). Grief response of parents after referral of the critically ill newborn to a regional center. *New Engl. J. Med.*, *294*, 975.

67. Hawthorne, J. T., Richards, M. P. M., and Callon, M. (1978). A study of parental visiting of babies in a special-care unit. In *Separation and Special Care Baby Units*, F. S. W. Brimblecombe, M. P. M. Richards and N. R. C. Roberton (eds), Clinics in Developmental Medicine, No. 68. London, SIMP/Heinemann Medical Books.

68. Rodholm, M. (1981). Effects of father-infant postpartum contact on the interaction 3 months after birth. *Early Human Developm.*, *5*, 79.

69. Parke, R. D. (1981). *Fathering*. London, Fontana.

70. Stinson, R., and Stinson, P. (1983). *The Long Dying of Baby Andrew*, Boston, Little, Brown and Co.

2 EVOLUTION OF SPECIAL CARE BABY UNITS

F. S. W. Brimblecombe

Everything has been thought of before.
The difficulty is to think of it again.
Goethe

Ideas are only as important as what you can do with them.
Bronfenbrenner

The development of special care for newborn infants and the recent application of advanced technology now used in intensive neonatal care units have their origins far back in history. Such topical issues as the methods of care of the pre-term infant and of sick full-term babies have been debated in the writings of philosphers, teachers and physicians for at least 3,000 years and there is archaeological and anthropological evidence that these were matters of concern in even earlier millennia.

Almost all the techniques currently used in special and intensive neonatal care have been described many centuries ago. For example, the value of early mother-child interaction was commended in the first century AD by Plutarch who specifically identified in *The Education of Children* the importance of bonding:

> It is the duty, I should say, of mothers to feed their children themselves and to give the breast; for they will have more sympathy with them and take more trouble in feeding them, in as much as they love their children, as the saying is, to their very finger tips, but the goodwill of foster mothers and nurses is counterfeit and assumed, they love for hire. Nature shews plainly that mothers ought to suckle and nurse those to whom they have given birth; this is the reason why she has provided every creature that gives birth with milk for feeding. A wise thing is the foresight; she has bestowed on women two breasts so that in case of twin births she shall have two founts of nourishment. But apart from all this, they are likely to be better disposed and more loving to their children, and by Jove not unnaturally, for the close association of suckling makes a bond of good feeling.

Mother-child Interaction and Infant Feeding

The controversy about maternal breast feeding and other methods of providing infant nutrition is apparent in historical treatises from very early times and has been well documented by Wickes.[1]

Archaeological discoveries have identified vessels for artificial feeding dating from 1000 BC. The Greek and Roman epochs were patriarchal in outlook and the status of children and the importance of breast feeding and close mother-child contact were accorded relatively low priorities.[2–3] Soranus of Ephesus, a contemporary of Plutarch, wrote that the main responsibility of the physician concerned with neonatal care was the selection of a suitable wet nurse. In many primitive cultures there was a taboo against the feeding of colostrum to newborn infants, and in others such as the Aztec culture[4] and the Mundugmor tribe in the Pacific Islands[5] close contact between mother and child was discouraged.

However, the general tendency throughout history has been to encourage breast feeding and mother-infant togetherness. Ishtar, the Sumerian goddess, is depicted in a delightful figurine of 5000 BC now displayed in the National Museum in Baghdad, breast feeding her small infant. During the Pharoanic dynasties, it was recommended that mothers should breast feed for six months. Babylon was in many respects a matriarchal society in which breast feeding was strongly encouraged. Susrata and Charaka in the Buddhist teachings of India of 600 BC emphasise the importance of antenatal care and infant care during the first ten days after birth. The Christian concept of Madonna and Child has been a constant reminder of close contact between mother and infant. The Koran (666 AD) teaches that mothers should suckle their infants for a full two months and that complete weaning should not normally take place before thirty months. The importance of suckling and of direct care by the mother of her infant was also a feature of the early culture patterns of China.

More recently, Thomas Phaire (1545) in his *Boke of Children* emphasises his belief in the importance of breast feeding. The heat of the controversy about infant feeding in the sixteenth century is clear from the writings of Pierre Tolet:

> I would have the mother to be the one and only feeder of her child lest some day the child seems if it had not a wet nurse but Hyrcanean or Arab tiger to suckle it . . . I see no room for drying up the sacred fount, the nurturer of man's body. When you knew not the

> child nor could see it, when there was no baby's cry and it was just a weight and mass in the womb, you nourished it with your blood; but now when it is alive, your very likeness, your own child, a human being imploring your help, you refuse, you destroy, you extinguish what nature has given you without cost. Wherefore if through fault of the wet nurses, as often happens, the infant is ruined by almost numberless diseases, do not rail against God in Heaven, He does not inflict evil; do not try to exorcise spirits, they live in graveyards. Let the child love thee as a mother; that he, your own child, may regard you for ever as his mother and not sink, as he often does, into the child of a stranger.

The need for this emotive exhortation is made clear by Harris, who in 1689 was told by the Rector of Hayes in Middlesex of his concern about the fashionable practice among both high- and low-born ladies of farming out their babies to irresponsible women. His parish, the rector told Harris, 'was filled with suckling infants from London and yet in the space of one year among 74 he buried them all except two'.

Jacques Guillemeau, whose book *The Nursing of Children* was translated into English in 1612, starts with an eight-page preface addressed to 'Ladies wherein they are exhorted to nurse their own children themselves'. Like Plutarch he emphasises the importance of not separating mothers and babies since natural affection may thus be lost. He relates the classical story of the boy, who when he was older, gave his nurse a present of gold, but gave one only of silver to his mother, saying that the mother had no alternative but to nourish him in her womb, whereas the nurse 'carried me three years in her arms and nourished me with her own blood'. Caulfield[6] rediscovered the book of repentance *The Countess of Lincolnes Nurserie* written by Elizabeth Clinton, Dowager of Lincoln, in 1662. The Countess herself had had 18 children, all of whom had been given to nurses. Only one, Theophilus, reached adulthood and became the fourth Earl of Lincoln. The book is dedicated to his wife Bridget, who breast fed her first child. It is to the credit of her mother-in-law that she admits the error of her ways and decided to write her book by way of atonement.

In a critical review of the history of infant feeding Brouzet (1755) wrote 'All that has been written on the choice of nurses and the nourishment of children is hardly anything more than a collection of prejudices.' To correct this and to provide some evidence of application of science to the subject Michael Underwood published in 1799 a detailed chemical analysis of milk. He contrasted the curdling properties and acidity of human and cows' milk and provided scientific advice about the nutritional requirements of infants.

By the early nineteenth century gavage feeding was recommended for pre-term and sick newborns and nasogastric tubes were in use. The debate about wet nurses continued well into the present century; Eden and Holland (1925) in their standard textbook *A Manual of Midwifery* state 'we commend a wet nurse as the best substitute for maternal breast feeding and cows' milk formula as a second best'.[7]

Resuscitation, Artificial Ventilation and an Enriched Oxygen Atmosphere

Positive pressure ventilation by mouth-to-mouth respiration was recommended by Paolo Bagellardo in 1472. Paracelsus (1493-1541) described the use of tracheotomy and the use of bellows for respiration in older children and adults in cases of laryngeal obstruction. Laryngeal intubation for the newborn was described by William Smellie[8] and positive pressure ventilation (IPPV) was again referred to by Petit in 1770. In 1774 Janin used a bellows apparatus to facilitate its application. The two methods of laryngeal intubation and positive pressure ventilation were again combined in the description by Kite in 1788. A further description of IPPV was provided by de Salle in 1823 (Figures 2.1 and 2.2). The discovery of oxygen in 1771 independently by Priestley and Scheele was soon applied to the newborn by Campbell and Poulton in 1934. Its use by face mask was described by François Chaussier (1780) who also used laryngeal intubation (Figure 2.3). The subsequent combination of incubators to maintain body temperature (the first reason for their introduction) with the provision of an enriched oxygen atmosphere is described below.

Artificial respiration, which during the eighteenth century had first been administered by positive pressure ventilation, was the subject of further experiments during the nineteenth century. There is little doubt that the initial efforts to use positive pressure ventilation had been found to be dangerous; almost certainly because excessive positive pressure was used which caused severe trauma to the fragile alveoli of the neonatal lung. The use of subcutaneous injections of oxygen was used for a brief period in the early years of this century. An equally abortive technique, namely intragastric oxygen, which for a few years was believed to be capable of being absorbed through the gastric mucosa, was devised by Akerren and Furstenburg in 1947.

Figure 2.1: Cannulae Used by de Chaussier for Neonatal Resuscitation (1806).

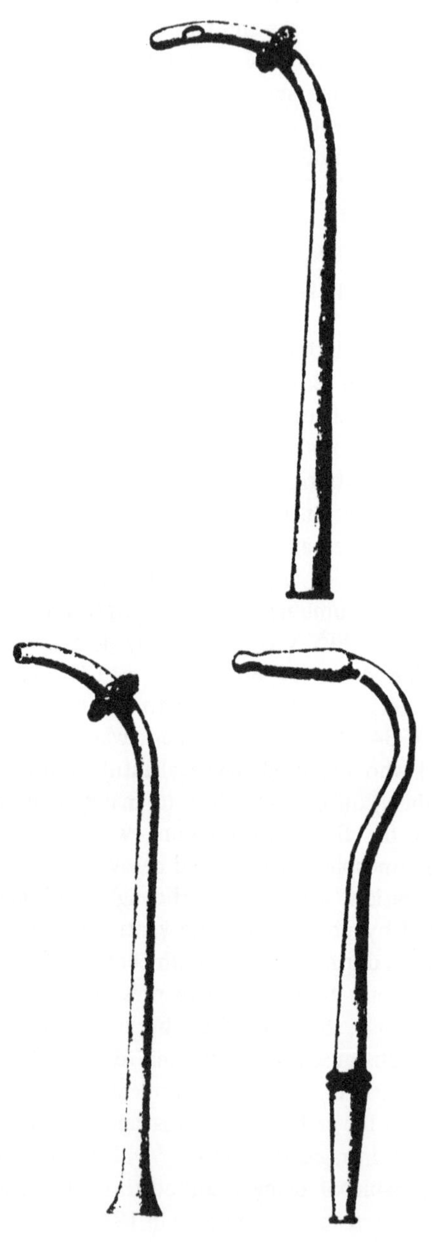

Figure 2.2: Instrument for Neonatal Resuscitation by Insufflation (de Pros, 1780).

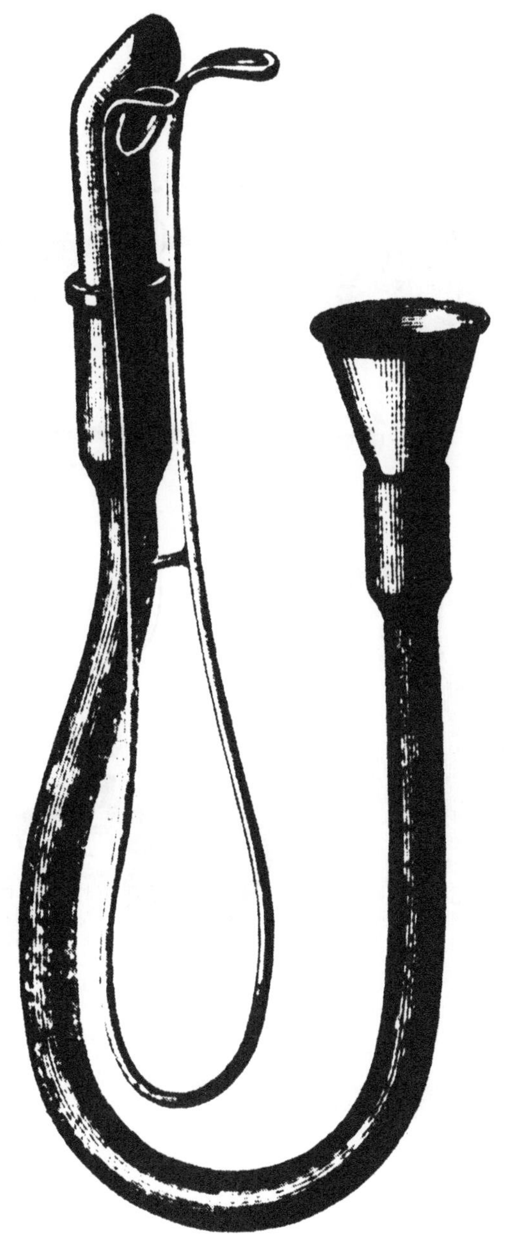

Figure 2.3: Use of Enriched Oxygen Atmosphere (Method as Used by de Chaussier, 1780).

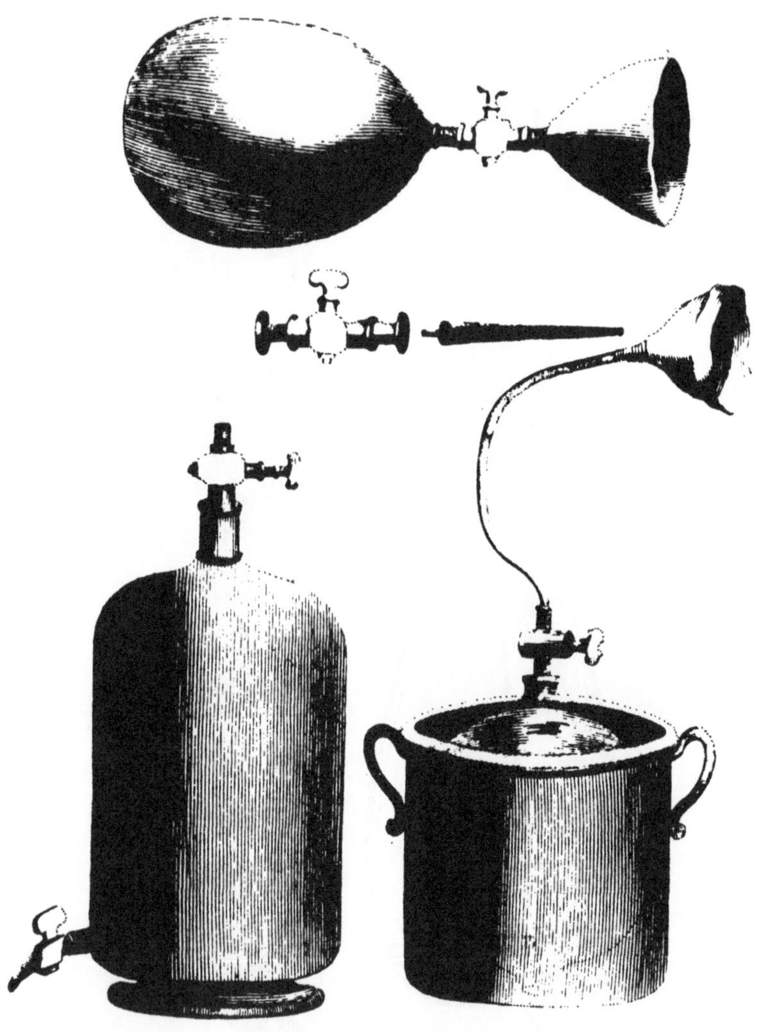

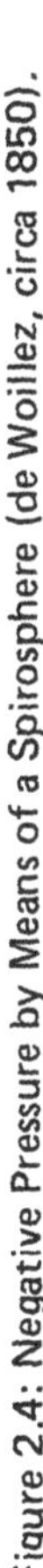

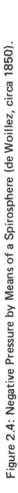

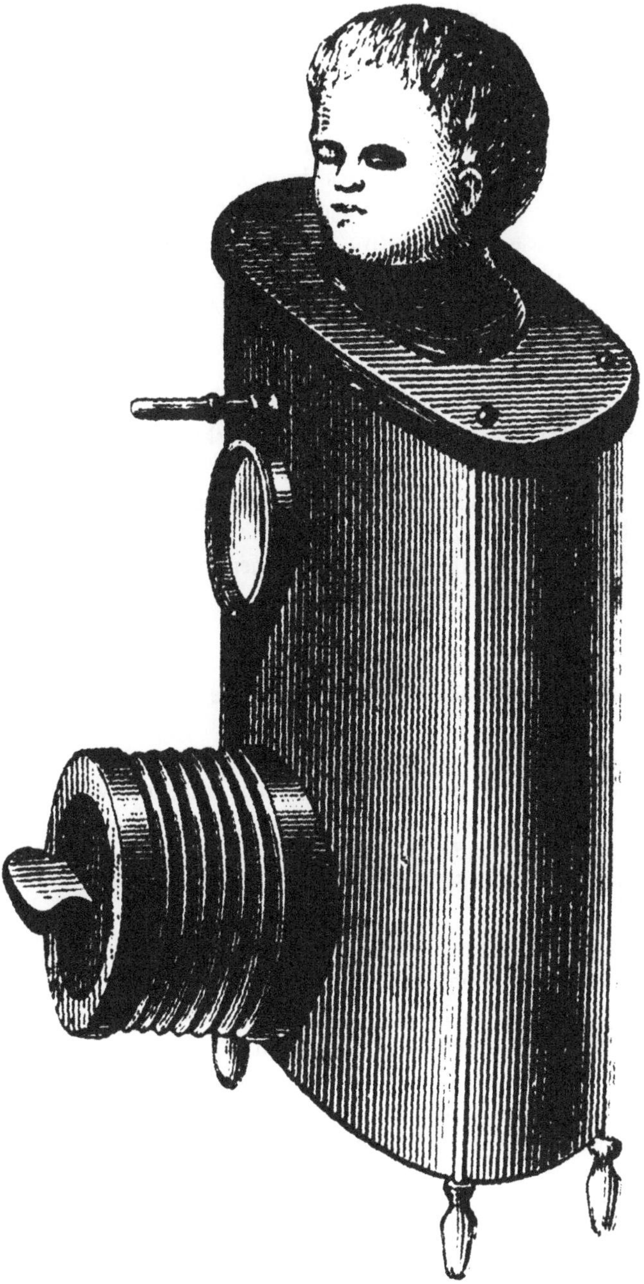

Figure 2.4: Negative Pressure by Means of a Spirosphere (de Woillez, circa 1850).

Experiments with external pressure ventilation included the use of the spirosphore devised by de Woillez (circa 1850 – Figure 2.4). A similar apparatus, the pneumotron, was used in Glasgow by Donald in the 1950s. During the same period Cross was experimenting with the use of electrical phrenic nerve stimulators, applied to the skin surface where the phrenic nerve passes through the neck, in an attempt to promote more powerful diaphragmatic contractions. By the 1960s it had become clear that positive pressure ventilation was the preferred method of artificial ventilation. This was soon followed by the use of continuous positive airways pressure (CPAP) introduced by Gregory in 1971, either alone or in combination with intermittent positive pressure ventilation.

Retrolental fibroplasia in pre-term infants was first described by Terry.[9] The scientific proof of its relationship to hyperoxia was provided by Ashton and his colleagues in 1953.[10] Subsequent progress in the attempt to reconcile the need for some pre-term infants to breath an enriched oxygen atmosphere and the risk of ocular damage which may result is described in the Supplement to Pediatrics edited by James and Lanman.[11]

Maintenance of Body Temperature and the Use of Incubators

Early evidence of attempts to prevent chilling in pre-term infants is illustrated by the peasants of Westphalia and Silesia who placed weakly newborn in jars of feathers. Laurence Sterne in the *Life and Opinions of Tristram Shandy* (1760) quotes the possibly apocryphal story of Licetus Fortuno 1597-1657:

> And for Licetus Fortuno, all the world knows he was born a fetus. He was no larger than the palm of the hand, but the father having examined it in his medical capacity, brought it living to Rapallo where it was seen by Jerome Bardi and other doctors of that place. They finding it not deficient in anything essential to life, the father undertook to finish the work of nature by the same artifice as is used in Egypt for the hatching of chickens. He instructed a wet nurse in all she had to do; and having put his son in an oven suitably arranged, he succeeded in rearing him and in making him take on the necessary increase of growth, by the uniformity of heat measured accurately in the degrees of the thermometer.

The development of purpose-built incubators for the human infant can be traced back to 1835 when Georg von Ruehl (1769-1846), physician in ordinary to the Czarina Feodorovna, wife of Czar Paul I, introduced a double-walled metal incubator containing warm water between its two layers at the Moscow Founding Hospital (Figure 2.5).[12,13] The first

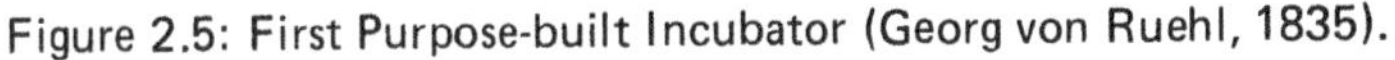

Figure 2.5: First Purpose-built Incubator (Georg von Ruehl, 1835).

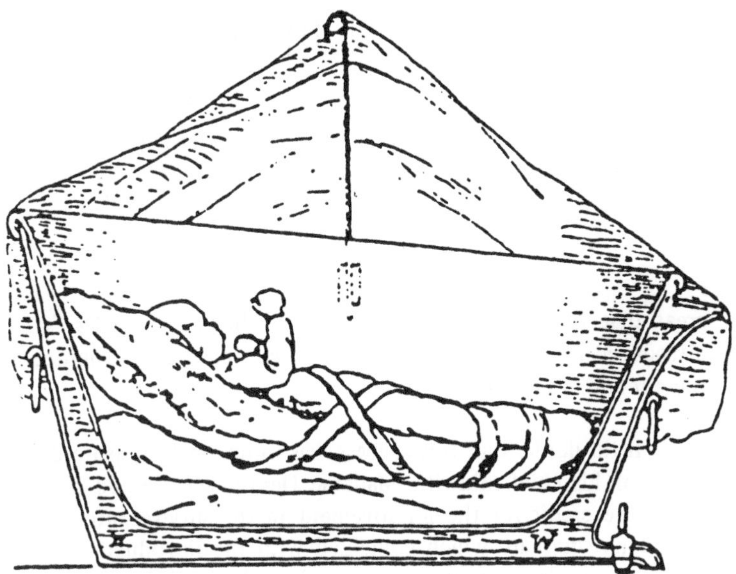

full medical reference to such an apparatus was by Denuce of Bordeaux[14] (Figure 2.6). In 1884 Carl Credé of Leipzig reported that treatment of 647 preterm or sick newborn infants using a similar apparatus.[15] Cone[16] provides a full account of the introduction of incubators and of the biographies of those who used them.

In Paris in 1878 Emile Stephane Tarnier, an obstetrician, visited an exhibition at the Jardin d'Acclimatation where he saw a warming chamber for the rearing of poultry devised by Odile Martin. Tarnier considered that the very high neonatal mortality rate among pre-term infants might be reduced by the introduction of incubators. By 1880 he had brought them into use at the Paris Maternity Hospital (Figure 2.7). In 1885 the Academy of Medicine reported:

> The minute and delicate care which these weakly prematurely born infants require, especially in winter, to protect them from cold is so

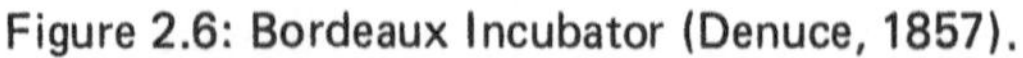
Figure 2.6: Bordeaux Incubator (Denuce, 1857).

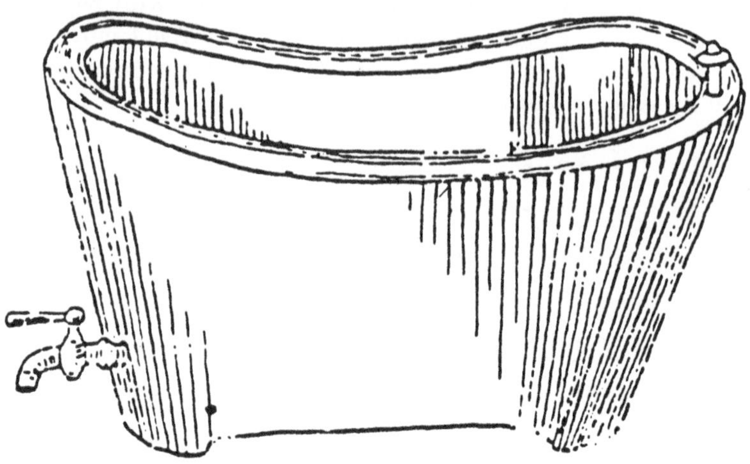

> great that till now many of them have died . . . since Dr Tarnier introduced the ingenious device called a couveuse, a large number of these infants have been saved.

There is little doubt that this success was in no small measure due to the skill of his chief midwife, Madame Henry, who should be given much of the credit for the improvement in the survival rate through improved nursing care which coincided with the introduction of the couveuse. Tarnier's assistants, Auvard and Berthod, produced statistical evidence of improved survival rates. In Berlin, Hearson introduced automatic temperature regulation into his incubators by means of an electrical alarm mechanism set off when the temperature in the incubator deviated from that which was required. In Montpellier, in 1896, Diffre added mechanisms to control ventilation and humidity.

In 1885 Pajot constructed a giant incubator more like a 'huge oven' in which congenitally feeble infants were entirely separated from their mothers and were cared for and fed by wet nurses, and Colerat (1896) in Lyons recommended a 'hot' room in which pre-term infants should be nursed. Tarnier appreciated that despite the provision of incubators the mortality among pre-term infants, although reduced, was still extremely high. He recognised that the vulnerability of immature infants to infection was a major factor. It is almost certain that he was influenced by the work on infection of Louis Pasteur at the Ecole Normale in Paris during the second half of the nineteenth century.

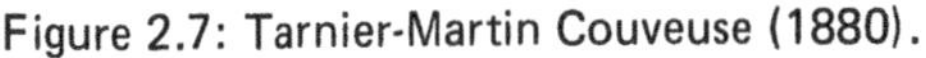
Figure 2.7: Tarnier-Martin Couveuse (1880).

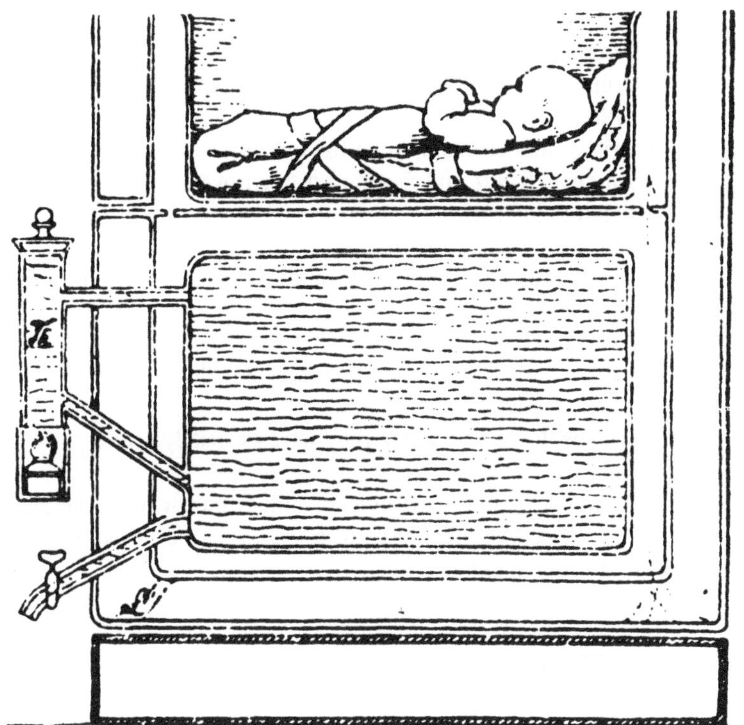

Tarnier and his pupil Budin therefore introduced in 1895 two new methods into their management of pre-term infants: special attention to hygiene in the feeding and care of infants and isolation from potential infection. This need for isolation from infection provided the main reason for the establishment of separate incubator rooms in Paris.

Special Care Baby Units

Thus the stage had been set in 1895 for the establishment of special care baby units. Tarnier encouraged Budin to establish a special care unit at the Maternity Hospital Porte Royal in Paris with the help of his chief midwife Madame Henry. In the same year a second unit was opened in Paris at the Clinique Tarnier. The principles on which these units were based included:

(1) Grouping together the healthy premature infants.
(2) The isolation of sick infants.
(3) The establishment of a special milk room.
(4) Sterilisation of milk and its retention in an ice chamber in hot weather.
(5) Provision of a changing room for wet nurses where they were 'to wash their hands and face and don an overall' before handling premature infants.

In a series of lectures in 1900 Budin[17] enunciated three basic principles of care for pre-term infants:

(1) Maintain body temperature and prevent chilling.
(2) Ensure adequate feeding.
(3) Treat the diseases to which they were especially prone.

He recommended feeding with human milk from birth. If the infant was unable to suck, the milk was expressed and either given by gavage or trickled into the infant's mouth.

Prevention of Infection by Isolation

To prevent infections to which pre-term infants were especially prone, Budin advocated their nursing in separate units and the isolation of those who showed evidence of infection. He recognised that contamination of feeds was a special source of infection and therefore recommended that milk should be sterilised and that nurses should apply a high standard of hygiene which involved hand-washing, use of overalls and the provision of a special milk room.

It can be further added that Budin, in commenting on the giant incubator used by Pajot in 1885, had observed that this carried the inherent danger that the natural mother would lose all interest in her infant. Presumably in his own unit he attempted to counteract this danger.

Dissemination of Information

News of these medical advances soon disseminated. Budin encouraged his pupil, Martin Couney, who had been educated in Breslau, Berlin and Leipzig to demonstrate the Parisian methods of neonatal care at international exhibitions. The first of these was in Berlin in 1896 where, with the support of Professor Czerny, an obstetrician, he brought six incubators to the World Exhibition and received much encouragement from Empress Augusta Victoria, the protectress of Berlin's Charity Hospital. Several 'batches' of pre-term infants who were otherwise considered to have had 'little chance of survival' were successfully reared during the course of the exhibition. A London promoter, Samuel Schenkein, was so impressed that he invited Couney to repeat the performance at Earls Court, London in 1887. The *Lancet*[18] commented that the advantage of the 'Couney' incubators (it appears that at this exhibition Couney in fact used the Altmann incubator devised in Berlin) was the automatic maintenance of temperature, that only air from outside the building was admitted to the incubators and that the only handling of infants was for their feeding and washing. A further demonstration was mounted at the World Fair in the Agricultural Hall, Islington, London in 1898. This prompted a further editorial in the *Lancet* which contained a note of criticism:

> Incubators are only useful for prematurely born children and especially for infants whose lives cannot be saved in any other way. Therefore constant medical supervision and the presence day and night of nurses trained in the use of incubators and of wet nurses is indispensable. To organise all this in a satisfactory manner necessitates outlay and cannot lightly be undertaken by inexperienced persons. We are informed at our visit to the World's Fair that the infants were fed by their mothers – but how can the mothers attend during the whole of the night at the Agricultural Hall and where is the sleeping accommodation?[19]

In 1898 Couney also undertook a similar demonstration at the Omaha Trans-Mississippi Exhibition, USA, and a further exhibition was given back in Paris in 1900. Couney subsequently worked in the United States until his death in 1950.

Considerable publicity was thus achieved by these exhibitions, but this does not appear to have resulted in an immediate response from the medical profession. In Paris, Budin, who had been involved in its instigation, may also have developed reservations about these public demonstrations of the care of pre-term infants which were called 'freak shows' by some reporters. He was also prompted to repeat the concern that he had expressed about the use of the giant incubator introduced by Pajot in 1885, 'the life of the little one has been saved, it is true, but at the cost of a mother'.

1900-50

It might have been expected that the first years of the twentieth century would have seen a period of further rapid expansion of neonatal care services. In practice progress was limited for a number of reasons. First, it needs to be emphasised that although much of the knowledge which would lead to better care existed, its effective application had to wait until scientific knowledge had provided safe methods for its use. Secondly, in the United Kingdom in particular and to a lesser extent in continental Europe and in North America, obstetricians rather than paediatricians continued to retain the major responsibility for the care of the newborn. Although some of these obstetricians, notably Ballantyne,[20] made major contributions, in many centres their primary attention was concentrated upon other crucial problems such as the very high maternal mortality.

It is not to be inferred that there were no changes in the promotion of special care baby units between 1900 and 1950.[21] Julius Hays Hess had established a special care unit at the Michael Reese Hospital, Chicago, by 1914. His publications[22-26] give a clear description of the progressive improvements that he initiated, including the use of portable incubators. The plan of his unit in the University of Illinois, which is illustrated in Figure 2.8, was designed in 1920. Both in the United States and in continental Europe, paediatricians in general were very much more involved with neonatal care than in the United Kingdom. To this rule V. Mary Crosse of Birmingham, England, was a distinguished exception. She established her special care baby unit at the Sorrento Hospital in 1931 and was without question the leading exponent of these units in Britain for the next fifteen years.[27] By contrast during the 1930s a large number of special care baby units were being established in the United States. A typical example was the A. N. Brady Hospital, Albany, New York.

It is not unreasonable to suggest that the shattering impact of World Wars I and II may have delayed the development of facilities in continental Europe and the United Kingdom during the period 1914-50. Even so, the initiatives at Maternité Port Royale, St Vincent de Paul and L'Hôpital des Enfants Malades continued to improve their facilities for special care for pre-term infants. The work of Yippo was also influential, not only in Finland but also in Sweden and Denmark.

Developments since 1950

After World War II the provision of special care baby units increased in all industrialised societies. This increase initially took place more slowly in some countries than in others. In the United Kingdom the increase did not occur until well after the establishment of the National Health Service in 1948, which had enabled specialist paediatricians to be appointed at each major centre in the country. In 1961 the Ministry of Health published *Prevention of Prematurity and the Care of Premature Infants*[28] which recommended the provision of special care baby units in all large and medium-sized maternity hospitals. Thus the general availability of special care baby units in the United Kingdom only became a reality just over twenty years ago. The subsequent development of intensive care facilities is of even more recent origin. It was only endorsed as national policy as recently as 1971 by the DHSS with the recommendation that regional and sub-regional intensive neonatal care units should be established.[29] In North America the widespread availability of both special care baby units and subsequently intensive care neonatal units had occurred a decade earlier than in the United Kingdom, these becoming increasingly available by 1950 and 1960 respectively.

The rapid advances in technology and the continuing application of new findings from basic scientific research tended to create an inbalance in the policies which governed the organisation of special care baby units. In the endeavour to make the best possible use of recent scientific advances and to avoid infection, some of the simpler basic human needs such as close mother-child contact received less attention. It is one of the more encouraging aspects of contemporary neonatology that, especially during the last 15 years, there has been a widespread and re-awakened awareness that the humanities must not be swamped by the sciences. This combined approach (unless it is again forgotten as has happened in past centuries) augurs well for the future.

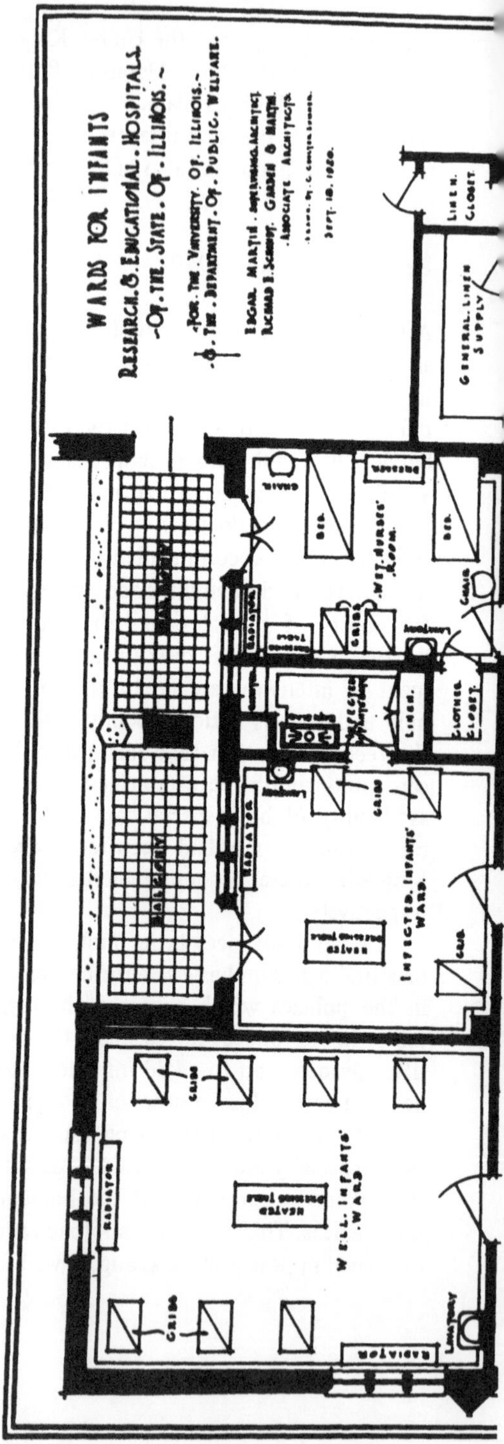

Figure 2.8: Design of Hess's Special Care Baby Unit, Chicago, 1920.

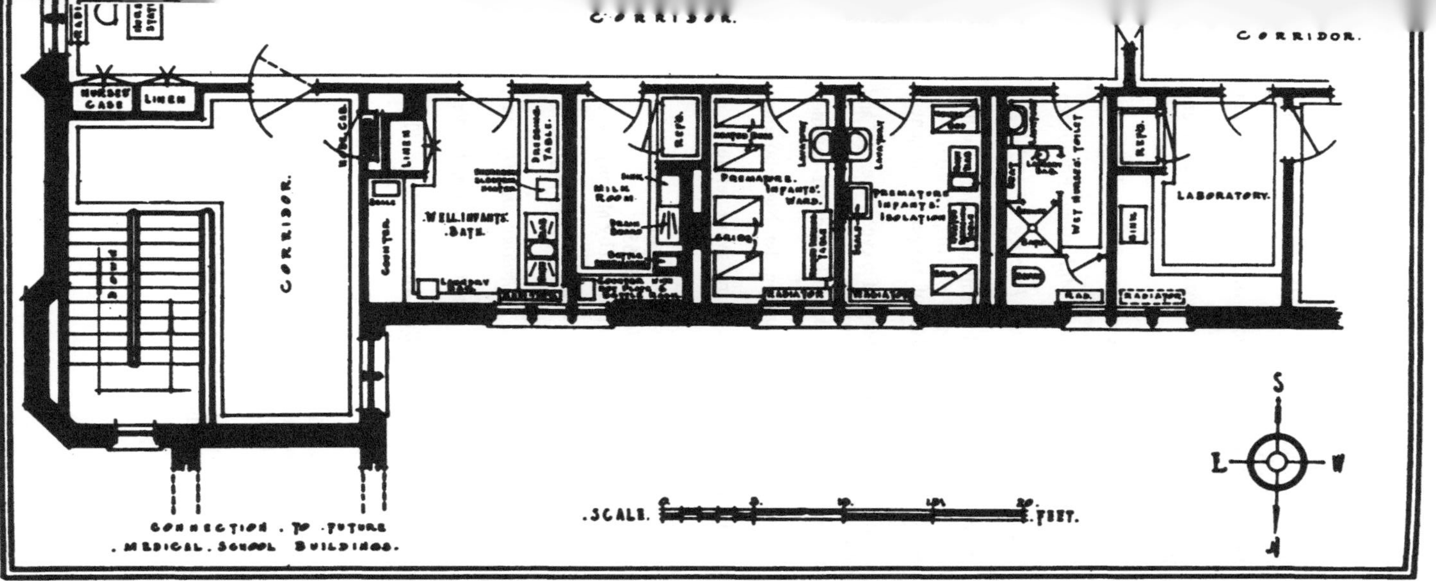

-Floor plan of infant ward for a general hospital with limited floor space. Wards for infected infants are equipped for complete isolation.

References

1. Wickes, I. (1953). A history of infant feeding. *Arch. Dis. Child.*, *28*, 151, 232, 332, 410, 495.

2. Pinchbeck, Ivy, and Hewitt, Margaret (1969, 1973). *Children in English Society*, 2 vols. London, Routledge and Kegan Paul.

3. Abt, I. A., and Garrison, F. H. (1965). *History of Pediatrics*. London, Saunders.

4. Vega., G. (1966). *Royal Commentaries on the Incas*. Austin, Texas, and London, University of Texas Press.

5. Mead, M. (1941). *Male and Female*, London.

6. Caulfield, E. (1931). *The Infant Welfare Movement in the Eighteenth Century*, with a Foreword by Still, G. F. New York, Hoeber.

7. Eden, T. W., and Holland, E. (1925). *A Manual of Midwifery*. Edinburgh, Churchill.

8. Smellie, W. (1752). *Treatise on the Theory and Practice of Midwifery*. London, Wilson and Durham.

9. Terry, F. L. (1942). Extreme prematurity and fibroplastic overgrowth of persistent vascular sheath behind each vascular lens. *Am. J. Ophth.*, *25*, 203.

10. Ashton, N., Ward, B., and Serpell, G. (1953). Role of oxygen in the genesis of retrolental fibroplasia. *Brit. J. Ophth.*, *37*, 513.

11. James, L. S., and Lanman, J.T. (1976). History of oxygen therapy and retrolental fibroplasia. *Pediatrics, 57*, Special Supplement No. 4.

12. Drepp, P. (1835). Bermerkungen uber einige krankheiten der saulinge. *Analckten, Kindek*, *3*, 150.

13. Clementovsky, P. (1875). Die Zellgewebsverpartung der Neugeborenen. *Oesterr. Jahl f. Paediatrik, 3*, 30.

14. Denuce (1857). Berceau incubateur pour les enfants avant terme. *J. de Méd. de Bordeaux, 2*, 273.

15. Crédé, C. S. F. (1884). *Arch. f. Gynak.*, *24*, 128.

16. Cone, T. E. (1981). The first published report of an infant incubator for use in the care of the premature infant. *Am. J. Dis. Child.*, *135*, 658.

17. Budin, P. (1900). *Le Nourisson*. Paris (English translation by Malony, W. J., *The Nursling*. London, Caxton Press, 1907).

18. *Lancet*, Editorials and Correspondence (1897), *i*, 1490, *ii*, 161, 744.

19. Ibid. (1898), *i*, 390.

20. Ballantyne, J. W. (1902). *Manual of Antenatal Pathology and Hygiene*. Edinburgh, William Green and Sons.

21. Dunham, E. C. (1957). Evolution of premature infant care. *Ann. Paediat. Fenmiae*, *3*, 170.

22. Hess, J. H. (1922). *Premature and Congenitally Diseased Infants*. Philadelphia and New York, Lea and Febiger.

23. Hess, J. H. (1928). *Feeding and the Nutritional Disorders of Children*. Philadelphia, F. A. Davis.

24. Hess, J. H. (1934). *The Physical and Mental Growth of Prematurely Born Children*. Chicago,The University of Chicago Press.

25. Hess, J. H. (1934). Oxygen unit for premature and very young infants. *Amer. J. Dis. Child.*, *47*, 916.

26. Hess, J. H., and Lundeen, Evelyn C. (1949). *The Premature Infant, Medical and Nursing Care*. Philadelphia, Lippincott.

27. Crosse, V. Mary (1945). *The Premature Baby*. Edinburgh, Churchill.
28. Ministry of Health (1961). *Prevention of Prematurity and the Care of Premature Infants*. London, HMSO.
29. DHSS (1971). *Report of the Expert Group on Special Care of Babies*. London, HMSO.

Further Reading

The following are not specifically referred to in the text, but serve as further reading on the history of neonatal care.

Amberg, S. (1934). The oxygen incubator. *Proc. Mayo Clinic, 9,* 134.
Anumonte, A. (1963). Some historical aspects on evolution of care for premature babies. *Dokita, Ibadan*, *4*, 31.
Berthod (1887). *La Couveuse et le Gavage à la Maternité de Paris*. Paris, Thése de Paris.
Booth, C. C. (1979). The development of clinical science in Britain. *Brit. Med. J.*, *i*, 1469.
— (1980). Clinical science in the 1980s. *Lancet*, *ii*, 904.
Boss, J. (1965). Birth in ancient and mediaeval societies. *Istanbul University Tip. Fak., Mec.*, *28*, 306.
Carnegie United Kingdom Trust (1917). *Report on the Welfare of Mothers and Children, England and Wales*. Liverpool, Carnegie Trust.
Crédé, C. S. F. (1880). *De Optima in Partu Naturali Placenta Amovendi Ratione*. Leipzig, Edelmannum.
Czerny, A. (1906). *Des Kindes Ernahrung. Ernahrungssturungen und Ernahrungstherapie*. Leipzig, F. Deuticke.
Fitzgerald, W. J. (1963). History of A. N. Brady Hospital and Infant Home 1915-1961. *New York State J. Med.*, *63*, 594.
Ghosh, S. (1965). Management of the newborn. *J. Indian Med. Assn.*, *45*, 71.
Guiart, J. (1933). L'accouchement au temps des Pharaons. *Aesculape*, *23*, 89.
Guillemeau, J. (1609). *De la Nourriture et Governement des Enfants*. Paris. Translated into English and published by A. Hatfield, London, 1612.
Henderson, J. L. (1953). The evolution of child care. *Lancet*, *ii*, 261.
Hinds, S. W. (1955). Child life in past times. *Med. J. Sthw.*, *70*, 199.
Huard, P., and Imbault-Huard, M. J. (1972). Stephane Etienne Tarnier (1828-1897 et les prématurés. *Gaz. Med. Fr.*, *79*, 6887.
Huard, P., and Laplane, R. (1979). *Histoire Illustrée de la Puericulture*. Paris, Roger Dacosta.
— (1981). *Histoire Illustrée de la Pédiatrie*. Paris, Roger Dacosta.
Jonas, R. (1540). *Byrth of Mankynde*. Dedicated to Katherine Howard, printed by Thomas Raynalde. Described by Ballantyne, J. W. (1906). *J. Obs. and Gynac. Brit. Emp.*, *10*(4), 297-325.
Kahn, E., Wayburne, S., and Fouche, M. (1954). The Baragwanath premature baby unit. *S. Afr. Med. J.*, *28*, 453.
Kite, T., (1778). *Laryngeal Intubation and Bellows*. London, Dilly.
Koch, R. (1881). Uber desinfection. *Mitt a.d.k. Gesundheitesante, Berlin*, *1*, 234.
Kubat, K., and Polisensky, J. (1962). Society and child care in Czechoslovakia from the end of feudalism to the present. *Ca. Pediat.*, *17*, 1112.

Lieberman, J. J. (1976). Childbirth practices; from darkness into light. *J. O. G. N. Nurs.*, *5*(3), 41.
McKinney, L. C. (1945). Primitive mediaeval incubator technique for premature babies. *J. Hist. Med.*, *1*, 483.
Marriott, W. McK. (1924). The food requirements of malnourished infants. *J. A. M. A.*, *83*, 600.
de Mause, L. (1974). *The History of Childhood*. New York, Psychohistory Press.
McCleary, G. F. (1945). *The Development of British Maternity and Child Welfare Services*. London, Nat. Assn. of Maternity and Child Welfare Centres.
Ministry of Health (1917). *Maternity and Child Welfare*. London, HMSO.
Newman, L. F. (1976). A bicentennial review of child rearing; notes of an anthropologist. *R. I. Med. J.*, *59*, 221, 241.
Pasteur, L. (1879). Septicémie puerpale. *Bull. Acad. de Med. Paris*, *8*, 505.
Paterson, D. (1937). *Sick Children*. London, Cassell.
Priestley, J. S. (1772). Observations on different kinds of air. *Phil. Trans. Roy. Soc. London*, *72*, 147.
Radbill, S. I. (1971). Child welfare in ancient Rome. *Clin. Pediat.*, *10*, 204.
Rousseau, J. J. (1762). *Emile ou de L'Education*, 1st edn, Paris.
Shore, M. F. (1976). The child and historiography. *J. Interdisc. Hist.*, *6*, 495.
Silverman, W. A. (1979). Incubator side shows. *Pediatrics*, *64*, 127.
Soranus of Ephesus (AD 98-138). *De Arte Obstetrica Morbisque Mulierum quae Supersunt*. Ex apographo F. R. Dietz (1838). Regimonto Pr. Graef et Vazer.
Still, G. F. (1931). *The History of Paediatrics*. Oxford, Oxford University Press.
Tarnier, E. S. (1883). Sie wurde in der Naternite aufgestellt und wohl zuerst in einer Arbeit von Auvard. *Arch. de Tocologie'*, October 1883.
Tarnier, E. S., Chantreuil, J., and Budin, P. (1888). *Allaitement et Hygiène des Enfants Nouveau-nés*. Paris, G. Steinheil.
Terry, F. L. (1942). Extreme prematurity and fibroplastic overgrowth of persistent vascular sheath behind each vascular lens. *Am. J. Ophth.*, *25*, 203.
Underwood, M. (1819). *Diseases of Children*. London, J. Matheus.
Yankaicur, A. (1966). An historical analysis of programs for the reduction of early childhood mortality in Latin America. *J. Trop. Pediat.*, *12*, 26.

3 ETHICAL ISSUES IN NEONATAL INTENSIVE CARE

John A. Davis

Introduction

Advances in science and technology have combined in recent years to put into the hands of doctors, for the first time in history, powers for cure commensurate with their responsibilities in care.[1] In consequence, although a hundred years ago the morality of medical practice seemed beyond question, the profession needs to re-examine its ethical presuppositions[2] rather than take them for granted. There now arise situations, some of them urgent and literally vital, in which our actions may no longer command the general assent necessary if we are to work for and with each other consistently and with public approval.[3-9] In these circumstances, if we do not put our own house in order, others will come forward with the offer to do it for us – as for example in Professor Kennedy's Reith lectures.[10]

Ethical problems occur particularly often and acutely in the perinatal period.[11] In such circumstances, the paediatrician cannot often help being emotionally involved if he is to meet adequately the needs of his patients and their parents. Among current issues are: the indications for inducing abortion[12-15]; whether priority is to be given to the mother or fetus when the right to life or well-being of one clashes with that of the other; the morality of resuscitating, on the one hand, or conniving at the demise of, on the other, extremely immature newborn infants[6,16-20]; when to treat or to withhold treatment of severe deformity or inborn metabolic error[21-23]; when to remove mechanical life support from a non-viable baby[24]; how to deal with rejecting parents; and the rights and wrongs of research procedures when the subject cannot give consent. In these circumstances if the means to do something is available, not to use them is as much a decision, and perhaps more of one, than to use them[25], but either course of action may entail an increase of suffering for the patient and the parents, either by allowing unnecessary handicap to develop or by prolonging a life which will never in fact remotely realise the human potential of the individual concerned.

Basic questions in neonatal care have been stated in these terms:

(1) Is it ever right not to resuscitate an infant at birth?
(2) Is it ever right to withdraw life support from a clearly diagnosed 'poor prognosis' infant?
(3) Is it ever right to intervene directly to kill a dying infant?
(4) Is it ever right to displace a poor prognosis infant in order to provide intensive care for a better prognosis infant?[2]

All these questions come up almost daily in neonatal practice[26] and are often dealt with on an *ad hoc* basis by relatively junior resident medical staff who may never have had the opportunity to think out all the possible implications of the actions they have to take. Not only do these decisions have to be made quickly but they need to be made with at least the tacit assent of all involved: the doctor who gives orders, the nurses who carry them out, the parents who are most deeply concerned and will have to bear most of the consequences of whatever decision is made, the hospital authorities who are ultimately answerable for the way resources are deployed, the ancillary staff who may be present as helpers, spectators or indeed critics, and the local community which the hospital serves.

Some of our problems will, of course, disappear or change in character with further advances in technology. Congenital central nervous system defects may prove to be preventable or genuinely treatable or they may become very rare because of early detection and abortion. In medical practice, however, new problems usually emerge as others disappear. It is therefore necessary for neonatal and paediatric intensive care units to develop some policy for dealing with their ethical problems based on a consensus which is unlikely to be challenged in the courts by the self-appointed tribunes of the people in newspapers or in the pulpit, does not offend the natural and professional ethics of any staff of the unit, and does not increase the sum of human misery, while yet enabling each baby to be considered individually.

Establishing Ethical Guidelines

In making life and death decisions when tired and overwrought, we need, like soldiers, a drill, since there is rarely time for argument or reflection until after the deed has been done. It would, therefore, be a relief to be able to fall back upon rules backed by law[27] as we could do were we all, for instance, orthodox Catholics as in the Middle Ages in Europe. In that case, any killing after conception would be murder, and the withholding of available and accepted standards of care would be negligence amounting to manslaughter, with those responsible having to accept the consequences as laid down in law. To take such inflexible attitudes in the twentieth century would be impractical.

Another attitude could be that since parents are responsible in every sense for their children they should dictate what is done or not done by their doctors, in the same way that feminists claim in relation to abortion that what a woman does with her own body is her moral business and not that of others. But both arguments ignore the crucial fact that they use someone else – the doctors and nurses with their own rights and feelings – to carry out their instructions; and moreover, at some time in his life the fetus or baby must be allowed rights of its own. It is the duty of the physician to respect these rights[28] even though his contractural arrangement may be with the baby's parents, who might be said, by sharing responsibility, to delegate some of their powers.

It would seem therefore that between the extremes of absolute adherence to external rules based on moral principles and absolute parental discretion, we should look for a middle ground in which decisions are made by consensus, even though the baby is excluded because he is not yet a truly separate being, but still absolutely dependent on his mother.

It is also very important, as we try to achieve this middle ground, for the public, who have to trust us and may not have much choice of doctor or hospital, to see us as reliable and trustworthy. That means our being able to give due weight to their point of view in the context of their whole lives – not solely to what they may say under the momentary pressures imposed by stressful situations. In addition, it behoves the staff of special or intensive care units to be familiar with the ethical stance of every other member of their team, and if at all possible with those of the parents whom they serve, as well as to take into account the law of the land and the moral mood of the community in which they work. It should be possible in these circumstances to judge each incident on its merits in relation to both the rights and needs of the baby, which include growing up in a caring family with biological equipment capable of enabling him or her to reach real maturity. When such a consensus view has been achieved it does not necessarily have to be made explicit, or to find its way into statute, for it is unlikely to correspond precisely with present law, which necessarily lacks discrimination and sensibility.

I believe that it is indefensible to act on presuppositions which have not been adequately discussed and shared in this way. To do so will bring about a muddle which only the law has the authority to resolve. The inevitable results will be a restriction on the freedom of action of those best able to make the sensible clinical decisions that are needed in each individual case.[29] The following presuppositions, I believe, express such a consensus and would probably command majority assent from those with bedside rather than armchair experience of the ethical issues involved in neonatal intensive care:

(1) Every baby possesses what could be called a moral value which entitles him or her to the medical and social care necessary to ensure as far as possible his or her well-being.
(2) Parents bear the principal moral responsibility for the well-being of their newborn infant.
(3) Physicians have the duty to take medical measures conducive to the well-being of the baby in so far as they have been entrusted by its parents to take professional responsibility for doing so.
(4) The state has an interest in the proper fulfilment of responsibilities and duties regarding the well-being of the infant, as well as an interest in ensuring the equitable apportionment of limited resources among its citizens.
(5) The *responsibility* of the parent, the *duty* of the physician and the *interests* of the state are conditioned by the medico-moral principle 'do no harm' without expecting compensatory benefit for the patient.
(6) Life-preserving intervention should be understood as doing harm to an infant who cannot survive infancy or will live on in intractable pain or cannot be expected to participate meaningfully in human experience.
(7) If a court is called upon to resolve disagreement between parents and physicians about medical care, the prognosis for the quality of life of the infant should weigh heavily in the decision as to whether or not to order life-saving intervention.
(8) If the infant is judged to be beyond medical intervention, and if it is judged that its continued brief life will be marked pain and discomfort, it may be ethical to hasten death by means consonant with our conception of the moral value of the infant and the duty of a physician.
(9) In cases of limited availability of neonatal intensive care, it may be ethical to withhold therapy from an infant with a poor

prognosis in order to provide care for an infant with a much better prognosis.

Common Practical Problems

There are a number of specific incidences in which moral and ethical problems commonly arise in neonatal intensive care.

Problem	Debatable course of action
(1) Babies born at the limits of extrauterine variability.	Should ventilatory support be embarked upon?
(2) Babies with major identifiable congenital defects of known prognosis and incompatible with development within normal limits, such as Down's sydrome or myelomeningocele, and particularly when there is a combination of abnormalities.	Should the infant be resuscitated and should he be operated upon in the neonatal period?
(3) Babies who have suffered, in the course of their illness, catastrophies which are likely to prove fatal or severely handicapping in the long term such as a large intraventricular haemorrhage.	Should intensive care be continued?
(4) Babies with major inborn metabolic errors likely to require extremely irksome and hazardous dietary management for the rest of their lives.	Should such treatment be started?
(5) Babies badly asphyxiated during birth and taking more than 20-30 minutes to establish regular breathing.	Should ventilation be continued as the future prognosis becomes more and more bleak?

Up to 50 per cent of the deaths in neonatal intensive care units, are likely to be the immediate consequence of withholding life support in such cases.[30] Thus, in 1981, of the 83 deaths in the Aberdeen Neonatal Intensive Care Unit (Campbell, pers. comm.) 40 occurred despite maximum intensive care, 25 were babies for whom intensive care was deemed inappropriate, and 18 were babies from whom such care was deliberately withdrawn.

Many complicating factors and influences have to be considered when deciding what treatment is appropriate in such cases. Because it is generally easier not to grapple with difficult ethical problems, it is all too easy to persist with treatment long after it has ceased to offer either hope or comfort. Conversely, it is equally easy to be influenced, often unjustifiably, by social factors such as the age, marital status, and socio-economic background of the mother and whether or not the baby was 'wanted'. Major difficulties can also arise when the parents quite reasonably drop hints to the staff that they hope a potentially damaged baby will not be allowed to survive, and then blame their doctors for going beyond what they would consider to be the calls of duty when it does. We have also met the converse situation. Another problem which can arise concerns the physician who is constrained to change his disinterested professional concern for the well-being of a particular patient and family for an interested concern related to, for instance, a wish to keep mortality figures as low as possible, or to establish in numerical terms whether a particular treatment is, or is not, advantageous in prolonging life or preventing handicap.

There is in fact no single universal criterion by which such matters can be decided; it may be necessary and justifiable to save the life of a deliberately and legally aborted fetus who turned out to be viable, and yet to allow a much wanted baby, who has suffered enough, to die. It is essential in these contexts for the doctor to be in full possession of the professional knowledge which enables him alone to give a reasonably accurate prognosis.

Much of our morality does in fact reside in our being good at our jobs and conscientious in acquiring and applying professional knowledge and skill; and some apparently ethical problems can be solved in almost technical terms when we are able to say yes to the following questions:

(1) Are we able to recognise brain death in a baby as our colleagues in adult medicine and surgery can in adults and older children?[31]
(2) Do we know enough about the diagnosis and prognosis in particular conditions, taking into account conceivable advances in science and technology, to be accurate in our long-run prognostic predictions?
(3) Do we know the parents of our patients well enough to understand the long-term consequences for them of their acquiescence in one course of action or another recommended by us, or taken on their behalf without consultation (and if not, should we not have arranged at least to meet them before we assume responsibility for their baby)?
(4) Do we understand the effect on the working of hospitals of apparent inconsistencies in attitudes or quality of care?

What the physician should never allow himself to do is to decide such an issue by reference to criteria other than those which stem from his professional knowledge and his obligation to his patient.

There is, therefore, no way out of any ethical dilemma other than reliance on our own and others' integrity. In a caring profession, it is carelessness that the public find hard to forgive; and it is possible to be morally, philosophically and legally as well as technically careless in the exercise of neonatal intensive care. This means that, in the future, as in the past, we will choose and value our colleagues as much for their moral sense as for their skill, learning industry and judgement in technical matters: indeed these will be seen to be part of a moral whole which makes the complete physician or nurse.

Ethical Problems in Research and Administration

Ethical dilemmas also affect those engaged in research and administration.[32] Nearly all of our established professional skills and knowledge are derived from research, and practical 'know how' becomes shared knowledge through the application of the scientific method. It is a large responsibility to carry out this task, which if ill done leads to the infiltration of error into the very citadels of truth. Therefore those who carry out and write up scientific work in the medical field have major ethical responsibilities relating to both the establishment of reliable theory and its sensible application. To acquire knowledge of reasonable certainty from experiments involving human subjects, it is crucial that studies are so designed that reliable results can be obtained from the smallest possible number of subjects and at the smallest cost to them in anxiety, discomfort or risk. This means an ability to use statistics wisely and correctly as well as to make sure that observations are accurate and therefore repeatable.[33] Careless research is as immoral as careless surgery, and is in the end likely to have even worse because more diffuse consequences. The ethics of research on babies is a controversial topic. To risk the well-being of one individual for the sake of others without consent is to arrogate to oneself moral decisions that belong to the individuals concerned. It is also clear that the parents do not have the right to volunteer their children, nor doctors their patients, as 'guinea pigs', unless they can be persuaded that the patient is likely to share in the benefit that increased knowledge is likely to bring and are certain that the research *will* add to knowledge by being well conceived and well planned. In this area, incompetence becomes immorality; but another form of incompetence is not to question established practice or at least to attempt to improve it.

Conclusion

To what general conclusions in relation to the particular problems of neonatal intensive care do these considerations lead us? Firstly, to maintain a respect for life according to its biological level and for our own and our clients' and colleagues' gut feelings. Secondly, to keep in mind that every act has public as well as private consequences that may reverberate down the years. Thirdly, to acknowledge that problems may be most easily solved when they are discussed and shared with colleagues and clients who are also involved: the more awkward the decision, the more reason that it should be taken by the most senior experienced and responsible member of the group on their behalf. Finally, that whatever is done should be done with what can only be called reverence. Perhaps the ventilator should not be turned off except in the presence of those – parents, siblings, possibly some friends, maybe an administrator, and desirably a clergyman – who might feel that they ought to be present at the moment of somatic death. While the person who actually turns it off feels himself publicly answerable for his act, it is in fact no different to withhold this kind of final life support than to refrain from risky surgical intervention on the grounds that the benefit is very unlikely to be comensurate with the cost to the patient. What we cannot withhold is good nursing care[34] and what we cannot condone is the prescription of drugs to kill rather than to comfort. We cannot play God, but only our professional part in real-life tragedies which can be ennobling or the reverse according to how they are experienced by all concerned.

References

1. Watt, J. (1980). Conscience and responsibility. *B. M. J.*, *281*, 1687-8.

2. Jonsen, A. R., Phibbs, R. H., Tooley, W. H., and Garland, M. J. (1975). Critical issues in newborn intensive care: a conference report and policy proposals. *Pediatrics*, *55*, 756-68.

3. Tomalin, C. (1981) Alexander – the cruel folly. *The Times* (June 12th, 1980).

4. Wick, S. (1981). Paul's story. In *The Premature Baby*, Helen Harrison (ed.). New York, St Martin's Press.

5. Silverman, W. A. (1981). Mismatched attitudes about neonatal death. *B. M. J.*, *ii*, 1313.

6. Ramsey, P. (1981). An ingathering of other reasons for neonatal infant-

icide. In *Ethics at the Edges of Life*. Bampton Lectures, New Haven, Yale University Press.

7. R. C. P. Study Group (1981). A thought from the Medical Services Study Group of the Royal College of Physicians. *Lancet*, *i*, 887-8.

8. Gustavson, J. M. (1973). Mongolism: parental desires and the right to life. *Perspectives Biol. Med.*, *16*, 527-9.

9. Whitehorn, K. (1981). Life on sufferance. *Observer* Newspaper (25 January), 34.

10. Kennedy, I. (1981). *The Unmasking of Medicine*. The Reith Lectures. London, Allen and Unwin.

11. Stahlman, M.T. (1979). Ethical dilemmas in perinatal medicine. *J. Paediatrics*, *94*, 516-20.

12. Fletcher, J. (1975). Abortion, euthanasia and care of defective newborns. *New Eng. J. Med.*, *29*, 75-8.

13. Bok, S. (1974). Ethical problems of abortion. *Hastings Centre Studies*, *2*, 33-52.

14. Goodhart, C. B. (1970). Abortion problems. *Proc. Royal Instit. Great Britain*, *43*, 378-93.

15. Christian, C. (1981). Life, liberty and the unborn child. *Hospital Doctor* (25 June), 7.

16. Revill, M. G. (1981). Implications of the Leicester trial. *Lancet*, *ii*, 1233.

17. Butler, R., and Butler, L. (1981). Deciding which child should live. *The Times* Newspaper (10 August).

18. Sherlock, R. (1979). Selective non-treatment of newborns. *J. Med. Ethics*, *5*, 139-43.

19. Aristotle, *Politics*: 'as to the exposure of children, let there be a law that no deformed child shall live'.

20. McCormick, R. A. (1974). To save or let die: the dilemma of modern medicine. *J. A. M. A.*, *229*, 172-6.

21. Lister, J., Waterson, D. J., and Zachary, R. B. (1981). Life of a child. *The Times* Newspaper (17 August).

22. Montgomery, J. N. (1981). Why Joanne didn't die. *World Medicine* (13 June), 33.

23. Heese, H. de V. (1971). Thoughts on the ethics of treating or operating on newborns and infants with congenital abnormalities. *South African Med. J.*, *45*, 631-2.

24. Absolon, M. J. (1981). The right way to live: the right to die. *B. M. J.*, *283*, 611-12.

25. Campbell, D. (1981). Sanctity of life. *The Times* Newspaper (5 January).

26. Campbell, A. G. M., and Duff, R. S. (1979). Deciding the care of severely malformed or dying infants. *J. Med. Ethics*, *5*, 5-7.

27. Robertson, J. A. (1975). Involuntary euthanasia of defective newborns – a legal analysis. *Stanford Law Review* (27 January), 212-69.

28. Paris, J. J. (1981). The New York Court of Appeals rules on the rights of incompetent dying patients. *New Eng. J. Med.*, *304*, 1424-5.

29. Cook, R. C. M., Evans, R., Goodhall, J., and Sanders, R. K. M. (1981). Paediatricians and the law. *B. M. J.*, *283*, 1543.

30. Diagnosis of Brain Death (1979). Conference of the Royal Colleges and Faculties of the United Kingdom – Appendix 5. *Lancet*, *i*, 261-2; *B.M.J.*, *i*, 332.

31. Puri, B., and O'Donnell, B. (1981). Outlook after surgery for congenital intrinsic duodenal obstruction in Down's Syndrome. *Lancet*, *ii*, 802.

32. Editorial (1981). Clouds over paediatric research. *Lancet*, *ii*, 771-2.

33. Altman, D. G. (1981). Statistics and ethics in medical research. *B. M. J.*, *ii*, 44-6.

34. McElroy, C. (1975). Caring for the untreated infant. *The Canadian Nurse*, *71*, 26-30.

4 THE DEVELOPMENT OF EX-SCBU BABIES

R. A. K. Jones

In recent years there has been a steady improvement in survival of low birthweight infants alongside a general decrease in perinatal mortality.[1] Much of this improvement can be attributed to greater understanding of the physiological needs of pre-term infants and better management of labour but, especially for the very low birthweight infant, much is due to the advent of successful intensive care techniques, particularly mechanical ventilation in the treatment of severe respiratory distress. Concern has been voiced that by keeping such babies, many of whom would otherwise undoubtedly have died, alive, there could be an increase in the number of handicapped survivors. There has thus been considerable interest in following these infants' progress into childhood and this chapter will review their long-term outcome. A child has been described as handicapped if he has a disability of body, intellect or personality proving to be a disadvantage in his environment.[2] Outcome will therefore be considered under three main headings: neurological and intellectual outcome, emotional and behavioural problems, and physical health and growth.

Neurological and Intellectual Outcome

Most studies of survivors from Neonatal Units (hereafter referred to as NNUs), classify children as normal or as having major or minor handicap. Unfortunately there is no agreement as to which disabilities should place a child in which category, but most authors classify as major handicap those conditions likely to necessitate special educational provision, namely IQ below 70, severe cerebral palsy, blindness and deafness. Some authors include all cases of cerebral palsy, although children with a mild diplegia and normal intellect may in practice be only minimally handicapped. The category of minor handicap tends to comprise children requiring extra help within normal schools, such as IQ 70 to 84 (or in some papers 70 to 89), partial vision or hearing loss, and sometimes includes children with mild cerebral palsy, clumsiness, learning difficulties or epilepsy. The full complement of minor handicaps will only be apparent if the children are followed well into school age and so, of necessity, such information only becomes available years after the infants leave NNU.

Infants of Birthweight Above 2 kg

As outlined in Chapter 5, few babies over 2 kg birthweight require admission to NNUs. Most of these will be larger pre-term infants needing tube feeds, though ideally they should be nursed on postnatal wards. Similarly in some hospitals term infants with mild or even no symptoms, such as those with moderate jaundice for phototherapy, infants of diabetic mothers or with mild birth asphyxia, are admitted to NNUs for observation. These relatively healthy infants should not be expected to have any more long-term handicap than the population as a whole. However, some full-term infants will require admission to NNUs because of serious illness. The outcome will largely depend on the specific conditions involved, too diverse for detailed discussion here. Permanent neurological handicap may result from conditions determined early in pregnancy, such as meningomyelocoele, hydrocephalus, chromosome anomalies or congenital infection, and for these infants modern intensive care may be unable to alter the outcome.

Conversely, potentially normal infants may sustain damage shortly before, during or after birth, particularly trauma and asphyxia, which may be considerably modified by the standard of perinatal care. Figures on the long-term effects of perinatal asphyxia are conflicting. Although a low Apgar score correlates with later outcome,[3] infants who appear to be severely asphyxiated may respond rapidly to resuscitation and have no subsequent neonatal symptoms, the majority of such infants showing no evidence of long-term damage. On the other hand, infants who despite prompt resuscitation do not establish regular respiration for a considerable period of time and/or have neurological symptoms persisting for several days, have a poor outcome. For example, Steiner and Neligan[4] found that following cardiac arrest, all of four survivors who took more than 30 minutes to start breathing were severely handicapped at follow-up, as compared with none of 18 survivors who established respiration before that time. Likewise, Mulligan *et al.*[5] found that 46 per cent of infants who developed seizures following birth asphyxia were later severely handicapped, compared with only 12 per cent of those who were seizure-free. Fortunately the number of infants sustaining severe birth asphyxia has declined in many centres, although it remains an important cause of handicap.

Infants of Birthweight 2 kg or Less

Although infants weighing 2 kg or less account for only 2 per cent of births in England and Wales,[6] they may supply 50 per cent of admissions to NNUs[7] and considerably more than half of the work load. Low birthweight in itself is associated with many adverse maternal factors, such as low socio-economic status, extremes of maternal age, poor maternal nutrition, illegitimacy[8,9] and heavy smoking,[10] all of which may themselves affect later development. These factors must be taken into account and the use of siblings or socially matched controls may help in trying to determine the effects of prematurity and neonatal illness *per se* or any effects that may arise from the admission to a neonatal unit.

In the early part of this century these infants had a high mortality, but the literature suggests that the survivors fared as well as their peers from similar social backgrounds.[11] In the 1930s to 1950s, paediatricians became involved in neonatal care and many premature baby wards were opened. New treatments such as oxygen therapy were associated with a dramatic increase in survival,[12] but unfortunately also with an epidemic of blindness from retinopathy of immaturity, a definite link between the two only being established some twenty years later.[13] Policies of withholding food, often for several days, may also have contributed to handicap amongst survivors, as did inappropriate doses of ototoxic antibiotics. This was espcially true for the very low birthweight infants (1.5 kg or less). The final toll of handicap reported from specialist centres ranged from 33 to 70 per cent.[14-17] These poor results came from centres with survival rates well above national figures at a time before specialised neonatal care was widely available. Conversely a cohort study of over 12,000 children born in one week in 1946 throughout England, Scotland and Wales, included only 14 surviving children of below 1.5 kg birthweight; none of these was later handicapped.[18]

Since that time there have been major advances in the understanding of neonatal physiology and in intensive care techniques, particularly successful mechanical ventilation in the treatment of hyaline membrane disease. Mortality has continued to fall steadily and major handicap has also fallen dramatically back towards the levels seen amongst the few lucky survivors from the days before specialised neonatal care. For example, University College Hospital, London, followed 259 survivors with birthweight 1.5 kg or less born between 1966 and 1975 and found that only 8.5 per cent had major handicap. Of 123 infants of birthweight above 1 kg who were ventilated for hyaline membrane disease only 6 per cent had major handicap.[19] Unfortunately not all centres have had such excellent results, particularly when infants are referred in from outlying hospitals in poor condition. For example, Fitzhardinge *et al.*[20] reported 30 per cent major handicap in very low birthweight infants, with 47 per cent major handicap amongst those surviving mechanical ventilation,[21] all infants being transferred to the hospital after birth and many being acidotic or hypothermic on admission.

Further falls in the percentage of handicapped survivors during the late 1960s and 1970s are partly explained by the steep fall in mortality, with a greater number of normal children diluting a 'hard core' of handicap.[22] Nevertheless many units are now reporting normal development in the majority of survivors.[23-27] Unfortunately most of these reports are from specialised referral centres and do not necessarily reflect what is happening within a total population. Recent geographically-based studies do show a slight but definite increase in the contribution of very low birthweight infants to cerebral palsy.[28,29] Several follow-up studies have emphasised the importance of social class and standards of maternal care on subsequent intellectual development.[18,30-32] Drillien states that 'the effect of low birthweight is seen to be most marked in children who have the added disadvantage of an adverse home background and a poor genetic endowment of intelligence'.[30]

Infants at Particular Risk

Although most low birthweight infants now do well, certain groups can be identified as being at higher risk of long-term handicap.

Light-for-dates Infants. Infants whose birthweights lie below the tenth (and particularly the fifth) centile for their gestation have lower IQ and more learning difficulties and neurological abnormalities than their appropriately grown peers.[32] Problems are especially likely if growth retardation starts during the second trimester[33] and is associated with poor head growth.[31] Cerebral palsy is also increased.[28,29] Many of these infants are apparently healthy in the neonatal period and their relatively poor outcome is thus the more disappointing. Those who are preterm as well as light-for-dates are at especially high risk, having more problems than appropriately grown infants of similar birthweight and hence low gestation.[20,31] In one study 12 out of 28 light-for-dates infants below 33 weeks gestation and below 1501g had major handicap compared with only 3 of 28 appropriate-for-dates infants matched for birthweight and perinatal complications.[20]

Infants of Birthweight 1 kg or Less

In recent years these extremely low birthweight infants have formed an increasing proportion of patients in regional neonatal units.[34] Their mortality has fallen from 85 per cent in 1965 to 76 per cent in 1978-9.[1] Although some of these infants have a relatively trouble-free course, some of the most immature may require prolonged periods of ventilation. Major handicap in this group remains high, ranging from 15 to 40 per cent[35-37] and their problems have been likened to those of survivors of 1-1.5 kg from the 1950s.[37] One earlier report had suggested major handicap rates as low as 7 per cent,[38] but the authors do not state how many had needed mechanical ventilation, which in the study of Cohen *et al.*[36] carried a 37 per cent risk of major handicap. Retinopathy of immaturity is re-emerging in these new tiny survivors despite careful monitoring of arterial oxygen levels.[39,40]

Infants with Neurological Symptoms. Recurrent apnoea is common amongst pre-term infants and usually responds well to stimulation or treatment such as methyl xanthine drugs, but for those who fail to respond to such measures and require assisted ventilation the outlook is poor.[19,41] Recurrent apnoea is a risk factor for later handicap[42] and specifically for retinopathy of immaturity[39] and sensori-neural deafness.[43] Birth asphyxia and fits are also risk factors for later handicap.[37,42]

The role of intraventricular haemorrhage in producing long-term damage is becoming clearer. Screening programmes using computerised axial tomography (CAT scanning) or real-time ultrasound have shown that subependymal and intraventricular haemorrhage are common amongst infants of very low birthweight,[44,45] much more so than overt neurological damage, suggesting that many of these bleeds do little or no harm. However, follow-up studies have shown that those bleeds involving either ventricular dilation or extension into cerebral substance are associated with high rates of handicap.[46-48] It is possible that the use of ultrasound may in future enable clinicians to predict those infants at greatest risk in whom withdrawal of intensive care might be considered.

Emotional and Behaviour Problems

Most of this book is devoted to discussing difficulties in maternal-infant relationships and ways of enhancing them to try to reduce long-term discord. Pre-term infants have long been recognised to have more than their fair share of behaviour problems and emotional maladjustment[11,30,32,49,50] and have been variously described as over-anxious, shy and passive, or aggressive. This has been partly attributed to prematurity *per se* and partly to over-protective attitudes by the parents.[49,50] More recently attention has focused on the possible role of early separation from the parents, especially the mother, in the genesis of such difficulties. This separation is especially common for sick preterm or term infants requiring transfer to a regional neonatal intensive care unit or even a supra-regional paediatric unit far from the parents' home. In a recent study from the North East Thames Region[34] surviving infants of 1 kg or less had a mean stay in a regional unit of seven weeks, likely to be followed by further weeks back at their local hospital. If possible, arrangements are made for the mother to be transferred with the infant to facilitate contact, but this may not be feasible if the mother herself is ill or if the baby is transferred to a children's hospital with no obstetric facilities. Even if the mother is resident in the hospital, visiting a sick infant surrounded by complicated equipment may be a daunting experience and despite a policy of unrestricted visiting at any time of day or night, visits are often very brief and may involve little direct physical contact with the baby. It is still not clear to what extent paucity of contact early on contributes to later behaviour problems.

Physical Health and Growth

Apart from the neurological and emotional sequelae of pre-term birth and neonatal illness, there may also be physical problems. Term infants with congenital abnormalities may, of course, have a host of defects which may or may not be fully correctible surgically. The family may have to learn to cope with a child with cyanotic heart disease who is slow to feed and thrives poorly. Care of special diets, colostomies, incontinence, etc., can put considerable strain on the family emotionally. Fortunately these sorts of problems are relatively rare.

Infants of low birthweight may also have problems, despite being physically normal at the time of their pre-term birth. Serious iatrogenic problems occasionally occur during intensive care,[51] such as thrombo-embolic damage to the legs from umbilical artery catheters, obstructive jaundice from intravenous feeding (fortunately usually reversible) and blindness from oxygen toxicity (not always avoidable). More minor problems, such as permanent scarring from extravasation of intravenous feeding solutions, pleural drainage tubes, etc., are common. Necrotising enterocolitis is a common problem amongst very low birthweight infants in some nurseries and seems likely to be partly iatrogenic in origin. Mortality is high and amongst survivors stricture formation and adhesions may later lead to gut resections and all the complications of prolonged intravenous feeding and malabsorption. Small babies also have more than their share of respiratory infections, otitis media, conductive deafness, strabismus and inguinal herniae.[30,32] Re-admission to hospital during the first year of life occurred in as many as one-third of one group of very low birthweight infants.[52] The risk of sudden infant death is also increased several-fold.[53]

Pre-term infants who have required mechanical ventilation may have permanent lung damage in the form of bronchopulmonary dysplasia.[21,35] These infants may require oxygen for many weeks or even months, preventing their discharge from hospital. Although the majority will gradually recover and leave hospital, a small number will die in chronic respiratory failure long after the immediate neonatal period. Those whose oxygen dependence has resolved, continue to be at greatly increased risk of lower respiratory tract infection and hence readmission to hospital.[21,52] Persistent changes in lung function tests may be demonstrated in school-age children who have survived pre-term birth, particularly if they suffered from respiratory distress neonatally.[54] Subglottic stenosis necessitating tracheostomy is another complication of prolonged endotracheal intubation for mechanical ventilation. In some of these infants a combination of tracheostomy, chronic lung disease and adverse social circumstances may lead to prolonged hospital care until such time as the tracheostomy can be closed, and even for those children whose parents can be taught to manage them at home, there is a considerable risk of sudden death.

Growth

Most larger pre-term infants will grow rapidly during the first few weeks and months to catch up fully with their peers. However very low birthweight infants, especially if growth-retarded *in utero*, may remain permanently stunted.[30,32,55] If head growth remains small this may be associated with intellectual impairment as discussed above. Similarly, infants appropriately grown at birth who have severe neonatal problems such as necrotising enterocolitis and bronchopulmonary dysplasia may have marked growth failure, with permanent stunting even after the initial complications have resolved. Marked impairment of body growth may increase parental anxiety and an over-protective attitude, and may be associated with emotional problems in the children. However its importance should not be over-emphasised by comparison with centile charts designed for children born at term.[55]

Summary

The vast majority of infants discharged from SCBUs can expect a healthy outcome, although there is likely to remain an irreducible minimum with varying degrees of handicap. Whether handicapped or not, the emotional impact of the time spent in hospital may have long-lasting effects on the family's adjustment. The pre-existing social disadvantage of many of the families into which such children are born must be remembered when considering ways to support them.

References

1. Pharoah, P. O. D., and Alberman, E. D. (1981). Mortality of low birthweight infants in England and Wales 1953 to 1977. *Arch. Dis. Child.*, *56*, 86.

2. Mitchell, R. G. (1977). The nature and causes of disability in childhood. In *Neurodevelopmental Problems in Early Childhood. Assessment and Management*, C. M. Drillien and M. B. Drummond (eds), Oxford, Blackwell.

3. Drage, K. S., Kennedy, C., Berendes, H., Schwarz, B. K., and Weiss, W. (1966). The Apgar Score as an index of infant morbidity. A report from the collaborative study of cerebral palsy. *Devel. Med. Child Neurol.*, *8*, 141.

4. Steiner, H., and Neligan, G. (1975). Perinatal cardiac arrest: quality of the survivors. *Arch. Dis. Child.*, *50*, 696-702.

5. Mulligan, J. C., Painter, M. J., O'Donoghue, P. A., MacDonald, H. M., Allen, A. C., and Taylor, P. M. (1980). Neonatal asphyxia. II. Neonatal mortality and long-term sequelae. *J. Pediatr.*, *96*, 903.

6. Chief Medical Officer. (1980). On the state of the public health for the year 1979. London, HMSO, 26.

7. Whitby, C., de Cates, C. R., and Roberton, N. R. C. (1982). Infants weighing 1.8-2.5 kg: should they be cared for in neonatal units or postnatal units or postnatal wards? *Lancet*, *i*, 322.

8. Drillien, C. M. (1957). The social and economic factors affecting the incidence of premature birth. Part I. *J. Obstet. Gynaecol. Br. Empire*, *64*, 161.

9. Baird, D. (1964). The epidemiology of prematurity. *J. Pediatr.*, *65*, 909.

10. Meyer, M. B., Jonas, B. S., and Tonascia, J. A. (1976). Perinatal events associated with maternal smoking during pregnancy. *Am. J. Epidemiol.*, *103*, 464.

11. Benton, A. (1940). Mental development of prematurely born children. *Am. J. Orthopsychiatry*, *10*, 719.

12. Hess, J. H., Mohr, G. J., and Bartelme, P. F. (1934). *The Physical and Mental Health of Prematurely Born Children*. Chicago, University of Chicago Press.

13. Ashton, N., Ward, B., and Serpell, G. (1953). Role of oxygen in the genesis

of retrolental fibroplasia; a preliminary report. *Br. J. Ophthalmol.*, *37*, 513.

14. Knobloch, H., Rider, R., Harper, P., and Pasamanick, B. (1956). Neuropsychiatric sequelae of prematurity. *JAMA*, *161*, 581.

15. Lubchenko, L. O., Horner, F. A., Reed, L. H., Hix, I. E., Metcalf, D., Cohig, R., Elliott, H. C., and Bourg, M. (1963). Sequelae of premature birth. Evaluation of premature infants of low birth weights at ten years of age. *Am. J. Dis. Child*, *106*, 101.

16. Drillien, C. M. (1967). The incidence of mental and physical handicaps in school age children of very low birth weight. II. *Pediatrics*, *39*, 238.

17. McDonald, A. D. (1967). *Children of Very Low Birth Weight*. London, Heinemann.

18. Douglas, J. W. B., and Gear, R. (1976). Children of low birthweight in the 1946 national cohort: behaviour and educational achievement in adolescence. *Arch. Dis. Child.*, *51*, 820.

19. Stewart, A., Turcan, D., Rawlings, G., Hart, S., and Gregory, S. (1978). Outcome for infants at high risk of major handicap. In *Major Mental Handicap: Methods and Costs of Prevention*, K. Elliott and M. O'Connor (eds), Ciba Found. Symp., No. 59. Amsterdam, Elsevier, 151.

20. Fitzhardinge, P. M., Kalman, E., Ashby, S., and Pape, K. E. (1978). Present status of the infant of very low birth weight treated in a referral neonatal intensive care unit in 1974. In *Major Mental Handicap: Methods and Costs of Prevention*, K. Elliott and M. O'Connor (eds), Ciba Found Symp., No. 59. Amsterdam, Elsevier, 139.

21. Fitzhardinge, P. M., Pape, K., Arstikaitis, M., Boyle, M., Ashby, S., Rowley, A., Netley, C., and Swyer, P. R. (1976). Mechanical ventilation of infants of less than 1,501 g birth weight; health, growth and neurologic sequelae. *J. Pediatr.*, *88*, 531.

22. Jones, R. A. K., Cummins, M., and Davies, P. A. (1979). Infants of very low birthweight: a 15-year analysis. *Lancet*, *i*, 1332.

23. Kumar, S. P., Anday, E. K., Sacks, L. M., Ting, R. Y., and Delivoria-Papadopoulos, M. (1980). Follow-up studies of very low birth weight infants (1,250 grams or less) born and treated within a perinatal center. *Pediatrics*, *66*, 438.

24. Shennan, A. T., and Milligan, J. E. (1980). The growth and development of infants weighing 1,000 to 2,000 grams at birth and delivered in a perinatal unit. *Am. J. Obstet. Gynecol.*, *136*, 273.

25. Peacock, W. G., and Hirata, T. (1981). Outcome in low-birth-weight infants (750 to 1,500 grams): a report on 164 cases managed at Children's Hospital, San Francisco, California. *Am. J. Obstet. Gynecol.*, *140*, 165.

26. Horwood, S. P., Boyle, M. H., Torrance, G. W., and Sinclair, J. C. (1982). Mortality and morbidity of 500- to 1,499-gram birth weight infants live-born to residents of a defined geographic region before and after neonatal intensive care. *Pediatrics*, *69*, 613.

27. Saigal, S., Rosenbaum, P., Stoskopf, B., and Milner, R. (1982). Follow-up of LBW infants with perinatal intensive care. *J. Pediatr.*, *100*, 606.

28. Hagberg, B. (1979). Epidemiological and preventive aspects of cerebral palsy and severe mental retardation in Sweden. *Eur. J. Pediatr.*, *130*, 71.

29. Dale, A., and Stanley, F. J. (1980). An epidemiological study of cerebral palsy in Western Australia, 1956-1975. II : Spastic cerebral palsy and perinatal factors. *Devel. Med. Child Neurol.*, *22*, 13.

30. Drillien, C. M. (1964). *The Growth and Development of the Prematurely Born Infant*. Edinburgh, Livingstone.

31. Francis-Williams, J., and Davies, P. A. (1974). Very low birthweight and later intelligence. *Devel. Med. Child Neurol.*, *16*, 709.

32. Neligan, G. A., Kolvin, I., Scott, D. M., and Garside, R. F. (1976). *Born Too Soon or Born Too Small*, Clinics in Developmental Medicine, No. 61. London, Heinemann.

33. Parkinson, C. E., Wallis, S., and Harvey, D. (1981). School achievement and behaviour of children who were small-for-dates at birth. *Devel. Med. Child. Neurol.*, *23*, 41.

34. Simpson, H., and Walker, G. (1981). Estimating the cots required for neonatal intensive care. *Arch. Dis. Child.*, *56*, 90.

35. Ruiz, M. P. D., LeFever, J. A., Hakanson, D. O., Clark, D. A., and Williams, M. L. (1981). Early development of infants of birth weight less than 1,000 grams with reference to mechanical ventilation in newborn period. *Pediatrics*, *68*, 330.

36. Cohen, R. S., Stevenson, D. K., Malachowski, N., Ariagno, R. L„ Kimble, K. J., Hopper, A. O., Johnson, J. D., Ueland, K., and Sunshine, P. (1982). Favourable results of neonatal intensive care for very low birth-weight infants. *Pediatrics*, *69*, 621.

37. Knobloch, H., Malone, A., Ellison, P. H., Stevens, F., and Zdeb, M. (1982). Considerations in evaluating changes in outcome for infants weighing less than 1,501 grams. *Pediatrics*, *69*, 285.

38. Stewart, A. L., Turcan, D. M., Rawlings, G., and Reynolds, E. O. R. (1977). Prognosis for infants weighing 1000 g or less at birth. *Arch. Dis. Child.*, *52*, 97.

39. Gunn, T. R., Easdown, J., Outerbridge, E. W., and Aranda, J. V. (1980). Risk factors in retrolental fibroplasia. *Pediatrics*, *65*, 1096.

40. Yu, V. Y. H., Hookham, D. M., and Nafe, J. R. M. (1982). Retrolental fibroplasia – controlled study of 4 years' experience in a neonatal intensive care unit. *Arch. Dis. Child.*, *57*, 247.

41. Jones, R. A. K., and Lukeman, D. (1982). Apnoea of immaturity. 2. Mortality and handicap. *Arch. Dis. Child.*, *57*, 766.

42. Kitchen, W. H., Ryan, M. M., Rickards, A., McDougall, A. B., Billson, F. A., Keir, E. H., Naylor, F. D. (1980). A longitudinal study of very low birth-weight infants. IV: An overview of performance at eight years of age. *Devel. Med. Child. Neurol.*, *22*, 172.

43. Abramovitch, S. J., Gregory, S., Slemick, M., and Stewart, A. (1979). Hearing loss in very low birthweight infants treated with neonatal intensive care. *Arch. Dis. Child.*, *54*, 421.

44. Burstein, J., Papile, L-A., and Burstein, R. (1979). Intraventricular haemorrhage and hydrocephalus in premature newborns: a prospective study with CT. *AJR*, *132*, 631.

45. Levene, M. I., Wigglesworth, J. S., and Dubowitz, V. (1981). Cerebral structure and intraventricular haemorrhage in the neonate: a real-time ultrasound study. *Arch. Dis. Child.*, *56*, 416.

46. Krishnamoorthy, K. S., Shannon, D. C., DeLong, G. R., Todres, I. D., and Davis, K. R. (1979). Neurological sequelae in survivors of neonatal intraventricular haemorrhage. *Pediatrics*, *64*, 233.

47. Papile, L-A., Munsick, G., Weaver, N., and Pecha, S. (1979). Cerebral intraventricular haemorrhage (CVH) in infants < 1500 grams: developmental follow-up at one year (Abstract). *Pediatr. Res.*, *13*, 528.

48. Palmer, P., Dubowitz, L. M., Levene, M. I., and Dubowitz, V. (1982). Developmental and neurological progress of preterm infants with intraventricular haemorrhage and ventricular dilatation. *Arch. Dis. Child.*, *57*, 748.

49. Howard, P. J., and Worrell, C. H. (1952). Premature infants in later life – study of intelligence and personality of 22 premature infants at ages 8 to 19 years. *Pediatrics*, *9*, 577.

50. Bjerre, I., and Hansen, E. (1976). Psychomotor development and school-

adjustment of 7-year-old children with low birthweight. *Acta Paediatr. Scand.*, *65*, 88-96.

51. Haas, R. H., and Davies, P. A. (1980). Iatrogenic hazards in the newborn intensive care unit. In *Topics in Perinatal Medicine*, B. A. Wharton (ed.). Tunbridge Wells, Pitman Medical, 104.

52. Hack, M., DeMonterices, D., Merkatz, I. R., Jones, P. and Fanaroff, A. A. (1981). Rehospitalization of the very-low-birth-weight infant: a continuum of perinatal and environmental morbidity. *Am. J. Dis. Child.*, *135*, 263.

53. Protestos, C. D., Carpenter, R. G., McWeeny, P. M., and Emery, J. L. (1973). Obstetric and perinatal histories of children who died unexpectedly (cot death). *Arch. Dis. Child.*, *48*, 835.

54. Coates, A. L., Bergsteinsson, H., Desmond, K., Outerbridge, E. W., and Beaudry, P. H. (1977). Long-term pulmonary sequelae of premature birth with and without idiopathic respiratory distress syndrome. *J. Pediatr.*, *90*, 611.

55. Kimble, K. J., Ariagno, R. L., Stevenson, D. K., and Sunshine, P. (1982). Growth to age 3 years among very low-birth-weight sequelae-free survivors of modern neonatal intensive care. *J. Pediatr.*, *100*, 622.

Part Two

PRACTICAL MANAGEMENT OF PARENT-BABY INTERACTION IN NEONATAL UNITS

INTRODUCTION

J.A. Davis, M.P.M. Richards and N.R.C. Roberton

In the preceding four chapters we have tried to outline the background to and the reasons for this book, by describing the rise and development of neonatal units and the growth in knowledge of how crucial early contact is, in caring for both parents and babies in the neonatal period. In addition we have dealt with two of the most important issues which lie behind the anxieties and stresses suffered by many parents, and indeed by the staff of neonatal units, namely, the prognosis for low birthweight infants, and the ethical issues involved in neonatal care.

A plethora of excellent books, both long and short, now exist describing the physical management of healthy infants, and the diagnosis and treatment of the many severe illnesses to which the low birthweight infant, in particular, is heir. But, as this aspect of care has become more and more sophisticated – and successful – we believe that more attention now needs to be given to providing for the emotional and physical needs of the parents whose newborn baby is a patient in a neonatal unit, and also to helping them to be with and be involved in the care of their sick baby. The eleven chapters in this section are an attempt to provide the ground rules for this vitally important area of neonatal care. We start with three chapters which aim to set the scene for the shorter and more practical chapters which follow. First we discuss how to keep babies out of neonatal units, since we believe that the most efficient way of coping with the topic of this book is prevention of neonatal unit admission. If at all possible, babies should be with their mothers on a postnatal ward or at home. There is then a review, written by Marshall Klaus and John Kennell – who in their seminal paper over one decade ago[1] first highlighted the problems of mother-infant separation in the neonatal period – of some of the many studies which have been done in an attempt to improve the care of parents in neonatal units. Thirdly, we have outlined the needs of the parents of babies on a neonatal unit as they have emerged in a series of studies carried out during the past few years.

The main meat of this section is, we believe, in the subsequent eight chapters written by nurses, sociologists, psychologists and physicians with a wide experience of neonatal care. These chapters aim to provide a practical guide to the management of what we see as the most crucial and important components of fostering optimal parent-baby interaction. Not only have we tried to cover specific problems like malformed infants, how the nurses handle first visits, the problems of a referral unit admitting neonates from a far-flung geographical area, and the particularly tricky and interrelated problems of establishing breast feeding in very low birthweight infants and at what weight they can be discharged, but we have also tried to show that professionals involved in providing this care and support do not need to be the more traditional care-givers – the nurses and doctors – but can be any interested and appropriately trained group including the unit's social workers, psychologists or even 'graduate' parents. We also discuss what we all hope to avoid, but must involve ourselves in with consummate efficiency and great tact and compassion: the management of the family whose newborn baby has died.

Reference

1. Klaus M. H., Jerauld R., Kreger N. C., McAlpine W., Steffa M., and Kennel, J. H. (1972). Maternal attachment – importance of the first post-partum days. *New Eng. J. Med., 286,* 460-3.

5 WHICH BABIES NEED ADMISSION TO SPECIAL CARE BABY UNITS?

D. M. Campbell, G. M. Gandy and N. R. C. Roberton

The decade up to 1977 saw a large increase in the number of babies admitted to neonatal units (NNUs) in England and Wales from a figure of 6 per cent of all liveborns in the mid 1960s to a peak of 20 per cent in 1977. However, in recent years the trend has reversed, with only 14.7 per cent of all infants being admitted in 1980.

There have been two important influences on the pattern of NNU admission. First, a series of reports starting with *Prevention of Prematurity and the Care of Premature Infants*[1], continuing with the important *Report of the Expert Group on Special Care Babies* ('Sheldon Report'[2]), and culminating in the House of Commons Social Services Committee *Report on Perinatal and Neonatal Mortality* ('Short Report'[3]), have focused attention on the problems of death and handicap arising in the perinatal period, and have made many recommendations, including the development of NNUs, with the aim of improving perinatal care. Secondly, in the last two decades the specialty of neonatalogy has appeared and special and intensive care baby units providing sophisticated care for critically ill, low birthweight infants have been developed, in part encouraged and supported by the official publications alluded to above. Having built, equipped and staffed these units, which in the interest of simplicity we will call neonatal units, there is a temptation to keep them full, otherwise they will constantly be under threat of closure; there is a clear correlation between cot provision and the number of infants admitted to NNUs.[4,5]

We believe that there is a major need to assess the reasons why babies are admitted to NNUs. We have done this by addressing ourselves to two questions, neither of which has been adequately discussed in the aforementioned official reports:

(1) Are there any disadvantages in being admitted to a NNU?
(2) Is it possible from an analysis of clinical data and the available literature to define a population of neonates who unequivocably would benefit from admission to a NNU?

The Disadvantages of Neonatal Unit Admission

In the last ten years it has become clear that separation from a mother of her newborn infant should be avoided whenever possible (Chapter 1); and the major cause of mother-child separation in maternity hospitals is admission of a neonate to a NNU.

NNUs are an unsafe environment because they contain the sickest infants in the hospital – many of whom are colonised or are actually infected by antibiotic-resistant, Gram-negative organisms. Even asymptomatic infants on NNUs are colonised by these organisms.[5] By contrast the infant on a postnatal ward (PNW) is usually colonised with organisms derived from his mother which are much less likely to be pathogenic.[7,8] Nosocomial outbreaks of serious infection are continually being reported in NNUs[9-11] and it is well recognised that the risks of cross-infection in any unit increase the busier and more crowded it becomes.[12]

Another hazard faced by babies on many NNUs is neglect. Only those who have worked on overcrowed units at night can appreciate how little time the few nurses on duty, pre-occupied with critically ill infants on ventilators, can give to asymptomatic infants who, if mature, and rooming-in with their mothers, would receive much more attention.

A further undesirable effect of keeping infants with minor or potential problems in NNUs is that expertise in the management of these problems is not disseminated amongst the nursing staff elsewhere in the maternity hospital, or indeed in smaller maternity hospitals without neonatal units. Nurses in lying-in wards used to cope expertly with feeding problems in small infants, and with hydrating jaundiced babies, and many were competent to manage the treatment of minor conjunctival and umbilical infections. But now, lacking experience and confidence, they press for such infants to be admitted to the NNU.

Validation of Criteria for Neonatal Unit Admission

We have addressed ourselves to this problem in three ways:

(1) Is the admission of large numbers of infants to a NNU likely to have any impact on neonatal mortality?

(2) Do infants admitted to NNUs for what might be considered, on theoretical grounds, to be unjustified reasons, in fact turn out to have a high morbidity or mortality?

(3) If admissions to the NNU are restricted, is there any excess morbidity in those infants admitted to a postnatal ward who might otherwise have been admitted to the NNU?

Effect of Neonatal Units on Neonatal Mortality

Malformation and birth asphyxia are currently the major causes of death in infants weighing more than 2.00 kg at birth (Table 5.1).

Table 5.1: Neonatal Deaths, Cambridge, 1978-80

Weight (kg)	Rds	Lethal Malfn	Infection	Asphyxia	Other	Total
Below 1.0	16	9	–	–	–	25
1.0 – 2.50	13[a]	11	6[b]	2	2[d]	34
Above 2.50	–	18	2[c]	4	1[e]	25

Notes: a. Only one infant, birthweight 1.52 kg, over 1.50 kg at birth, b. E. coli (3), Pseudomonas, Enterobacter, Str. viridans. c. GBS, Coxsackie B4. d. Pulmonary haemorrhage, kernicterus. e. Persistent fetal circulation.

Whether or not an infant dies from or is handicapped by these problems may well depend on the expertise and skills within the NNU, but his basic problem cannot be *prevented* by NNU admission. Furthermore the absolute number of such infants is small. There were only 42 of them (1.3 per cent) among over 3,000 infants weighing 2.00 kg delivered in Cambridge in 1974 (Table 5.2).

The major causes of neonatal death in pre-term infants are the respiratory distress syndrome (RDS) and its complications (particularly in infants weighing less than 1.50 kg at birth), a small persisting residuum of severe infections and, as with bigger babies, malformations and birth asphyxia (Table 5.1).

Could it be that many of the infants weighing more than 2.00 kg at birth currently admitted to NNUs are gravely ill and only survive because of the treatment they receive? The evidence does not support this view. The British Births Survey,[13] analysing all births in April 1970, a year in which only 12 per cent of infants were admitted to NNUs, noted that 42.5 per cent of all babies admitted to NNUs on the first day of life – many of whom must have weighed more than 2.00 kg – had no illnesses recorded. In 1974, 3,032 infants weighing more than 2.00 kg at birth were delivered in Cambridge. Some 828 (27 per cent) were at some stage admitted to the neonatal unit (Table 5.2). In a retrospective analysis,[4] 623 (75 per cent) of these admissions were

Table 5.2: Infants Greater than 2.00 kg Born in the Cambridge Maternity Hospital, 1974. Indications for admission to neonatal unit at birth or subsequently.

Unjustified	Total	% of all Live Births 2.0 kg
Abnormal delivery (LSCS, forceps, breech, twin, etc.)	293	9.7
Jaundice	57	1.9
Mild birth asphyxia (less than 10 mins artificial ventilation; Infant in good condition afterwards)	54	1.8
Small for dates	53	1.8
Low birthweight	52	1.7
Minor medical problems (e.g. odd glucose tolerance test, past medical history of mother, infant rhesus negative)	45	1.5
Feeding problems, vomiting	29	1.0
Apparently blue (i.e. traumatic cyanosis, blue hands and feet etc.)	26	0.9
Miscellanea	14	0.5
Total unjustified	623	20.5
Justified		
Lung disease	93	3.1
TTN 72		
Apnoea 12		
RDS 5		
Miscellanea 4		
Severe asphyxia	23	0.8
Malformation 19	19	0.6
Other significant illness	48	1.6
Prematurity 33/52	22	0.7
Total justified	205	6.8
Total Admitted to NNU 828		
Total Live Births 2.00 kg 3,032		

thought to be unjustified in that the infants remained asymptomatic, and none of them died. It was thought that 205 (25 per cent) of admissions were justified, including 13 babies who died (ten from lethal malformations, two from severe birth asphyxia and one from respiratory distress syndrome). Respiratory disease occured in 93 babies, and a further 90 babies were admitted suffering from one or other of the many illnesses which afflict newborn babies (Table 5.2). There were no infants with septicaemia; only six infants, including the three who died of birth asphyxia or RDS, required assisted ventilation; and only eight other infants with respiratory disease required umbilical artery catheterisation. This shows that symptomatic disease occured in no more than 6-7 per cent of infants weighing greater than 2.00 kg at birth, and that serious disease was rare.

More recently (Table 5.3) we found that only 2.7 per cent of infants weighing 2.00 kg or more at birth needed admission to the NNU immediately after delivery, with a further 1 per cent needing admission later in the first week.

There are two major implications of these data. First, that component of neonatal mortality (RDS and infection) which is amenable to improvements in neonatal care requires neonatal *intensive care* and is almost entirely limited to the 2 per cent of infants weighing less than 2.00 kg at birth. Secondly, neonatal mortality and morbidity are unlikely to be influenced by admitting for routine neonatal care large numbers of normally formed, unasphyxiated infants weighing more than 2.00 kg; such infants are highly unlikely to die in the neonatal period.

Morbidity and Mortality in Infants Unjustifiably Admitted to NNU

In evaluating unjustifiable reasons for admission, peripheral or traumatic cyanosis misdiagnosed as lung disease (Table 5.2, group 8), and admission for minor medical problems (Table 5.2, group 6), which we believe can be managed satisfactorily on the postnatal wards, will not be considered further: we will concentrate on malformations and criteria 1, 2, 3, 4, 5 and 7 in Table 5.2.

Instrumental and Caesarean Section Deliveries. Today, the vast majority of instrumentally or Caesarian section delivered infants will be in good shape at birth and subsequently, since the intervention will have been aiming to prevent a crisis rather than responding to one. Thus, to admit all infants so delivered to the NNU can only be justified if an increased risk stems from the procedure itself, or if serious symptoms are likely to occur sometime after birth in a large number of infants so delivered, who show no clinical abnormality by 10-15 minutes after delivery.

There are only two problems, not obvious at birth, which might arise in the two or three days following Caesarean section and forceps delivery and which are specifically related to the mode of delivery

Table 5.3: Reason for Admission in Infants of 2.00 kg or over Birthweight, Born Cambridge Maternity Hospital, 1977-80 (figures in parentheses = deaths). Total born of 2.50 kg or over = 14, 274; total born 2.0-2.49 kg = 748.

Diagnosis	Number Admitted Immediately			Number Admitted from Postnatal Ward		
	Birthweight 2.50 or over	Birthweight 2.00–2.49	Total	Birthweight 2.50 or over	Birthweight 2.00–2.49	Total
Transient tachypnoea	82	38	120	23	6	29
Respiratory distress syndrome	26	44(1)	70(1)	4	4	8
Other lung disease	28	1	29	11(1)	–	11(1)
Rhesus incompatibility	10	3	13	4	1	5
ABO incompatibility	–	–	–	8	–	8
Physiological jaundice	–	–	–	10	1	11
Malformation	35(16)	10(6)	45(22)	12(4)	5(2)	17(6)
Apnoeic attacks	–	2	2	9	–	9
Hypoglycaemia[a]	–	–	–	1[a]	2[a]	3[a]
Feeding problems	–	–	–	6	12	18
Miscellanea	14	1	15	3	–	3
Birth asphyxia	25(3)	8(1)	33(4)	–	–	–
Convulsions	–	–	–	12	–	12
Other CNS symptoms	1	–	1	3	–	3
Normal infant	7	66	73	1	4	5
Infections	7	2(2)	9(2)	11(2)	–	11(2)
Total	235(19)	175(10)	410(29)	118(7)	35(2)	153(9)
% of all live births at that birthweight	1.6	23	2.7	0.8	6.2	1.0

Note: a. Two infants who presented with hypoglycaemic fits are included under fits.

(after all any neonate is at risk from congenital heart disease or urine infection). The infant could suffer some asphyxia or traumatic insult which was neither severe enough to cause problems at birth or to make him neurologically abnormal in the first 10-15 minutes of life, but which might nevertheless cause irritability, jitteriness or even a fit in the first 48-72 hours. Secondly, infants born by Caesarean section may have an increased incidence of mild respiratory disease compared with vaginally delivered infants,[14] and these symptoms may take an hour or two to develop after birth. The evidence suggest that neither of these conditions is either common or a problem.

In 1974 in Cambridge[3] there was no morbidity or mortality (Table 5.2) among the 293 infants admitted to the unit only because they were surgical or instrumental deliveries. In 1977-80 when the majority of such infants were routinely admitted to the postnatal ward, delayed onset respiratory disease was not only rare but mild (Table 5.4). However, five of the eight infants who developed RDS on a PNW in the four years of that study (Table 5.4) were delivered by caesarean section, including all four whose birthweight was greater than 2.50 kg. However, they do not constitute a justification for admitting to the NNU, during the same period, over 1,700 other infants delivered by caesarean section who weighed more than 2.00 kg at birth and went safely to the PNW with their mothers.

There was no excess of infants with fits, apnoea or hypoglycaemia among those delivered abnormally (Table 5.4).

A similar result was obtained in a recent survey carried out in Peterborough District Hospital.[5] In early 1979, the routine policy in that unit was to admit all caesarean and breech births to the NNU immediately after delivery. Moreover the majority of forceps deliveries (except for 'lift-out' procedures) were also admitted to the NNU. In 1979 the unit's policy was changed so that by 1980 infants weighing more than 2.00 kg were admitted only if they were ill.

Two six-month periods starting on 1 January 1979 and 1 January 1980 were studied. Except for a significant increase in the use of general anaesthesia and narcotic antagonists in the second six-month period the obstetric antecedents of the infants in the two six-month periods were judged to be comparable, as were their birthweight and condition at birth. The subsequent course of these infants is shown in Tables 5.5-5.7. Symptomatic illness was rare in all groups in both years and in 1980 the staff apparently successfully identified at birth those infants requiring admission to the unit. Illness was rare in infants admitted initially to the PNW, and if it did develop there was no

Table 5.4: Outcome of Infants, Birthweight Greater than 2.00 kg, by Delivery, Cambridge Maternity Hospital, 1977-80.

Route of Delivery	Caesarean Section	Forceps	Breech	Spontaneous Vertex Delivery
Total delivered 2.00 kg or over	1,861	2,024	256	10,877
Number admitted immediately to NNU	110 (5.9%)	44 (2.12%)	14 (5.5%)	290 (2.7%)
Number trans. to PNW with mother	1,751	1,980	242	10,587
Number subsequently admitted to SCBU	40 (2.3%)	18 (0.9%)	5 (2.1%)	91 (0.9%)
Diagnoses of the infants admitted subsequently[a]				
Transient tachypnoea	7	3	–	19
RDS	5	1	–	2
Other pulmonary disease	4	3(1)	–	4
Fits and other CNS disease	4	1	1	9
Malformations	7(4)	1	–	9(2)
Infections (Sepsis, meningitis PUO, NEC, etc.)	4(1)	2	–	7(1)
Hypoglycaemia[b]	–	–	–	3
Jaundice including rhesus and ABO disease	1	3	2	18
Apnoeic attacks	–	2	–	7
Feeding problems	4	1	2	11
Other	2	1	–	3

Notes:
a. Numbers in parentheses are deaths.
b. Two infants who presented with hypoglycaemic convulsions are included under fits.

evidence that it caused the infants any harm.

Jaundice. Jaundice is one of the commonest conditions which develops in the neonate. The significance of jaundice of first day onset and/or rapid rise occurring in infants with severe septicaemia or haemolytic disease is vastly different from (so called) physiological jaundice which rises gradually to a maximum on the fourth day in an otherwise entirely asymptomatic mature infant. The former may cause kernicterus; the latter is benign. There is no evidence that conjugated bilirubin levels of

Table 5.5: Comparison of Number and Clinical Reasons for Admission to NNU, Caesarean Section Deliveries of Babies 2 kg or over, January-June 1979 and January-June 1980, Peterborough District General Hospital.

	Jan-June 1979	Jan-June 1980
Caesarean section total	114	151
Number of admissions to NNU	110	40
Main reasons for admission		
Observation	88	15
Asphyxia	12	7
Respiratory problem	8	13
Severe congenital malformation	1	0
Neurological problem	1	1
Other	0	4[a]
Deaths following admission	1[b]	1[c]
Reason for subsequent admission from the postnatal ward		
Respiratory problem	0	3[d]
Vomiting	0	2[e]

Notes:
a. Two cases admitted because of vomiting, two cases because shocked.
b. Hydrocephalus.
c. Severe asphyxia.
d. One apnoeic and cyanotic, two grunting } none received CPAP, IPPV or
e. One cause unclear, one infection } were catheterised.

up to 25 mg% (430 mmol/1) have ever harmed an otherwise healthy term infant.[15]

If the bilirubin level exceeds 15-16 mg% (250-270 mmol/1) in a mature infant on the third-sixth day, it is wise to exclude urinary infection and rhesus, ABO or other mild blood group incompatibility. If physiological jaundice is diagnosed, phototherapy, with its side effects of diarrohea, poor weight gain, rashes, sticky eyes, maternal anxiety and mother-child separation is not necessary until the bilirubin is 18-20 mg% (310-340 mmol/1). If phototherapy is necessary, it can be given on the PNW where the mother can continue to care for her baby.

Small-for-dates Infants. When it was recognised that asymptomatic and symptomatic hypoglycaemia were common in infants below the third centile for weight for their gestational age,[16,17] and that untreated

Table 5.6: Comparison of Number and Clinical Reasons for Admission to NNU, Instrumental Deliveries of Babies 2 kg or over, January-June 1979 and January-June 1980, Peterborough District General Hospital.

	Jan-June 1979	Jan-June 1980
Instrumental delivery total	233	254
Number of admissions to NNU	93	38
Main reason for admission		
Observation	66	10
Asphyxia	6	5
Respiratory problem	12	13
Haematological problem	0	1
Infection	1	1
Malformation	2	0
Neurological problem	3	4
Other	3[a]	4[b]
Deaths following admission	1[c]	0
Reason for subsequent admission from the postnatal ward		
Respiratory problem	3[d]	2[e]
Congenital malformation	1	0
Infection	0	1
Neurological problem	0	1

Notes:
a. Shocked.
b. Three described as shocked, one mucosy.
c. Intracerebral haemorrhage.
d. Two apnoeic and cyanotic, one grunting.
e. Two grunting.

symptomatic neonatal hypoglycaemia could cause severe brain damage[18,19] small-for-dates (SFD) infants became a focus for anxiety and concern. There is no doubt that such babies must have an adequate intake of calories – from formula if necessary – in the first 48 hours, and that their blood glucose levels must be monitored by the nurses every 6-8 hours using Dextrostix. In Cambridge, SFD babies weighing 1.80 kg or over are successfully kept on the PNW. If the mother intends to breast-feed, the babies suckle at the usual feeding times during the first 48 hours to give them colostrum and to stimulate lactation. In addition, the infants receive 60 ml/kg of formula on day one and 90 ml/kg on day two. With this regime, even asymptomatic hypoglycaemia is very rare.[20]

Table 5.7: Comparison of Number and Clinical Reasons for Admissions to NNU, Breech Vaginal Deliveries of Babies, 2 kg or over, January-June 1979 and January-June 1980, Peterborough District General Hospital.

	Jan-June 1979	Jan-June 1980
Breech vaginal deliveries	41	28
Number of admissions to NNU	33	2
Main reason for admission		
Observation	28	0
Asphyxia	2	1
Respiratory problem	2	1
Neurological problem	1	0
Deaths following admission	1[a]	0
Subsequent admission from the postnatal ward	0	0

Note: a. Fits and infection.

Normal Pre-term Infants Weighing 1.80-2.50 kg. Infants of this birthweight are, in many hospitals, routinely admitted to and kept on the neonatal unit, presumably in Britain in deference to the Sheldon Report.[2] However, serious illness in infants of this birthweight is rare. In 1978-81, the non-malformation neonatal mortality in the Cambridge Maternity Hospital for infants weighing 2.0-2.50 kg was 1.3/1000: one death (from group B streptococcal sepsis) in 749 live births. In the same period, only 35 per cent of infants weighing 1.80-2.50 kg at birth needed admission to the NNU at any time; the majority of these stayed on the the unit for less than five days and went home with their mothers after spending a few days with them on a postnatal ward. The other 65 per cent were cared for successfully by their mothers on the postnatal ward.[20]

Intubation at Birth. As the understanding of the sequence of events in neonatal asphyxia has grown, and with it the benefits of prompt, efficient resuscitation, more and more infants are intubated and receive artificial ventilation in the first 2-3 minutes after delivery with the express intention of establishing respiration as soon as possible, and of keeping the infant in good condition. That having been done, and the endotracheal tube removed, most infants cry lustily and are obviously in good condition clinically. They do not require any further special neonatal care.

Feeding Problems. The reasons for feeding difficulties are many. If the difficulties stem from the actual feeding process, the infants should stay with their mothers so that both can solve their mutual problems. If other diagnoses, such as infection or intestinal obstruction, are suspected, preliminary investigation can be carried out successfully on the postnatal ward without separating the baby and mother.

Infants with Malformations. Although there are only a small number of such infants, their postnatal management merits special mention. Infants with a life-threatening malformation likely to require urgent surgery, such as myelomeningocoele, gut atresias or congenital heart disease, need admission to the NNU. However, infants with non-life-threatening malformations, such as hare lip, cleft palate and Down's syndrome, should be with their mothers. Not only does she need to adjust to and cope with her abnormal baby, but the evidence is clear that a mother's fantasy about her malformed infant is usually worse than the reality (Chapter 13).

Morbidity Resulting from a Restrictive Admission Policy.

Since the mid-1970s, we have introduced rigorous admission criteria for our NNU. To establish whether or not our policy is safe and/or practicable for infants greater than 2.00 kg we have:

(1) Observed how many infants not initially admitted to the NNU at delivery were subsequently admitted; this assesses the efficiency of selection criteria based on the condition of the infant at birth.
(2) Assessed whether illness developing on the PNW might have been prevented by earlier admission to the NNU, and whether the severity and outcome of the illness was worse because it presented on the PNW rather than on the NNU.

The details for babies born in 1977-80 are given in Table 5.8. Only 6 per cent of infants weighing 2.0-2.50 kg, and only 0.8 per cent of those weighing more than 2.50 kg at birth, who were initially admitted to a PNW, subsequently required admission to the NNU. The diagnoses in all infants admitted who weighed more than 2.00 kg are given in Table 5.3. Babies admitted after they had been in the PNW for some time can be divided into three diagnostic groups:

Table 5.8: Admissions to NNU, Cambridge Maternity Hospital, 1977-80.

	Birthweight 2.0-2.50 kg	Birthweight 2.5 kg or more	Total over 2.0 kg
Total live births	748	14,274	15,022
Total admitted to NNU	210(28%[a])	353(2.5%[a])	563(3.7%[a])
Admitted at once to NNU	175(23%[a])	235(1.6%[a])	410(2.7%[a])
Admitted to post-natal ward after birth with mother	568	14,042	14,610
Admitted to NNU later in puerperium	35(6.2%[b])	118(0.8%[b])	153(1.0%[b])

Notes:
a. As a % of total births.
b. As a % of infants admitted to the PNW.

(1) Those suffering from conditions which, from their very nature, normally present sometime after delivery in infants who are not identifiably different at the time of birth: e.g. cardiovascular, gut and renal tract malformations; postnatally acquired infections; ABO and mild rhesus haemolytic disease; physiological jaundice and feeding problems. There were 70 (45 per cent) babies with these diagnoses out of the 153 late admissions (Table 5.3).

(2) Infants with mild respiratory disease such as transient tachypnoea of the newborn (TTN), mild RDS or pneumomediastinum, may not develop symptoms until 2-3 hours of age. A small number of infants with these conditions are bound therefore, to be recognised some – hopefully short – time after admission to the PNW with their mother, and since this type of illness is likely to be mild, they are very unlikely to come to harm. There were 48 (41 per cent) such cases (Table 5.3: see also page 232).

(3) Infants who develop an illness for which a case could be made that it might have been prevented by early admission to the NNU. The four conditions in Table 5.3 which might be included in this category are fits, CNS symptoms, apnoeic attacks and hypoglycaemia. There are 30 such infants in Table 5.3, 29 over 2.50 kg birthweight and only one weighing between 2.00 and

2.50 kg. In both groups this constitutes 0.2 per cent of the infants who were admitted after delivery. Because of the potential importance of this group of infants they will be discussed in greater detail.

Infants with Fits (Table 5.9; see also p. 232). Out of 14,610 infants of greater than 2.00 kg birthweight admitted to the PNW with their mothers in 1977-80, twelve were subsequently admitted to the NNU with fits, an incidence of 0.08 per cent or 1:1200. Although the Apgar scores were in the middle range, no infant required active resuscitation by either bag and mask or endotracheal intubation, and they were all vigorous and in good condition by five minutes of age. All the infants presented on the PNW with short fits which stopped spontaneously. The infants were all then admitted to the NNU. In nine of them the fits were easy to control, and did not require long-term anticonvulsants; these babies, including the two infants with isolated subarachnoid haemorrhage, and the two infants who had seizures with hypoglycaemia, have progressed normally on follow-up. One infant has a very mild left hemiparesis which has delayed his motor milestones in comparison with his twins; other aspects of his development are normal. One other infant has a right-side hemiparesis secondary to a CT diagnosed left side infarct. No cause for this could be found in the perinatal period. The twelfth case, despite a normal pregnancy and delivery and apparently being in good condition at birth, presented aged 15 hours with a large left temporal lobe haemorrhage which progressed to hydrocephalus which required shunting. The infant was profoundly retarded on follow-up and died following acute shunt blockage aged 16 months. Careful retrospective review of his notes failed to demonstrate any factor, which, if avoided, could have improved the outcome.

Apnoeic Attacks. Nine infants on the PNW went transiently blue and had irregular breathing; in seven cases this occurred just after feeds. All nine were admitted to the NNU; no cause was found for their symptoms and subsequent apnoea was rare. After an average stay of four days they were all reunited with their mothers on the PNW. Eight had no problems on follow-up but the ninth has developed the same as-yet-undiagnosed degenerative neurological disorder from which her older sister died at the age of five years.

Neurological Abnormalities. Only three infants out of 14,610 were admitted because they were hypertonic, hypotonic or obviously

Table 5.9: Infants with Fits.

Baby	Delivery	Apgar	Resuscitation	B'wt	Gestational Age	Fits	Age Diagnosed	Diagnosis	Follow-up
C	SVD[a]	9	nil	3.89	42	right focal	6 hrs	CT scan – left sided cortical infarct	right hemiplegia
La	SVD	8 5 mins	facial O_2 only	3.06	40	multiple focal	12 hrs	no cause found	normal
Le	SVD (twin 2 after EVC[f])	8	facial O_2 only[c]	3.01	38	single tonic	30 hrs	? SAH[e]	normal
W	SVD	5-6	facial O_2	3.93	41	3 clonic	6 hrs	no cause found	normal
D	SVD	9	nil[c]	3.51	35	multiple clonic tonic	14 hrs	large intracerebral bleed, hydrocephalus	severe damage: decreased DQ: death 16 months, blocked shunt
R	breech twin 2	7	nil[c]	2.64	36	7 clonic	15 hrs	SAH; transient increased intracerebral pressure on day 2	mild left hemiplegia, no overt handicap aged 2 yrs
Lei	LSCS[d]	4	facial O_2 only[c]	2.51	38	single clonic	52 hrs	blood sugar 0.1 mmol/l	normal
T	LSCS	8	nil	3.40	38	8 clonic	4 days	blood sugar 0.7 mmol/l	normal
Ma	LSCS	8	nil[c]	3.46	40	multi-focal clonic	3 days	Mg 0.4 mmol/l	normal
Mo	SVD	8	nil	3.81	40	right focal x 3	16 hrs	? SAH	normal
A	Forceps	7	nil	2.71	42	single tonic	34 hrs	no cause found	normal
Co	SVD	8	nil	3.85	40	single clonic	7 days	Ca 1.7 mmol/l	cataract (?congenital)

Notes:
a. Spontaneous vertex delivery.
b. This child had many fits.
c. Paediatrician present at delivery.
d. Lower segment caesarean section.
e. Subarachnoid haemorrhage.
f. External cephalic

neurologically abnormal on the PNW. Both the hypertonic infants were spontaneous vaginal deliveries, but the hypotonic one was delivered by caesarean section. None of the infants caused any concern at birth.

Two of these infants were only transiently abnormal, both were reunited with their mothers after 48 hours on the NNU, and both have made normal developmental progress. The third infant presented aged 30 hours with irritability, a tense fontanelle and hypertonicity, attributed to cerebral oedema secondary to severe fetal distress and hypoxia during a spontaneous vertical delivery – even though he was vigorous after delivery and had a good Apgar score. In the NNU his condition rapidly improved and he was thought to be neurologically normal at seven days of age and was discharged, breast-feeding well. He was readmitted aged one month with an enlarging head which on the evidence of a CT scan was thought – despite a positive family history – to be due to a communicating hydrocephalus secondary to a perinatal intracerebral bleed in the right frontal cortex. He was shunted, but his milestones are delayed on follow-up.

Hypoglycaemia. Five infants were admitted with hypoglycaemia. Two presented with convulsions (Table 5.9), one being borderline SFD and the other normally grown although he had probably been underfed. Both were treated with IV 10% dextrose, made a complete recovery and were normal on follow-up. Two other SFD infants (2.26 kg and 2.29 kg at term, and a full-term infant who had suffered mild intrapartum asphyxia, were transferred from the PNW to the NNU with asymptomatic hypoglycaemia. In one of the SFD infants the blood glucose level rose following extra feeding; the other two babies required intravenous 10% dextrose to maintain a blood glucose of 1.0 mmol/l. All three babies are also normal on follow-up.

Deaths. There were nine deaths in infants admitted initially to the PNW and subsequently transferred to the NNU. Six of these had lethal abnormalities, three being inoperable forms of congenital heart disease, two being untreatable inborn errors of metabolism – one with methylmalonic acidemia, the other with non-ketotic hyperglycinaemia – while the sixth had trisomy 21 with multiple malformations. Two others died of viral infections. One, who had disseminated herpes infection, was a spontaneous vertex delivery to a woman not known to have genital herpes. The other was the index case in the Echo 11 epidemic which has been described fully elsewhere.[10] Clearly none of these eight deaths was preventable.

The ninth case merits more detailed assessment. He weighed 3.55 kg at 41 weeks gestation and was delivered by Neville Barnes forceps for delay in the second stage. At ten minutes of age he was noticed to be slightly cyanosed with irregular respiration, but his respiratory symptoms rapidly resolved. Eight hours later he was admitted from the PNW with central cyanosis but only mild dyspnoea. Arterial blood gas analysis suggested cyanotic congenital heart disease. He was transferred to a regional cardiac unit, where a diagnosis of persistence of the fetal circulation was made. He died aged three days. It is doubtful whether earlier admission of this baby to the neonatal unit would have altered the outcome.

Conclusions – Which Babies to Admit?

On the basis of the data presented in this chapter and elsewhere (Chapter 1 and 4, 5, 20), the only absolute indications for admitting a baby to a neonatal unit are clinically apparent disease and a birthweight of less than 1.80 kg. Our grounds for these conclusions are:

(1) Admitting asymptomatic babies 1.80 kg or over for observation is highly unlikely to reduce neonatal mortality and morbidity.
(2) Admitting infants to a neonatal unit exposes them to a definite risk of nosocomial infection.
(3) There is no evidence that infants weighing more than 1.80 kg who are asymptomatic immediately after delivery come to any harm on a PNW with their mothers irrespective of the mode of delivery, or whether they needed transient resuscitation.
(4) There is no evidence that infants who develop symptoms on a PNW come to any greater harm than infants who develop the same symptoms on a NNU.
(5) PNW nurses can cope with Dextrostix testing and extra feedings in SFD neonates.
(6) There are evident disadvantages to the nursing couple from any separation in the neonatal period.

With the admission policy suggested here, the proportion of infants admitted to NNUs could be cut by at least 50 per cent in England and Wales. The current data for Cambridge show that 6 per cent of all neonates admitted to our NNU (Table 5.10) compared with more than twice that number nationally.

Table 5.10: Inborn Admissions to Cambridge SCBU, 1979-80.

Birthweight	Number Delivered	Number Admitted to SCBU at Any Time in Neonatal Period	Per cent
Below 1.50	120	120	100
1.5 – 2.0	171	136	80
2.0 – 2.5	380	85	22
2.5 or over	7,695	163	2.1
Total	8,366	504	6

References

1. Ministry of Health (1961). *Report of the Sub-committee on the Prevention of Prematurity and the Care of Premature Infants*. London, HMSO.

2. DHSS (1971). *Report of the Expert Group on Special Care for Babies* Chairman, Sir Wilfred Sheldon). Reports on Public Health and Medical Subjects, No. 127. London, HMSO.

3. House of Commons (1980). *Second Report of the Social Services Committee. Perinatal and Neonatal Mortality* (Chairman, Mrs Renee Short). London, HMSO.

4. Richards, M. P. M., and Roberton, N. R. C. (1978). Admission and discharge policies for special care units. In *Separation and Special Care Baby Units*, F. S. W. Brimblecombe, M. P. M. Richards and N. R. C. Roberton (eds). London, Spastics International Medical Publications/William Heinemann Medical Books, 82-110.

5. Campbell, D. (1982). *The Evaluation of Aspects of Neonatal Paediatric Services*. PhD dissertation, University of Cambridge.

6. Goldmann, D. A., Leclair, J., and Malone, A. (1978). Bacterial colonization of neonates admitted to an intensive care environment. *Journal of Pediatrics*, *63*, 288.

7. McCallister, T. A., Given, J., Black, A., Turner, M. J., Kerr, M. M., and Hutchinson, J. H. (1974). The natural history of bacterial colonisation of newborn in a Maternity Hospital. *Scottish Medical Journal, 19*, 119.

8. Bullen, C. L., Tearle, P. V., and Stewart, M. G. (1977). The effect of 'humanized' milk and supplemented breast feeding on the fecal flora of infants. *Journal of Medical Microbiology, 10*, 403.

9. Aber, R. C., Allen, N., Howell, J. T., Wilkenson, H. W., and Facklam, P. R. (1976). Nosocomial transmission of group B streptococci. *Pediatrics*, *58*, 346-53.

10. Nagington, J., Wreghitt, T. G., Gandy, G., Roberton, N. R. C., and Berry, P. J. (1978). Fatal Echovirus 11 infections in outbreak in special care baby unit. *Lancet*, *ii*, 725.

11. Townsend, T. R., and Wenzel, R.P. (1981). Nosocomial blood stream infections in a neonatal intensive care unit. *American Journal of Epidemiology*, *114*, 73.

12. Goldmann, D. A., Durbin, W. A., and Freeman, J. (1981). Nosocomial infections in a neonatal intensive care unit. *Journal of Infectious Diseases*, *144*, 449.

13. Chamberlain, R., Chamberlain, G., Howlett, B., and Claireaux, A. (1975). *British Births 1970. Volume I. First Week of Life*. London, Heinemann Medical Books, 175, Table 6.20.

14. Roberton, N. R. C. (1980). Caesarean section – paediatric outcomes. In *Outcomes of Obstetric Intervention in Britain*, R. W. Beard and D. B. Paintin (eds). London, Royal College of Obstetricians, 107.

15. Bengtsson, B., and Vernholt, J. (1974). A follow-up study of hyperbilirubinaemia in healthy term infants without iso-immunization. *Acta Paediat. Scand., 63,* 70.

16. Raivio, K. O., and Hallman, N. (1968). Neonatal hypoglycaemia. I. Occurrence of hypoglycaemia in patients with various neonatal disorders. *Acta Paediat. Scand., 57,* 517.

17. Lubchenco, L. O., and Bard, H. (1971). Incidence of hypoglycaemia in newborn infants classified by birthweight and gestational age. *Pediatrics*, *47*, 831.

18. Anderson, J. M., Milner, R. D. G., and Strich, S. J. (1967). Effects of neonatal hypoglycaemia on the nervous system. A pathological study. *J. Neuro., Neurosurg. Psychiat., 30,* 295.

19. Pildes, R. S., Cornblath, M., Warren, I., Page-El, I., Di Menza, S., Merritt, D. M., and Peeva, A. (1974). A prospective controlled study of neonatal hypoglycaemia. *Pediatrics*, *54*, 5.

20. Whitby, C., De Cates, C. R., and Roberton, N. R. C. (1982). Infants weighing 1.8-2.5 kg: do they need neonatal unit or postnatal ward care? *Lancet*, *i*, 322.

6 AN EVALUATION OF INTERVENTIONS IN THE PREMATURE NURSERY

Marshall Klaus and John Kennell

In recent years investigators have studied the unusual and confusing environment parents of a premature infant encounter as they try to meet the needs of their sleepy, fragile and unpredictable infant. Observations based on recently completed studies suggest a number of promising interventions that may reduce parental anxiety and stress, and which deserve further study on the traditional hospital environment. This chapter will integrate these investigations in an attempt to develop new and more positive environments for both parents and infants.

Background

Since parental visiting has been permitted in the intensive care nursery a number of studies[1-4] have revealed that most parents continue to suffer severe emotional stress. Harper noted that even when parents have close contact with their infants in the intensive care nursery they experience prolonged stress.[1] Most parents felt that holding their infant made the infant feel more loved. Benfield and associates also noted that most parents experienced grief reactions.[2] Interestingly, the level of their response was unrelated to the severity of the baby's problems.

From interviews and observations it has been suggested that early parental reactions predicted how the mother would manage with her infant in the early weeks at home.[3-5] From interviews early in the course Mason[5] found that if the mother expressed a moderately high level of anxiety, actively sought information about the condition of her baby, showed strong maternal feelings for the baby, and had strong support from the father, there was usually a favourable outcome. If the mother showed a low level of anxiety and activity, the chances were that her relationship with her child would be poor.

Newman noted variations between families in their individual coping styles.[4] She described 'coping through commitment' as the label given for an intense yet variable involvement in the care of a low birthweight infant. In contrast, 'coping through distance' was a slower acquaintance process where the parents expressed fear, anxiety and at times denial before they accepted the surviving infant. Minde, in observations and interviews,[3] noted that the most important variable was the mother's relationship to her own mother, her relationship to the father and whether or not the mother had a previous abortion. Highly interacting mothers in the nursery visit and telephone the nursery more frequently while the infants are hospitalised and stimulate their infants more at home. Mothers who stimulate their infants very little in the nursery also visit and telephone less frequently and provide only minimal stimulation to them at home. However, Minde noted perceptively that mothers who touched and fondled their infants more in the nursery had infants who opened their eyes more often.[3] He observed the contingency between the infant's eyes being open and the mother's touching and also between gross motor stretches and the mother's smiling. He and his associates could not determine to what extent the sequence of touching and eye opening was an indication of the mother's primary contribution or whether it was initiated by the infant. Thus from interviews and observations, Mason, Newman and Minde predict that mothers who become involved, interested and anxious about their infants in the intensive care nursery will have an easier time when the infant is taken home.[3-5]

Field[6] has demonstrated the close connection between what a mother does and her infant's arousal level. While most mothers of full-term babies adopt a moderate level of activity which is associated with optimal arousal in their babies, some mothers of 'prems' either over or under react. Field found that mothers of premature infants who were overactive during early face-to-face interactions were more likely to be overprotective and over-controlling during interactions with their infants two years later.[6]

Infant Stimulation or Imitation

In the last fifteen years numerous studies have revealed that if small premature infants are either touched, rocked, fondled, or cuddled daily during their stay in the nursery, they may have significantly fewer apneic periods, show increased weight gain, pass fewer stools and manifest a possible advance in certain areas of higher central nervous system functioning which persists at least for a short time after discharge from the hospital. As a result, parents and caretakers have often engaged in additional stimulation of the infant after discharge from the hospital.

As a result of studies by several perceptive researchers our conceptual framework about stimulation of the infant after discharge home and possibly before discharge needs to be reconsidered and may have to be altered drastically.

From observation of normal full-term mothers and infants, Winnicott noted that what babies observe in their caretaker's faces in the early months of life helps them to develop a concept of themselves.[7] He suggested that ordinarily the baby sees himself or herself: 'In other words, the mother is looking at the baby and what she looks like is related to what she sees there.' The mother imitates the infant's face. He noted that there are some mothers who do not imitate their babies and thus the babies do not see themselves. He postulated that in these situations the infant's own creative capacity is in some way atrophied and they look around for other ways of getting to know themselves from the environment. The significant observation noted by Winnicott[7] was that in normal mother-infant couples the mother was often following or imitating the infant. Trevarthen[8] confirmed these observations in mothers and infants using filming techniques and observed that mothers imitate their babies during spontaneous play. From this and other evidence he concluded that the mother's imitation of her infant's behaviour, rather than the reverse, sustained their interaction and communication. Detailed analysis revealed that mothers were studiously imitating the infant's expression with a lag of a few tenths of a second, and thus the infant was choosing the rhythm. Pawlby[9] also found that both mothers and infants imitate each other and she observed this occurring during the entire first year of life.

Lastly, in the series of creative experimental manipulations of infant-mother face-to-face interactions referred to above, Field[6] found that the mother and the normal *full-term* infant are each interacting about 70 per cent of the time in their spontaneous play (Figure 6.1). However, when the mother is asked to increase her attention-getting behaviour (stimulation), her activity increases to 80 per cent of the time and, strikingly, the infant's gaze decreases to 50 per cent. When such mothers are told only to imitate the movements of their infant, which reduces their activity, the infant's gaze time greatly increases.

Field[6] noted that in the spontaneous situation mothers of *high-risk infants* are interacting up to 90 per cent of the time, whereas their infants are only looking 30 per cent of the time. If the mothers are told to use attention-getting gestures their activity increases even above 90 per cent of the time, but their infants' gaze decreases further. If the mother's interactions are decreased by asking her to imitate the baby's

Figure 6.1: Relationship between Maternal Activity and Infant Gaze in Three Maternal Situations: (1) Attempting to Get the Infant's Attention (Attention Getting), (2) Spontaneous Interaction, and (3) Mother Imitating the Baby.

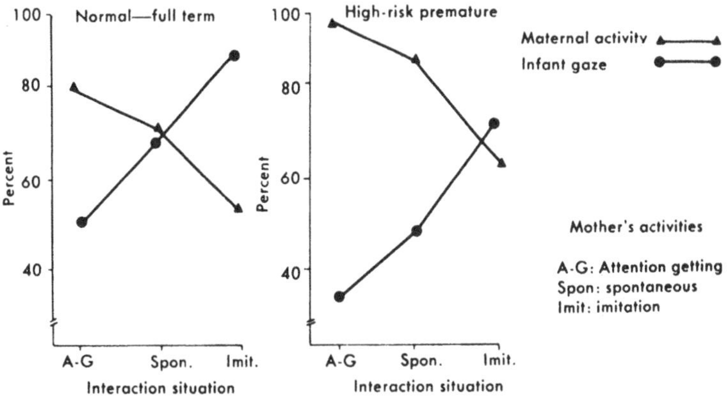

Source: Adapted from Field[6]. Copyright The Society for Research in Child Development, Inc.

movements, there is then a striking increase in the infant's gaze. These experiments show that while much of the parent's activity is aimed at encouraging more activity or responsivity from the premature infant, their approach may be counter-productive, leading to less instead of more infant responsiveness.

Thus by three separate and different techniques it appears that mothers of normal infants follow or mirror their infant's behaviour for significant periods of time.

We have noted a few nurses who seem especially adept at increasing an infant's responsivity. When they take infants out of the incubator, and interact with them, these nurses often seem to move imperceptibly. It would appear from the work of Winnicott, Trevarthen and Field[6-8] that they may be intuitively following, very slightly behind, movements of the infant and allowing the infant to find himself or herself. Since the infant is moving very little these nurses also move infrequently.

Once a person has a well-integrated self, any imitation is an invasion of that individual's integrity. However, during the early months when the infant's self is incompletely formed, imitation of the infant's gestures and facial expressions appears to be a help in the process of self-discovery. All these observations suggest that we should be careful about recommending increased stimulation for the premature infant. Instead, it would appear to be more appropriate to suggest that the mother attempt to find her infant and move at her infant's pace.

There is thus a great deal to be studied and defined about the mother's efforts to increase interaction with her premature infant. How should it be provided? By whom? When? Stimulation or imitation? In addition there is the question of its long-term significance.

Interventions

In recent years there has been special interest in studying how to help parents become attached to their small babies and how to provide support for mothers and fathers during their difficult days of hospitalisation and prepare them for the early stressful weeks at home. Some of the results are discussed in Chapter 7. In the next section interventions that seem to be of most value are discussed.

Transporting the Mother to be Near her Small Infant

With the development of high-risk perinatal centres there have been an increasing number of mothers who are transported to the maternity division of hospitals with a neonatal intensive care nursery just prior to delivery or shortly after. We believe this trend is helpful for both parents, since the father is not distracted by having members of his family in two hospitals and others at home. If there is not sufficient time to arrange for her transport prior to giving birth, we strongly recommend that the mother be moved during her early postpartum period. As yet we know little about how transportation of the mother may influence her relationship with her baby.

Rooming-in for the Parent of a Premature Infant

Baragwanath Hospital in South Africa provides another model of successful premature infant caretaking. Mothers of premature infants used to live in a room adjoining the premature nursery, and each feeding time they entered the nursery to feed and handle their babies. Now the modern unit is run somewhat differently (see Chapter 19). Dr Kahn[10] originally instituted this arrangement because of a shortage of nurses, but his solution has multiple benefits. It allows the mother to continue producing milk, permits her to take on the care of the infant more easily, reduces nursing time and allows mothers time for mutual discussion and support.

When Tafari and Ross[11] in Ethiopia permitted mothers to live within their crowded premature unit 24 hours a day, they were able to care for three times as many infants in their premature nursery and the number of surviving infants increased 500 per cent. Mother-infant pairs were discharged when the infants weighed an average of 1.7 kg and most infants were breast-fed. Previous to this most of the infants had gone home bottle-feeding and usually died of intercurrent respiratory and gastrointestinal infections. When the cost of prepared milk amounts to a high proportion of the parents' weekly income, policies in support of mother rooming-in and breast-feeding in premature nurseries have a direct relation to infant mortality. This procedure is probably appropriate for 50 per cent of the world.

Torres,[12] in a special care unit in the slums of Santiago, Chile, has also achieved an excellent, low perinatal mortality and morbidity by placing special care units for low birthweight infants on the maternity unit and maintaining babies under professional observation for only as long as is necessary (see also Chapter 18).

Donald Garrow,[13] at a general hospital in High Wycombe, England, opened a new 20-bed special infant care unit that can accommodate eight mothers at a time and 250 admissions each year. No matter how seriously ill they may be, some 70 per cent of the babies have their mothers with them from the first few hours of life. Six of the mothers' rooms open directly into the infant special care unit so that the parents can easily see or care for their infants. This unit is described in detail in Chapter 16.

Whitby, De Cates and Roberton[14] have described a Unit in Cambridge where a large proportion of infants over 1.80 kg can be cared for by the mothers on the postpartum wards (see also Chapters 5 and 17).

Nesting

In the United States, James[15] first described the successful introduction of a care-by-parent unit to provide a homelike caretaking experience. Nursing support was available for parents of premature infants prior to discharge if they needed help. Earlier Crosse[16] in England had provided a small room for mother and infant to live together before discharge.

For several years we have been studying 'nesting', namely permitting mothers to live in with their infants before discharge. When babies reach 1.72-2.11 kg, each mother is given a private room with her baby where she provides all caregiving. Impressive changes in the behaviour of these women are observed clinically. Even though the mothers had fed and cared for their infants in the intensive care nursery on many occasions prior to living-in, eight of the first nine mothers were unable to sleep during the first 24 hours. However, in the second 24-hour period the mothers' confidence and caretaking skills improved greatly. At this time, mothers began to discuss the proposed early discharge of their infants and, often for the first time, began to make preparations at home for their arrival. Several insisted on taking their babies home earlier than planned. The mothers were not satisfied with the living-in nesting procedure until we established unlimited visiting privileges for the father and provided him with a comfortable chair or a cot.[17]

When 'nesting' is started, the role of the nurse and the mother must be clarified, or there will be tussles over who makes decisions. In our unit the mother makes the decisions with the nurse serving as the consultant. We suggest that early discharge, preceded by a period of isolation of the mother-infant dyad, may help to normalise mothering behaviour in the intensive care nursery. Encouraging the increasing possibilities for mother-infant interaction and total caretaking may reduce the incidence of mothering disorders among mothers of small or sick premature infants.

Early Discharge

Berg and associates, Dillard and Korones, and Davies and associates discharged premature infants when they weighed about 2 kilograms.[18-20] Dillard found no deleterious effects associated with this early discharge.[19] Experienced personnel should visit the home to organise the families and after discharge help supervise infant care. Recent studies of early discharge have not revealed any gross adverse effects on the physical health of the infants, but there have been no systematic observations of maternal behaviour and anxiety or later infant development.

Parent Groups

In recent years a number of neonatal intensive care units have formed groups of parents of prematures who meet together once a week, or more often, for 1-to-2-hour discussions. Documented clinical reports from these centres suggest that parents find both support and considerable relief from being able to talk with each other and to express and compare their inner feelings.

Minde and colleagues, in a controlled study of a self-help group, reported that parents who participated in the group visited their infants in the hospital significantly more often than did parents in the control group.[21] The self-help parents also touched, talked and looked at their infants more in the *en face* position and rated themselves as more competent on infant care measures. These mothers continued to show more involvement with their babies during feedings and were more concerned about their general development three months after their discharge from the nursery.

Additional Contact and Reciprocal Interaction

The parents' affection and enthusiasm are stimulated and sustained by seeing the baby's open eyes. Therefore it is helpful to explain that as premature babies develop they will be awake for increasingly longer periods of time. Often parents will stroke or pat their babies who respond by opening their eyes. If mothers are able to meet their special needs, the babies they take home will be more responsive and closer in behaviour to the full-term infant they hoped for.

Over many years we have gained the impression that the earlier a mother comes to the premature unit and touches her baby, the more rapidly her own physical recovery from the pregnancy and birth progresses. As a result of these observations and other experiences, we have studied the effect of an early intervention programme to maximise the attachment of mothers and fathers to their premature infants. The study was designed to determine if mothers who (1) follow a pattern of stroking their infants, (2) are involved in caretaking such as feeding and changing diapers, and (3) are given special guidance on how to understand their infant's needs and responses, will develop a closer attachment to their infants than will mothers who are not given these three experiences during the first two weeks of life. Mothers in both groups were allowed and encouraged to come into the nursery and were given a description and an explanation of all treatments. Only the experimental group was given the special experiences during the first two weeks after the baby's birth. After the programme ended, both groups received the same care.

Following the intervention, both groups were similar in the hospital aside from slight differences in visiting rates. One month after the discharge of the baby, mothers in the control and experimental groups behaved similarly during physical examination. Their response to a questionnaire concerning their adjustment to the premature infant and their perception of the baby showed no significant differences between the two groups.

The lack of differences in our study has forced us to examine further the needs and problems faced by the parents. First, even the most sensitive interventions may fail if the parents view their infant as weak and unlikely to live. Secondly, for years we had been thinking along one track when devising interventions for premature infants. We had been bringing parents into the intensive care nursery. However, the milieu in the nursery makes it difficult for parents to be confident about their infant's viability. With these factors in mind, we took a different approach in designing a new intervention for parents of premature infants.

Transporting the Healthy Premature Infant to the Mother – a New Intervention

Rather than bringing mothers into the neonatal intensive care unit with its frightening sounds, strange equipment and unfamiliar faces, we are studying the effects of bringing the baby to the mother in her own room in the maternity division of the hospital. In this way the mothers have an opportunity to become acquainted with their premature newborns under circumstances similar to those experienced by mothers of full-term infants. The results of studies of early maternal contact with healthy full-term infants served as a guide for the design of this intervention.

We included healthy infants whose birthweight was between 1.50 and 2.10 kg, whose gestational age was between 32 and 36 weeks, and whose medical status during the first day permitted the infant to stay with his mother (for example, no continuing respiratory distress or hypoglycaemia).

The early contact consists of 0.5-1 hour of mother-infant contact on each of the first, second and third days after birth. A research nurse brings the baby to the mother's room in a transport incubator. The baby, clothed only in a diaper, is placed in the mother's bed with a radiant heat panel overhead. The research nurse is present during the visit but seated out of the mother's view above the head of her bed. During the visit the nurse observes the infant's condition, particularly his colour and respirations. Resuscitation equipment is carried on the transport incubator for use in the event of apnoea. As part of our research protocol, the nurse also made detailed observations of the mother's behaviour during each of the three one-hour visits. Verbal interaction between the mother and nurse was limited to a standard statement and answers to the mother's questions.

We have monitored the babies' temperatures frequently and found that on a single occasion one baby had a temperature less than 36°C, but that was the only episode of hypothermia. With the use of a heat panel and transport incubator there have been no significant problems with temperature control. In addition, we have had no episodes of apnoea, bradycardia, vomiting, or other unusual behaviour. We appreciate that there may be times when difficulties with premature babies may occur, so the nurses continue to monitor them closely. So far it appears to be a safe procedure; however, one infant died with late streptococcal septicaemia. We have found that this procedure is increasingly acceptable to the nurses caring for the premature infants.

Figure 6.2 presents a summary of the behaviour of mothers on the first and second visit of the premature infant in the early contact study compared with mothers visiting their pre-term baby in incubators and mothers who have their undressed, full-term infants in their own beds on the maternity unit. In the first and second visits there was far more touching activity than we have previously found in parents of premature infants. However, it should be noted that in our past research the infants were in incubators in the premature nursery and the mothers walked to the incubator. At that time the total amount of touching during any observed period was 20 per cent during the first visit and 36 per cent during the second visit compared with more than 80 per cent when the infant was in the mother's bed. Therefore bringing the infant to the mother significantly increased her physical contact with her infant, and touching the infant's trunk occurred more rapidly.

When the infants visited their mothers, the mothers spent a striking amount of time looking at them – 84-90 per cent of the time. These results are of special interest since in our study of premature infants

Figure 6.2: Fingertip and Palm Contact on the Trunk or Extremities in Three Groups of Mothers: (1) Twelve Mothers of Full-term Infants at their First Visit; (2) Nine Mothers who Visited their Premature Infants in Incubators in the ICU; and (3) Fourteen mothers Whose Premature Infants Were Brought to their Maternity Rooms and Placed in their Beds.

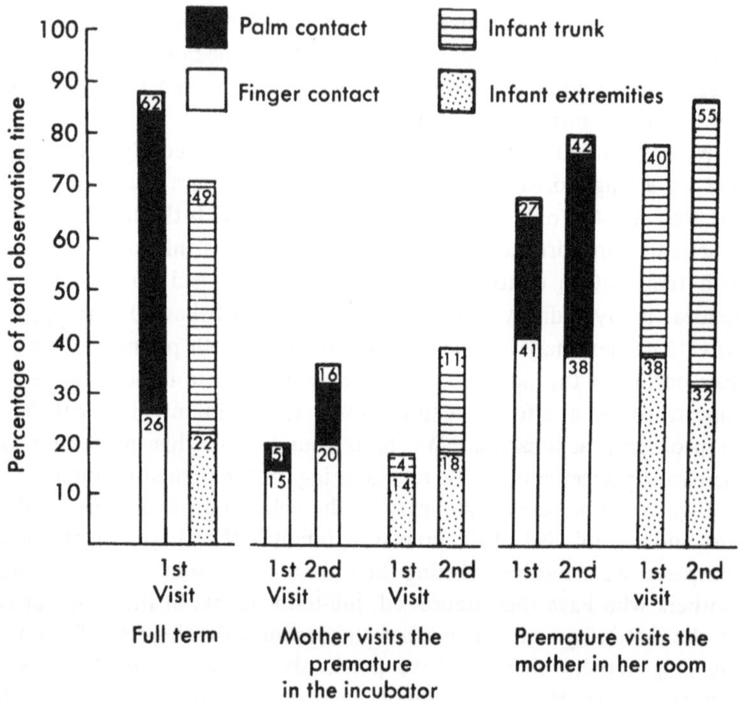

several years ago there was a strong correlation between the amount of time a mother looked at her infant during a feeding at discharge from hospital and the baby's development at 42 months.

When the mothers visited their babies in incubators in the intensive care nursery, we were greatly impressed by the observation that parents of premature infants rarely spoke to them. However, in the current study, such communications have occupied almost 40 per cent of the time at the first and second visits. The full impact of this intervention will await the results of long-term studies presently underway.

Summary

(1) The intensive care nursery should be open for parental visiting 24 hours a day and be flexible about visits from others such as grandparents, supportive relatives and on certain occasions, siblings. Providing proper precautions are taken, infection will not be a problem.

(2) When an infant weighs between four and five pounds and appears to be doing well without grunting and retractions, we have found it safe for the mother to have the baby placed in her bed for 20 to 30 minutes in the first hours of life with a heat panel above both of them. We do not recommend this unless the physician (and mother) feels relaxed and sure about the infant's health.

(3) Mother and infant should be kept near each other on the same floor if possible. It is helpful if the mother can have some private sessions with her infant in a separate room close to the unit.

(4) Transporting the mother and baby together to the medical centre that contains the intensive care nursery is now occurring more frequently and should be encouraged for its immediate and long-term benefits.

(5) We should continue to study interventions such as rooming-in, nesting and early discharge as well as transporting a healthy premature infant to be with his mother. It is necessary to try out these various interventions in different hospital settings and evaluate their ability to reduce the severe anxiety that many parents experience during the prolonged hospitalisation and the early days following discharge.

(6) In all these interventions it is critical that nurses take mothers under their wing, especially supporting and encouraging them during these early days and weeks. The nurse's guidance in helping a mother with simple caretaking tasks can be extremely valuable in helping to overcome some of her anxiety. In this sense the nurse assumes the role of the mother's own mother and contributes much more than teaching her basic techniques of caretaking.

(7) To begin an intervention with parents early, it is necessary to identify high-risk parents who are having special difficulties in adapting. Generally these parents will visit rarely and for short periods, appear frightened, and do not usually engage the medical staff in any questionning about the infant's problems. Sometimes the mothers are hostile or irritable and show inappropriately low levels of anxiety.

(8) As we develop a further understanding of the process by which normal mothers and infants interact with each other during the first months and year of life, it appears that recommendations for stimulation may be detrimental to normal development. Rather than suggesting

stimulation, it may be important for a mother naturally and unconsciously to use imitation to learn about and find her own infant.

It is probable that in the future several of these interventions will be combined so that a mother may both have early contact with her premature infant if it is healthy, and have the baby brought to her bedside in the maternity unit on several occasions early in the course of the infant's stay in the hospital. In addition, she will be living-in with the baby for three or four days before early discharge.

References

1. Harper, R. G., Sia, C., Sokal, S., and Sokal, M. (1976). Observations on unrestricted parental contact with infants in the neonatal intensive care unit. *J. Pediatr.*, *89*, 441.

2. Benfield, D. G., Leib, S. A., and Reutor, J. (1976). Grief response of parents following referral of the critically ill newborn. *N. Engl. J. Med.*, *294*, 975.

3. Minde, K., Trehub, S., Corter, C., Boukydis, C., Celhoffer, L., and Marton, P. (1978). Mother-child relationships in the premature nursery: an observational study. *Pediatrics*, *61*, 373.

4. Newman, L. F. (1980). Parent's perceptions of their low birth weight infants, *Paediatrician*, *9*, 182-90.

5. Mason, E. A. (1963). A method of predicting crisis outcome for mothers of premature babies. *Public Health Rep.*, *78*, 1031.

6. Field, T. M. (1977). Effects of early separation, interactive deficits and experimental manipulations on infant-mother face-to-face interaction. *Child. Dev.*, *48*, 763.

7. Winnicott, D. W. (1971). The mirror role of mother and family in child development. In *Playing and Reality*, London, Tavistock Publications.

8. Trevarthen, C. L. (1977). Descriptive analyses of infant communicative behaviour. In *Studies in Mother-infant Interaction*, H. R. Schaffer (ed.). New York, Academic Press.

9. Pawlby, S. J. (1977). Imitative interaction. In *Studies in Mother-infant Interaction*, H. R. Schaffer (ed.). New York, Academic Press.

10. Kahn, E., Wayburne, S., and Fouche, M. (1954). The Baragwanath premature baby unit – an analysis of the case records of 1,000 consecutive admissions. *S. Afr. Med. J.*, *28*, 453.

11. Tafari, N., and Ross, S. M. (1973). On the need for organized perinatal care. *Ethiop. Med. J.*, *11*, 93.

12. Torres, J. (1978). Personal communication.

13. Garrow, D. H. (1979). Personal communication.

14. Whitby, C., De Cates, C. R., and Roberton, N. R. C. (1982). Infants weighing 1.8-2.5 kg; should they be cared for in neonatal units or postnatal wards? *Lancet*, *i*, 322.

15. James, V. L., Jr, and Wheeler, W. E. (1969). The care-by-parent unit. *Pediatrics*, *43*, 488.

16. Crosse, V. M. (1957). *The Premature Baby*, 4th edn. Boston, Little, Brown & Co.

17. Kennell, J. H., Chesler, D., Wofe, H., and Klaus, M. H. (1973). Nesting-in the human mother after mother-infant separation. *Pediatr. Res.*, *7*, 269.

18. Berg, R.B., and Salisbury, A. (1971). Discharging infants of low birth weight: reconsiderations of current practice. *Am. J. Dis. Child.*, *122*, 414.

19. Dillard, R. G., and Korones, S. B. (1973). Lower discharge weight and shortened nursery stay for low birth-weight infants. *N. Engl. J. Med.*, *288*, 131.

20. Davies, D. P., Herberts, S., Haxby, V., and McNeish, A. S. (1979). When should pre-term babies be sent home from neonatal units? *Lancet*, *i*, 914.

21. Minde, K., Shosenberg, B., Marton, P., Thompson, J., Ripley, J., and Burns, S. (1980). Self-help groups in a premature nursery – a controlled evaluation. *J. Pediatr.*, *96*, 933.

7 PARENTS AND THE SUPPORT THEY NEED

Nicola C. S. Jacques, Joanna T. Hawthorne Amick and Martin P. M. Richards

Introduction

Research on the effects of early parent-baby (most often mother-baby) separation has tended to focus upon the consequences for the later relationship and for the development of the infant. Comparatively little attention has been paid to parental reactions to the separation itself, still less to the great variation in the responses of individual parents and to their differing vulnerability to the adverse effects of separation. Our main concern in this chapter will be with the period of separation itself, the reactions of parents, especially mothers, during this time and some of the ways in which the distress that many feel may be reduced.

In considering this, it is important to realise that the birth of a pre-term baby and the postnatal period that follows constitute a series of events which may have a profound effect on both parents. We are dealing not simply with effects that may stem from the separation of parent and child which is likely to occur at this time, but also with the consequences of giving birth to a baby too soon, or one who is inadequately grown, or both. The baby may be seriously ill and, as we saw in Chapter 1, becoming a parent is itself an important psychological and social event, and the more so with the added difficulties of a premature baby.

Widespread publicity and interest concerning fetal malformations in recent years may have served to increase parental anxieties about the possibility of a defective child. If a baby is not completely normal at birth a mother may be confronted with what she had most feared. Solnit and Stark,[1] for instance, have commented on the narcissistic blow she may experience in this situation. In a society that may tend to judge a woman's competence by her ability to become an adequate mother the inability to grow a normal child may be seen as a fundamental failure. It is not surprising therefore that Kennell and Rolnick[2] have reported that even minor health problems in newborns can give rise to considerable feelings of anxiety and guilt. The mother's own psychological make-up may be much more important in determining her reaction than the magnitude of the impairment in her baby.[3] The care of parents who do have a handicapped child is discussed in detail in Chapter 13.

When an infant is born prematurely, a mother may not be as emotionally or physiologically prepared for childbirth as she would have been had the pregnancy gone to term, quite apart from any unpreparedness in terms of practical arrangements. She may experience a sense of failure, guilt and loss of self-esteem not only because she did not carry the infant to term but also because the baby differs from the one she had anticipated.[4,5,6] Kaplan and Mason[6] have listed the psychological tasks which they suggested must be surmounted by a mother of a premature infant if their relationship is to progress in health: grief for the loss of the wished-for child, acknowledgement of failure, resumption of active relating to the baby, and seeing its prematurity as a temporary state yielding to normality. These authors described premature birth as an acute emotional crisis for parents. If the baby is removed before the mother has had a chance to see him or her properly (or at all) her fears concerning the baby's health and appearance may increase out of all proportion to the actual situation. Richards[7] has pointed out that separation may be viewed as a punishment when feelings of guilt attend the birth. Sometimes parents react to their feelings by a form of denial and infrequent visiting of a baby in the neonatal nursery may indicate that the problems have not been resolved.[8] Monitoring parental visiting patterns is one means by which staff can be alerted to the possibility of underlying unresolved difficulties. Minde[8] has observed great variety in the individual reactions to the birth of a pre-term or sick baby, some parents becoming highly anxious and over-concerned and others distancing themselves from the infant. Separation from the baby may not have a similar effect in these two situations.

In addition to the emotional trauma of giving birth prematurely, extra stresses are likely to be associated with caring for a low birthweight infant. Low birthweight babies may be unresponsive and difficult to feel close to.[9,10] Their cries and appearance may be more off-putting than those of full-term babies and so parents may be less eager to interact with them.[11] This may have important implications for the understanding of some cases of child abuse.[12]

Multiple-birth infants are commonly of low birthweight and so are particularly frequent among those who are admitted to neonatal units. While clinical experience suggests that the practical and emotional problems of multiple births may be particularly daunting for parents and these children may be especially prone to behavioural problems, there has been little systematic study of the topic. Because of this lack and not from any belief that the topic is unimportant, we will not discuss the particular problems of parents who have twins, triplets or higher multiple births.

In this chapter we will first describe a study which was designed to investigate the feelings of mothers who gave birth to a pre-term baby who was admitted to a neonatal unit. We will then go on to discuss some of the interventions that have been used to try and alleviate the psychological problems for parents of a baby who goes to a neonatal unit and some of the ways in which parent-infant relationships may be improved in this situation. Other intervention studies have been described in Chapter 6. In this chapter we will not deal with the important problems of births that result in a handicapped child; these are discussed in Chapter 13.

The Exeter Study

Between 1974 and 1976 a study was carried out by one of us[13] at the Royal Devon and Exeter Hospital, England, to explore the effect of mother-infant separation after a pre-term delivery and the infant's removal to a neonatal baby unit. The investigation was designed to assess two different modes of care: the normal procedures as they then were, in which mother and baby were separated, and an extended contact rooming-in. (It is important to note that there have been great changes in the care provided by this unit since this study was completed, with a view to fostering closer parent-infant contact.) While this unit was not specially designed for rooming-in, an arrangement was created which is not unlike that described by Garrow in Chapter 16.

Babies in the sample had a mean gestational age of 35 weeks (range = 33-7) and the two groups of primiparous mothers and their babies were matched as far as possible on a variety of variables. Normal hospital procedures applied to the first group (n = 10). These mothers usually left hospital within a few days of giving birth. They and their partners were free to visit their infants in the neonatal unit at any time and returned to collect them at a later stage when the babies were judged fit to be discharged. In contrast, mothers in the extended-contact group (n = 10) were able to remain in hospital throughout their babies' stay. Each baby (whether in incubator or not) was left in his mother's single room during the day and sometimes also at night, and the mothers were able to participate in the care of their infants to a greater extent than was possible in the normal procedure group.

The experience of the two groups of mothers were described in detail, and a case study approach was used so that individual variations in response could be explored. The questions posed by this project included the following: was there a difference betweeen the groups in expressed feelings and attitudes indicative of closer relationships between the extended-contact mothers and babies in hospital? What factors were cited by the mothers as important in helping them to feel close to their babies? Which aspects of the hospital environment facilitated or inhibited the developing relationships?

The mothers had very different hospital experiences according to their allocation to the two groups and this had important consequences for the developing mother-baby relationships in the hospital period. For example, by the time of discharge all the extended-contact mothers, but only half of the normal-procedure mothers, said they felt emotionally close to their babies. Extended-contact mothers were more likely to say that their infants could recognise them and they were less inclined to feel depressed into the second week after birth. They had much more success at breast feeding and they were also more likely to feel confident at the prospect of taking their babies home. Babies in the extended-contact group were discharged earlier than normal-procedure babies and according to the Nursing Officer this was because their mothers were judged to have become proficient in caretaking more rapidly than the normal-procedure mothers.

'Rooming-in' met with an enthusiastic response from all the mothers assigned to the extended-contact condition and mothers in this group were able to fulfil the maternal role which they had been expecting to perform after giving birth. Their position in the hospital was relatively close to that of mothers of full-term infants, i.e. of the normal, anticipated pattern of events. In contrast, normal-procedure mothers were unable to behave as they thought a new mother should. This often gave rise to feelings of confusion and inadequacy.

Mothers in both groups cited visual and especially tactile contact as very important in helping them to get to know their babies, while caretaking was felt to play an even more fundamental role. One mother thought:

> Well, how long is it going to be before I can actually *do* something for him? . . . I think it takes touching them and handling them, doing something, to get to know them.

This mother had been surprised at her absence of feelings for the baby but said,

> I just accepted it. I thought to myself it was because I hadn't had any contact with her . . . I just accepted that I would have to wait till I could have bodily contact with her before I actually felt this motherly instinct . . . it wasn't until I started changing her bottom and wiping her face over and things like that, that I sort of got this feeling 'Well, she's mine' . . . When they first took her out of the incubator I felt as if she was mine more.

The mothers needed to feel that their babies really belonged to them. Extended-contact mothers had their babies beside them all day in the privacy of their own room and they therefore had far more opportunity than normal-procedure mothers for all forms of contact. They were more quickly able to build up confidence that they could meet their infants' needs and to develop a sense of responsibility for them. This feeling of being 'in charge' of their own babies played a vital part in helping the mothers to feel emotionally close to them. Since extended-contact mothers were soon encouraged to take over day-to-day caretaking, they were able to develop the feeling that they knew their infants better than did anyone else and that their babies were depending on them rather than on the nurses. Again, this helped the mothers to feel that their infants were really their own and that they had a special relationship with them. Several extended-contact mothers started to resent the nursing staff for interfering with what they did with their own babies. They began to feel that the nurses were less sensitive to their babies' needs than they were themselves and became reluctant to leave them to the care of the nurses. One mother commented:

> I used to get terribly agitated when one of the little nurses used to come in and say you ought to do it like this – and I'd been dealing with him for 2 or 3 days on my own.

It is significant that none of the extended-contact mothers was willing to leave hospital without her baby, although they could have chosen to do so.

Among normal-procedure mothers there was a tacit assumption that they were unable to care adequately for their own babies, and since the nurses were acting as primary caretakers it was difficult for mothers in this group to feel a sense of responsibility for their infants. The staff were undeniably in charge and the mothers played a subordinate role. For example, some mothers felt that they had to obtain the nurses' agreement before they handled or fed their own babies. In this situation it was by no means easy for them to feel that they had a special relationship with their babies and that the infants needed them; indeed, many found it difficult to believe that they had actually had a baby. Feelings of anxiety, confusion and even resentment could result when they did not experience the motherly feelings which they had expected and wanted to feel.

Jeffcoate[14,15] has drawn attention to the frustration and loss of self-esteem often felt by mothers in this type of situation. She observed that a sample of mothers of low birthweight babies overwhelmingly perceived their role as giving love and essential care to their infants, but that they were unable to perform this role in the neonatal unit. Mothers experienced a greater emotional crisis than fathers and this was attributed to their differing role expectations. Fathers did not suffer such a catastrophic violation of their expectations.

Leiderman and Seashore[16] suggested that mothers who had handled their babies in incubators and who had participated in their care felt more confident in being able to look after them and felt emotionally closer to their infants for the first few weeks after discharge. However the link between maternal self-confidence and early close mother-infant contact is obviously rather complex. There is some suggestion that close contact with a sick or frail infant could lead to maternal anxiety and over-protectiveness. Working with babies born in 1946 when admittedly conditions were very different, Douglas and Gear[17] compared children of low birthweight who had been born and cared for at home with children who had been born in hospital and discharged after a minimum of 21 days. At 13 and 15 years those born at home were rated as more nervous and troublesome by teachers and the authors suggested that close contact with a frail infant could serve to heighten maternal anxiety. Indeed, Harper *et al.*[18] reported that increased contact in a neonatal nursery was associated with heightened parental anxiety. The direction of the effect is uncertain and it is important to note that 90 per cent of the parents said they would have opposed any restriction of contact. The relationship between early contact and maternal over-protectiveness is unclear; some workers[19] have suggested that exaggerated concern may be reduced rather than increased by early contact and it would seem that the advantages of contact probably compensate for the possible disadvantages. As has been pointed out before[7] the extent to which parents *believe* that separation is important could be a significant factor in determining the effect on them of early separation from their baby. The issues of parental anxiety and over-protectiveness are important as over-feeding of infants and repeated calls on doctors in cases of trivial illness have not infrequently been observed in the follow-up of ex-neonatal unit babies.

The possible connection between close contact with a sick infant and maternal nervousness was not investigated in the Exeter study. Certainly extended-contact mothers voiced more positive comments about their situation than did the normal-procedure mothers about theirs. Extended-contact mothers had a relatively private and relaxed setting in which to relate to their babies; for instance, they could cuddle and talk to them without feeling self-conscious and they could learn to handle them unobserved by the nurses. The privacy and freedom from routine in the mother and baby rooms afforded a considerable degree of autonomy. Winnicott[20] has emphasised the importance for new mothers to feel responsible and in charge:

> How can a mother learn about being a mother in any other way than by taking full responsibility? If she just does what she is told, she has to go on doing what she is told. But if she is feeling free to act in the way that comes naturally to her, she grows in the job. (p. 25)

Extended-contact mothers were able to maintain stronger links with the outside world than mothers on the postnatal ward, and they were better able to sustain a sense of personal independence in the hospital setting. This was particularly important in view of their comparatively long hospital stay. It was quite feasible for them to make trips into town, to go out with their husbands or even to pay visits home and this provided a welcome variation to the relatively monotonous life in hospital. Open visiting, allowed in their single rooms, gave these mothers the benefit of extra support and recognition in their maternal role since visitors could watch them attending to their babies; it also enabled fathers to have extended contact with their infants in private.

Normal-procedure mothers accommodated on the postnatal wards sometimes felt upset if all the other mothers in the ward had their full-term babies beside them:

> At the moment I'm feeling a bit down in the dumps because everybody else has got their baby. You see them nursing them and feeding them and that, and I feel like crying . . . I do feel like a mother and I don't if you see what I mean.

Another mother commented:

> I feel sad when the other babies are up in the ward and I wish mine was too . . . I feel ever so strongly, ever so sad about that . . . when I go down there they do let me cuddle her quite a bit but when I can only look at her I feel ever so sad then.

Normal-procedure mothers could only walk along to the neonatal unit intermittently because of the hospital routine, and visiting in the period after delivery was sometimes restricted by their physical condition as some were unable to walk as far as the unit without discomfort. Not surprisingly mothers in this group had reduced contact overall with their babies and, in addition, the setting in which contact took place was comparatively formal and clinical, allowing little maternal autonomy and affording no real privacy. In this, as in most neonatal units, all the internal partitions are glazed, presumably to allow staff maximum visibility. The effect on parents can be very inhibiting. Some mothers felt self-conscious in full view of the staff and they were unable to relate to their infants in a natural way. One remarked: '. . . they said you should speak to the baby but I was afraid to because I thought people might think I'm mad.' This mother would like to have spent more time with her baby:

> . . . but I don't because I feel I am getting in the way. She has got three other babies in the room with her and the nurses are in and out looking at those and the mothers come up too, so I feel I can only go up now and then.

Normal-procedure mothers had a rather tenuous role in the unit and were less inclined to approach staff with questions:

> I do feel that once I am home on my own I can feel more relaxed, it will be just her and me getting on with it . . . whereas here you have to fit in with a routine and a procedure, you feel sometimes that you are a bit of a bother . . . now and again I felt that I wished we could be left alone . . . there is always a lot of hub-bub going on around.

> I think they'll tell me off in a minute because I wander in and out . . . I shall be glad when I can do what I want when I want.

A third mother commented: 'I don't do nothing unless the nurses say I can pick it up . . . they'd turn round and snap I expect.' Despite their greater need for information and reassurance, frustration over lack of information was a greater problem for mothers in the normal-procedure group:

> No particular person had responsibility for her . . . and I didn't know who to ask to find out . . . you felt you were being a nuisance keeping on . . . I just felt more than anything that I'd like to know when she's coming home.

As already noted, violation of expectations was a primary cause of the disturbance experienced by normal procedure mothers. Without a proper role in the hospital setting they often began to feel superfluous, bored and inadequate: 'There's nothing to do in here really, is there?' Some became anxious to leave in order to escape from a situation in which their absence of maternal feeling was increasingly unacceptable:

> I was pleased to have a rest to be honest . . . it's a bit unrealistic, you've gone through your birth and everyone's saying 'Well done!' and 'Oooh it's a girl' and people come in, you're all chattering but you don't seem to realise that the bond between mother and baby isn't quite. . .

In addition, as several normal-procedure mothers commented, husbands seemed to need them at home whilst their infants seemed to have no need of them in hospital. A small minority described the beginning of the development of maternal feelings and these mothers found it more difficult to leave their infants; one reaction was to try to guard against these feelings by shunning contact with the babies in an attempt to reduce the upset caused by the separation. Very significantly, while mothers in the extended-contact group were beginning to feel that their babies really belonged to them, some normal-procedure mothers were having actually to guard against those feelings in order to try to minimise the hurt imposed by a looming separation. One such mother said: 'I think it would be better to go now – I certainly wouldn't be able to stay here until Emma can come out and the longer I stay the worse it's going to be.' She was trying not to think about the baby in order to avoid missing her: 'I'm trying not to feel so attached. . . I think tomorrow morning I'll feed her at 6 a.m. and then I probably won't go down again, I'll go straight out.' Another mother said, 'I think that depending on how much I see her I will try and forget most of the time.'

While most normal-procedure mothers had welcomed hospital discharge, once at home they often experienced an intensification of their sense of failure and deprivation. Despite very frequent visits to the hospital many were still unable to feel emotionally close to their babies, and visiting itself could be upsetting since they had to leave the infants behind each time. Mothers commonly felt 'lost' during this period and some found it difficult to believe that their babies would ever be discharged:

> I thought, fancy coming home without your baby, what a thing. . . I felt lost, I thought, Well I did have a baby I suppose . . . I wonder if he's alright, I wonder if he'll die . . . I wonder if he'll ever come home.

> Having carried her for eight months and then being in hospital a full week and then coming home – and nothing. And just sort of popping down to see her – it didn't seem right at all. . . I didn't feel as though she was ever going to come home.

> I think the whole thing of coming out without your baby is confusing . . . you sort of felt in a way that you didn't have a baby.

One strategy in the face of this disturbance was to try to avoid thinking about the infants and to reduce visiting.

Some mothers who could not respond to their babies with warmth and affection felt guilty. If they were unable to feel and act as they felt a mother should, this could give rise to a sense of failure and frustration:

> The separation mucked me about a hell of a lot really . . . it could be an utter stranger really after being in there all that time, in a way.

> I feel almost like she'll be adopted.

> I certainly didn't feel she was mine when I was visiting her. . . I think it was being at home pregnant and then coming into hospital and then going home and having *nothing*. I didn't feel as though she was mine at all.

Mothers who *did* feel maternal were similarly likely to experience frustration when they were thwarted in their urge to have a close involvement with their babies. Feelings of guilt, frustration or failure arising in the context of separation could result in resentment directed towards the infants as the cause of the upset. Two mothers in the normal-procedure group expressed resentment towards their babies in their confusion and sense of failure. Both said bitterly during the course of the separation that since visiting made them even more upset they did not want to visit the babies. (Only one of these did actually restrict her visiting.) The first commented:

> Well, I got tired, and when I did get tired like after coming up I even felt resentful. Sometimes I even felt like saying *no* I am *not* going up . . . I got cross, tantrummy even . . . you sort of felt in a way that you didn't have a baby. . . And then you would go the opposite, you would really feel that you had one and you had been missing her. Then I would resent her . . . all mixed up really.

She had felt guilty about her negative feelings and had been pleased that she had read about other mothers 'not feeling this great motherly thing for a while'.

The second mother felt upset and inadequate because the separation prevented her from doing things for her baby and she felt worried in case this would affect their feelings for each other later. She resented the fact that other people were looking after her baby and that the infant had no need of her and did not know her. She said bitterly:

> I knew that where she was going was by far the best place for her and that I couldn't cope with her – can't cope with her now I'm sure. . . I appreciate she's being well looked after, she doesn't really need me and she doesn't know me when she sees me . . . well it sort of affects also my feelings about how often I should see her – should I see her every day? Well, she wouldn't know me. Also it would upset me. I feel seeing her more would upset me more.

Later when this mother came to collect her baby she said, 'It's a lovely feeling to be needed.' These two mothers who had experienced negative feelings towards their babies both voiced concern that the separation might influence their later relationships with them. It might have been expected that they would wonder whether their feelings of resentment would persist even after they had been reunited with their babies:

> Since I've been thinking about it I've felt that the first bond between a mother and a child is very important – you know, the getting to

> know each other. And to think that I probably won't have this until she's say a month old. . . I feel worried – that first bond – how will it affect us both later on seeing as we weren't able to forge it? Me more than anything being separated from her.

This is a salutary warning against over-dramatising the effects of separation and therefore reinforcing or creating the expectation for parents of persistent difficulties following this experience. This mother also expressed concern about the fact that her baby was being looked after not by one person as is the usual pattern, but by many caretakers:

> I wonder how differences in handling will affect her? With one person you have a bit of continuity in handling, but there's different nurses and I should think different ways of handling, and I wonder if she notices this and how she feels about it?

After the period of separation from their babies a proportion of mothers who had originally thought it best to go home decided instead that this had been a mistake. The separation had not simply been a 'waiting out' period but one of increasing upset. One mother noted that it was upsetting seeing the baby and 'having nothing'; on the other hand it was also distressing having to leave her after visiting: 'When I was in hospital first I wanted to come home and feed Alan and when I got home it didn't seem right being here without her.' Attention has already been directed towards the emotional barriers that may inhibit parental visiting of sick and/or low birthweight infants in hospital. However, we must not forget the many practical or circumstantial barriers which may also play a very significant role in preventing or reducing early close parent-infant contact. Neonatal units serve large catchment areas and may not be easily accessible to many parents. Factors such as the cost of visiting, the distance involved, the mother's health, and whether she has to rely on public transport may all have an important bearing on visiting patterns.[21]

During a period of separation the father's involvement and support may be particularly vital. The importance of father-baby contact must not be underestimated; if the father feels a high sense of involvement with his infant this is likely to influence family relationships all round, in addition to his own special relationship with the child. He will be less likely to feel left out and may give his wife increased practical help and emotional support. In a study of parental visiting in a neonatal unit, mothers of very sick babies appeared to be particularly dependent on their husbands to accompany them during visits and to maintain contact with the unit by telephone.[22] There was some evidence that fathers were less intimidated by the technical equipment in the unit, and they may also be less affected by feelings of guilt and failure after an abnormal delivery.[23] In addition, if the mother herself is unable to visit the unit due to ill health or confinement elsewhere, the father can provide an important link with the baby.

Mason[24] and Blake *et al.*[25] have stressed the importance of the father's role in supporting the mother of a low birthweight baby after hospital discharge.

Some normal-procedure mothers were more susceptible than others at the time of the separation to feelings of distress and inadequacy. Those who seemed most vulnerable tended to belong to a 'special risk' group identified on the basis of their home backgrounds and current difficulties. Mothers with personal and social problems may be less able to withstand the normal frustrations accompanying separation, and in addition they may be more likely to have special needs, fears or expectations which cause the separation to be particularly upsetting. Interestingly, Seashore *et al.*[25] found that the separation had a negative effect on maternal self-confidence, but that those initially low in self-confidence were most vulnerable to this effect.

It is worth remembering that low birthweight infants are more likely to be born to women who are already in stressful situations,[26] who may be least in a position to cope with additional strain. The number of vulnerable women may be much greater than is commonly realised. Baum and Howat[27] reported that 10 per cent of families with babies admitted to the neonatal unit in Oxford had social and emotional problems serious enough to require continuing social work support after discharge. One aim of future research should be to identify the women most vulnerable to the adverse effects of separation so that they may be offered special support. There is some evidence that vulnerable mothers may visit their babies in the neonatal units less often than other mothers; in other words that separation is greatest for those mothers who may be most in need of close early contact with their infants.[28,29]

Many of the difficulties encountered by parents of small or sick infants are created or exacerbated by hospital care practices which could be altered. Efforts to increase visiting will meet with little success unless neonatal units provide the sort of environment in which parents can feel relaxed rather than clumsy and superfluous. Detailed examination of the effects of existing procedures is necessary to determine which aspects of the neonatal situation pose problems for the parent-infant relationship and how closer contact can be fostered in a more rewarding setting.

The Cambridge Study

In the previous section, we have seen some of the reactions of mothers who have been separated from their low birthweight babies at birth. These mothers suffer from a lack of confidence in their caretaking abilities and may feel inadequate if they have only restricted contact with their babies. Increased contact and early contact may enhance a mother's feelings of closeness to her baby. As we have mentioned earlier, some studies suggest that contact with ill or low birthweight babies increases parental anxiety.[18] But despite their increased anxiety the parents favoured unrestricted access according to this evidence. This is consistent with the view argued in Chapter 11 that parental anxiety is normal in this situation and may be a precondition of a satisfactory parental relationship.

Another problem parents may face in a neonatal unit is their feelings of self-consciousness and inhibition in front of the staff. The staff may seem to care very adequately for the babies and possess all the skills and confidence that parents would like to have. In the face of this, parents feel helpless and useless. These problems can be overcome only by a change in staff attitude towards the inclusion of parents in the care of their neonatal babies and a greater sensitivity to and sympathy with their situation.

We now report an intervention study which attempted to improve conditions for mothers in the neonatal baby unit in Cambridge, England, by fostering their contact with their babies. Two groups of low birthweight babies who stayed in the neonatal unit for more than three weeks after birth were followed up for one year. The parents in one group received the normal treatment that was standard in the Unit prior to the second phase of the study. The second group received an intervention treatement designed to increase parent-infant contact and support for parents. The procedures introduced in this intervention phase of the project were:

(1) An explanatory booklet (see Appendix at the end of this volume) was distributed to parents which described procedures employed there as well as some of the more usual problems faced by pre-term babies.

(2) Parents were provided with a Polaroid photograph of the baby taken soon after admission to the neonatal unit.
(3) Parents were given increased encouragement to visit, touch, cuddle, change nappies, clothes and cot blankets, tube feed, breast feed, bottle feed and bath their babies in the unit.
(4) All parents had at least two discussions with a paediatrician, one on the baby's admission to the unit and a second at discharge.
(5) Mothers were asked to stay for two nights in the mother-and-baby room near the neonatal unit before they went home with their baby.
(6) Health visitors were asked to visit mothers at home: (a) once a week before the baby came home, (b) once a day for the first five days the baby was at home and (c) once a week until the baby had been home for a month.

These procedures were chosen because they were considered to be changes that could be relatively easily introduced, and seemed likely to provide support for parents (especially mothers) and increase contact with the babies and communication with the staff in the hospital and community. The control group received the usual treatment which included freedom to visit at any time and some contact with the baby but no tube feeding. Primiparous mothers were offered the possibility of staying in the mother-and-baby room near the neonatal unit for one night before their baby was discharged home.

The changes between phases of the study are probably more subtle than those which are described by listing the new procedures that were introduced. During the transition between phases one and two many discussions were held with the staff about ways in which parents could be given better support. Very quickly things 'took off' so that staff themselves began to initiate measures and this led to a very noticeable change in the whole atmosphere of the unit.

Booklet (see Appendix, p. 298)

The explanatory booklet was designed to increase the amount of information for the parents and to serve as a supplement to the information given by the staff. An important point was that parents could refer to it as they wished. They could discover what they wanted as and when the question arose even when they were not in the unit. The information contained in the booklet that the parents seemed to find most helpful described visiting, the appearance of the unit, the mother-and-baby room, types of medical procedures, the sorts of feelings the parents may have, how parents can look after their baby in the unit, description of the various staff, tube feeding, breast feeding, bottle feeding, weight, what the prem baby looks like, procedures for transferring babies from other hospitals, what happens on and after discharge from the unit with common questions and answers, follow-up clinics and how parents may feel when the baby comes home. In the back of the booklet is a conversion chart of grams into pounds and ounces and of centimetres into inches, as well as a glossary of medical terms. The conversion table was important for many parents who were unused to metric units.

It was found[30] that the predominantly middle-class mothers said that the booklet helped them to understand their baby's problems better and put them into perspective. The parents also felt informed and more confident in speaking to the staff about their baby. The booklet explained the developmental abilities of low birthweight babies and what to expect when a baby is very ill. This information helps to acquaint parents with their babies and to feel closer and more involved in their care.

In a study by Jeffcoate,[14,15] a booklet was introduced to improve the communication in a neonatal baby unit serving a poor, urban population. Before the book was introduced, 78 per cent of the sample of 18 mothers had been worried by inadequate explanation about apparatus, procedures and tests used for their baby and conditions such as jaundice and minor infections. Ten mothers complained that they had difficulty in finding the unit and gaining access to their baby, even though the policy was for the parents to visit at any time. Jeffcoate also reported that, during the first week, seven mothers had not been told that they could touch their baby and only five mothers felt free to handle their baby as often as they wanted.

When Jeffcoate introduced her (3,500 words) explanatory booklet, a short questionnaire was given to the parents. These were returned by 73 per cent (30) of parents, all of whom said they understood the text, did not find the booklet too lengthy and did not feel that any item should be omitted. All these parents said they found the booklet helpful and 47 per cent (14) added a positive written comment.

Jeffcoate also stressed the need for a section in such booklets which discussed parental emotional distress, as many parents feel helpless and unable to form a close relationship with their baby who they feel is the hospital's property. Parents may be reassured to know that their feelings of anxiety, depression, guilt, anger and often disgust at the appearance of their infant are common. The Cambridge study found that parents' anxiety about their neonatal baby was great and parents welcomed as much information and reassurance as possible. The use of the booklet in the Cambridge study may also have contributed to the finding that the intervention-group mothers who received the booklet felt less inhibited with the staff, felt closer to their babies in the neonatal unit and more confident about coping at home after the baby was discharged. Although these mothers also had more contact with their babies and had received other supports, a booklet does seem to provide support. However, as Jeffcoate points out, the booklet can only cover basic and routine matters and other information about the baby's condition must be provided by the staff.

Experience has shown that the suggestions of introducing booklets of this kind may provoke resistance from some staff members. They may be concerned that parents may be made unneccessarily anxious by descriptions of medical problems which may not even arise with their baby. However, the two studies that we have described have shown that worries of this kind are unfounded and that the overall impact of such literature is reassuring and has a very positive effect on relationships between staff and parents. Booklets may also serve to foster contacts between the parents of the various babies in the unit, as they help to explain what is happening to other babies parents may see on their visits.

Photographs

A photograph taken soon after the baby's admission to the neonatal unit is another way of improving contact between mother and baby. In Hawthorne Amick's study,[30] a polaroid colour photograph was given to the intervention-group mothers. The mothers were all pleased to have the photograph and often showed it to other mothers on the ward, as well as nurses, siblings and friends who might not be permitted to visit the baby in the neonatal unit. The photograph is a tangible symbol of the baby and seems to be reassuring for mothers perhaps because, in the baby's absence, it may help to dispel some of the worst fantasies about the baby's condition and appearance. It may also be seen as a statement from the hospital staff that can help to make the mother feel that the staff want to include her in the care of her baby. The photograph also should be taken early so that it shows the baby as the parents first saw him or her. This may help them to adapt to their baby's looks and to see the difference as their child develops.

Other units[19] have used this technique and it now seems to be becoming fairly general practice.

Visiting and Contact with the Baby

In order to reduce the effects of separation, units must provide free access for parents to their babies at all times. More than this, not only must visiting be encouraged, but parents will often need help and support to make contact with their baby during a visit. The staff have to be aware that the parents may feel that their baby belongs to the hospital, and can be feeling anxious, guilty, angry and depressed. Contact with the baby may help parents to feel that their responsibilities are not being usurped by the hospital. Physical contact may allow parents a chance to develop their parental feelings. However, it must always be remembered how off-putting a small and sick baby enclosed in an incubator and surrounded by medical equipment may be. Apart from the very mixed and complex feelings parents may have about a baby in this situation, there may be fears that to touch the baby may cause damage or infection. Other parents may be afraid that they will upset the equipment and so prejudice their baby's chances. Particularly in the early stages of visiting it is essential that staff are present for some of the time to demonstrate what the parents can do and to encourage parents in making contact with their babies in whatever ways the parents find most comfortable.

Following the early reports from such centres as Kennell and Klaus's unit in Cleveland, Ohio, and at University College Hospital, London, it is now usual practice to encourage parents to touch and hold their babies as soon as their medical condition permits. In most situations, it should be expected that visiting rates and the amount of contact during visits will increase with time. Rosenfield[31] found that the increase in maternal visits was related to the improvement in the physical condition of the baby, the mother's greater certainty that the infant would survive, increasing familiarity with the neonatal unit and the improving appearance of the infant.

As we have noted earlier, there is evidence that visits may increase some parental feelings of anxiety,[18,32] but anxiety engendered by visiting does not seem to inhibit further visiting in a supportive unit and is probably a normal and unavoidable part of parental feelings in this situation.

It is not sufficient to open the doors to parents to ensure that parental relationships with the babies will be improved. Once parents are in the unit they need to be able to exercise a normal parental role as far as possible. This means being much more than a spectator of their baby and being involved in caretaking and decision making. As soon as the baby's condition permits it, parents should be involved in such activities as changing nappies and bedding, washing and bathing, tube, bottle or breast feeding. Parental involvement in caretaking activities can cause conflicts among staff. It does require a modification of role for staff and we must recognise that it is not always easy for an experienced caretaker of sick babies to watch an inexperienced parent fumble and make a mess of things. But it is vital that the parents remain parents. After all, in the end they will be left holding the baby (as the expression goes).

Breast Feeding

Apart from any nutritional arguments, breast feeding has a particular role in the care of pre-term and sick babies because it is a tangible way in which a mother can care for and quite literally provide for her child. It gives the mother, who is likely to have feelings of being inadequate and superfluous, a unique role in the care of her child. For these reasons, it is especially important that mothers of babies in neonatal units are provided with all the help and support they need to establish lactation, if they choose to breast-feed. For those that do not, it is obviously vital not to increase their bad feelings by dwelling on their choice.

If the unit has a milk bank where breast milk can be frozen, mothers can bring in their expressed milk in the bottles provided by the unit. Breast feeding should take place as soon as possible both for maternal psychological reasons and because it may be the most effective way of establishing lactation (see Chapter 12). Some units put the baby to the breast even before he can suck so that the mother gets some stimulation. Normally babies can suck at about 35 weeks of gestation, depending on their condition.

The Cambridge study found that in a unit that promoted breast feeding there was very little information for the mothers on how to maintain lactation. It was difficult for these mothers to find an electric breast pump to hire and these were expensive. The mothers who did hire them and used them consistently had better success with maintaining lactation than those who used manual breast pumps. Some mothers did not know that their breasts had to be expressed every four hours and needed to be given factual information as well as reassurance that it was possible to breast-feed their baby at home. As in an earlier study it was found that mothers who breast-fed visited more, probably because they had to bring in their milk.[22,28]

It may be a good idea to have a nurse or midwife who is a specialised breast-feeding counsellor attached to the neonatal units, as this may be the best way of giving mothers individual help and support. The counsellor can be responsible for giving mothers correct information about expressing their milk. Whether or not a specialist staff member is employed it is important that the advice given by all staff members is consistent.

Bottle Feeding

Mothers who do not want to breast-feed are likely to feel guilty if they are told that breast milk is the best milk for their ill or small baby. If mothers prefer to bottle-feed, they should be supported in their decision.

Feeding their baby is an event of great significance to mothers with babies in neonatal units, as it makes the mothers feel they are doing something positive for their babies and it helps them to feel emotionally closer to them. Parents should be given the chance to bottle-feed the baby as soon as the baby is ready. They should be given guidance in how to do it, but not made to feel that the nurses can do it better than they can. Bottle feeding may take longer than tube feeding and so there may be a tendency to prolong the latter beyond the period necessary. This may be undesirable for at least two reasons. It may not be good for a baby to be denied the experience of sucking any longer than is strictly necessary and, from a parent's point of view, seeing a baby making positive sucking movements can be very encouraging. Bottle feeding may help to emphasise the similarity between a pre-term baby and a normal full-term one.

Tube Feeding

In the Cambridge study routines were changed so that the mothers were asked to hold the tube and pour the milk down if their baby needed tube feeding. Most parents wanted to be involved in this way, although some preferred just to have physical contact with their baby or wait until the baby was ready to bottle- or breast-feed. Where parents want to do it, tube feeding is important, as it is one of the tasks they can start doing almost immediately the baby is born. A mother may be particularly pleased to be able to tube-feed if her own milk is being used.

Bathing

This is another activity which gives the parents a chance to get to know their baby and to be involved in caretaking. Washing the baby with cream, or whatever is used in a particular neonatal unit, can be done until the baby is well enough to have a water bath. During washing, parents can begin to see their baby responding to different forms of stimulation which may give them a growing sense of reciprocity in their relationship.

Early Transferral to Cots

Once the baby is out of the incubator, parents visit more frequently,[30-32] and may feel closer to the baby as he or she becomes more accessible. When the baby is in a cot, parents are able to perform a wider range of caretaking activities and, again, it may serve to emphasise the normality of the baby. During the Cambridge study the policy changed and some babies were dressed warmly and put in cots at a lower weight (an average of 1.50 kg instead of 1.70 kg). Not only did parents seem to appreciate this, but more incubators were available for the babies who needed them.

Other Policy Changes

Parents or siblings often want to bring in soft toys or other objects for their baby. Providing these are reasonably clean there is no reason why they should not be placed in the incubator or cot. This may help the family to welcome their new baby in a more natural way and can emphasise the individual and personal in an otherwise rather institutional atmosphere. Some units have music boxes, mobiles, rocking chairs and pictures on the walls which make the unit cheerful and comfortable and can soften the clinical atmosphere.

Several units dress the babies in colourfully patterned gowns or use colourful sheets which help to make the unit less clinical. A mother one of us once interviewed spoke at length of her resentment at having her baby dressed in smocks which said 'Property of the Royal . . . Infirmary' in large red letters. She, like the interviewer, found it hard to understand why she could not provide her own clothes for her baby. The mother's interpretation was that the lettering symbolised the staff's attitude to the babies in this particular unit.

The baby's first name can be written on a card attached to the incubator for everyone to see and notes for the parents about feeding, bathing, or other things to do with the baby can also be put up.

Another way to help parents is to show them photographs of babies when they are very small or ill as well as photographs of the same baby taken later (three months, six months, one year, etc.) to show how infants changed and developed. Most units have a bulletin board covered with photographs of babies they have looked after, or photograph albums the parents can look at. Our feeling is that it is important not to 'censor' pictures that parents provide for the unit and that collections should include some in which the children have obvious handicaps.

Doctor-parent Communication

Studies have universally pointed to the need for good communication between parents and staff.[14,33,34] Taylor and Hall, for instance, point out how easy it is to talk *at* the parents rather than *with* them. It is important for the paediatrician to find out how the parents are perceiving their ill baby and how their individual experiences with past pregnancies, illnesses and fears will play a role in their reactions to the present child. Hawthorne Amick[30] found that parents of very ill babies felt relatively well-informed about their babies' progress, while parents of small, healthy pre-terms had almost no contact with doctors and felt uninformed. Parents in the intervention group always spoke to a paediatrician on the baby's admission to the unit and on the baby's discharge, as well as at other times in many cases. Many parents are likely to feel more reassured by talking to the most senior medical staff but, as an ideal, parents should have contact with all the medical staff who deal with their child. In each case doctors must introduce themselves and explain their role. Booklets can help by describing for parents the various kinds of doctors and other staff parents may encounter on a neonatal unit, including such people as opthalmologists and radiographers. Parents feel more at ease if they can identify the staff in the neonatal unit and know them by name.

Most parents want to know exactly what tests, procedures and medicines are being used for their baby and the reasons for their use. As far as possible they need to feel involved in decision-making and not simply informed after the event. If the mother is ill or unable to visit the baby, it is helpful for the paediatrician to visit her in person in the ward even though the baby's father may pass on information from the doctor to the mother. It always seems parents are helped by direct contact with the person who has direct contact with their child.

Some units encourage a degree of specialising among nursing staff so that a particular nurse on each shift has responsibility for the same baby (or babies). This can help parents as they get to know this nurse and know who to ask about what their child has been doing since they last visited. The feeling that some staff members really know or understand their baby can have a very positive effect on parents.

Counsellors, Psychotherapists and Psychiatrists

As we have seen, parents of neonatal babies may suffer a great deal of anxiety and conflicting feelings as well as other emotional difficulties and some may be helped through counselling. The role of psychotherapy and other specialist counselling is described in Chapter 11.

The counsellor should meet the parents as each baby is admitted. In this way, parents will know who to turn to when in difficulties.

Discussion Groups for Parents and Staff

The counsellor (psychotherapist, psychologist or psychiatrist) can lead a discussion group for parents where they can discuss their feelings. Parents often feel better able to cope when they express their feelings and find that other parents feel the same way. Minde[35] reports the establishment of a self-help group for parents in his nursery where a 'veteran' mother or father who has had an infant in the unit in the last twelve months leads a discussion group. Minde found that the parents who participated in these groups visited significantly more frequently, showed more affectionate behaviour and reported more satisfaction.

Staff may also benefit from supportive groups amongst themselves (see Chapter 11). Working in a neonatal baby unit can be very stressful. It is an environment which is noisy and busy, with incubators and machinery and fluorescent lighting on for 24 hours a day.[35] In addition, it is an environment in which death and tragedy are frequently seen. Several people have suggested that nurses and medical staff should have an outlet for discussing their feelings such as individual conferences or group discussions.[37] Until they come to terms with their own feelings about the job it may be difficult for nurses and doctors in neonatal units to understand parental attitudes and to cope with parents' feelings.

Mother-and-baby Room

Some units have rooms where the mother can stay with her baby overnight before they both go home. Facilities of this kind give parents a chance to be alone with their babies and to get to know them and look after them without staff necessarily being present. Other family members can visit so that the family has time to be alone together.

The room should be furnished in the style of a bedroom with a comfortable chair and a radio, TV and so on. There is usually a bathroom nearby and a kitchen where the mother can make herself a snack or a drink. Some hospitals have several rooms for mothers with a sitting room nearby.

Although the policy varies between units, it appears beneficial if the mothers come to stay for at least two nights with their baby before taking him home. The first night they often do not sleep very well as they are excited and may be unused to the baby's schedule. Mother and baby need time to adapt to each other while the mother still has the support of hospital staff.

Mothers who are breast feeding often need to stay a few days in the room in order to establish this. These mothers can be asked to come and stay for a few days when they first start breast feeding, even though their baby might not yet be ready to go home. Mothers say that staying with their baby makes them feel much closer and more confident about taking their baby home. In the Exeter study mothers stayed with their pre-term babies for up to five weeks in hospital, but not all hospitals have enough room for this and not all mothers will want it. The new maternity hospital in Cambridge will have six mother-and-baby rooms, a sitting room and kitchen in a unit which is designed to have 18 special care and 6 intensive care cots. A unit with more extensive facilities for parents is described in Chapter 16.

Health Visitor Contact

Mothers who have babies in neonatal units may be very isolated if they go home leaving their baby in hospital, and may benefit from talking to people in their community who can give them supportive help and advice. Health visitors (in Britain) or other community workers can play a role here as they can visit the mother at home and may be able to see the baby in hospital. Some hospitals have a health visitor liaison system where a hospital health visitor informs the mother's local health visitor about the baby's condition weekly or as necessary. If the local health visitor cannot visit the baby in hospital, she can still be informed about the baby which makes it easier for her to talk to the mother.

In the Cambridge study mothers in the intervention group seemed to appreciate the extra contact they had with health visitors as their morale was boosted and they were often able to share their worries. There are suggestions that health visitors (or visiting nurses) might be able to reduce problems on follow-up.[38]

The health visitor should arrange to visit the mother as soon as she goes home without her baby, visiting at least once a week. When the baby comes home, it is important that the health visitor visits every day for the first five days or longer and then once a week for as long as is necessary. In communities where there is no health visitor system, neonatal units may have their own visiting nurses who go into the home.

Contact with the General Practitioner (or Family Doctor)

The family doctor should be informed as soon as the baby is born. According to our studies the GP often may not know about the baby's birth until the baby is at home, which can be several months later. If the GPs know sooner, they can lend support to the parents and provide medical attention if necessary. Once the baby comes home, the GP can help in providing follow-up, particularly if there are no other provisions for follow-up by health visitors, visiting nurses or local clinics.

Several studies have reported high rates of hospital readmission of ex-special care babies.[39,40] Some of this seems to stem from parental anxieties which are not adequately dealt with by the general practitioner. Some GPs seem to regard ex-special care babies as 'paediatric property' so that they will get them admitted to hospital with relatively minor illnesses which in other babies would have been dealt with at home. Often parents take their ex-special care babies home with the message 'come back if you are worried about anything'. So they may do just that and there is not always sufficient guidance given to parents on what is and what is not a situation in which medical advice is appropriate. Frequent calls to doctors may be an indication that the parents' anxieties about their baby are not being listened to and dealt with adequately. It is also vital that parents are given clear instructions about the roles of the various medical and nursing services in their community so they know who the right person is to consult in a particular situation.

Clinics

Local (Community) Clinics. In Britain, mothers can visit community clinics with their babies every week in order to weigh their babies and see the health visitor or the doctor. Mothers generally find these clinics supportive as they can ask questions and they meet other mothers with whom they can share experiences. However, some mothers need more support than they seem to receive, and clinics should be able to provide mothers with information on baby's sleeping, feeding or crying problems, all of which are common with low birthweight babies. Parents may be unclear about the role of the numerous professionals that they are likely to encounter and it is often helpful if they are told about the people who may be involved in the follow-up and their various roles.

Hospital Clinics. Neonatal baby units in Britain arrange a hospital follow-up for babies who have been ill and some see all babies discharged about six weeks later. The mothers in the Cambridge study returned to the hospital clinic three times in the baby's first year for the purpose of the study and seemed to like to see the doctors who knew their baby's medical history, and they felt reassured, even if their baby had not been very ill in the neonatal unit.

Sensory Stimulation

So far in this chapter we have concentrated on interventions which are designed to support and modify parent-child relationships. Other intervention programmes have been used which have been directed at the infant in the hospital and have been intended to modify sensory stimulation. These have been based on varied and conflicting rationales, including attempts to simulate the intrauterine environment, to make good supposed sensory deprivation in the incubator or reduce its supposed overload. Other programmes are designed to give the baby's sensory input a pattern rather than the unvarying conditions that may exist in an incubator. Some workers have been concerned about the lack of contingency in what the baby is doing and the caretaker response. A very wide range of stimuli have been applied, including such things as stroking of the baby's body, patterned coloured lights, heart beat sounds and baroque music, pulsating water beds and lambswool bedding. It is not our intention to discuss these kinds of programmes here as their primary aim is not to support parent-child relations. Indeed, a possible criticism of some of the interventions is that they completely ignore the parents and seem to be based on the premise that only a physical environment is needed by a developing child. Interested readers are referred to reviews of the field.[41,42]

While one may be critical of some of the intervention programmes, there is every reason to look carefully at the physical environment of the newborn pre-term infant and to do all we can to make sure that it is optimal for social as well as physical development. As yet, little work has been done to assess the ways in which particular medical or nursing interventions may inhibit or enhance parental relationships. For instance, it is not uncommon for babies on ventilators to be paralysed. Two points arise here for the psychologist: what is the impact for parents of seeing a baby who is unable to make any movements and what consequences, if any, are there for the infant? It is interesting to note that when such techniques are used with adults, it is usual practice to render the adult unconscious as it is felt that to be conscious and paralysed would be (or is, according to case reports) a terrifying experience. Does the same hold for a baby? What would the effects of the narcotic drug that would be used to create unconsciousness? Similar questions arise over many aspects of treatment used in neonatal intensive care.

There may be some very simple techniques that can be used to enhance the baby's environment. One such may be nursing on lambswool. Preliminary studies[43] have shown that this may increase the growth rate of pre-term babies. Additionally, this may improve the 'image' of the baby in the eyes of the parents and other caretakers. Certainly mothers report their babies were 'more cuddly' as well as more comfortable when on lambswool. In a pilot study adults rated pre-term babies more positively when shown pictures of them on lambswool rather than in traditional bedding.[44]

Conclusion

In this chapter we have outlined some of the complex feelings that the birth of a pre-term baby may engender in parents. We have described the potential that neonatal units may have for interfering with parent-child relations in what is already often a fraught situation and ways in which this potential may be reduced or removed. This is a field in which we still have much to learn and the growth of knowledge of neonatal physiology has far outstripped that of neonatal and parental psychology. However, as was plain to Pierre Budin, the inventor (or one of its inventors; see Chapter 2) of the incubator, to save the life of a pre-term baby at the expense of the relationship with the parents would represent little advance.

References

1. Solnit, A. J., and Stark, M. H. (1961). Mourning and the birth of a defective child. *Psychoanal. Study Child.*, *16*, 523.

2. Kennell, J. H., and Rolnick, A. (1960). Discussing problems in newborn babies with their parents. *Pediatrics*, *26*, 832.

3. Lax, R. F. (1972). Some aspects of the interaction between mother and impaired child: mother's narcissistic trauma. *Internat.J.Psychoan.*, *53*, Part 3.

4. Korones, S. B. (1972). *High Risk Newborn Infants*. St Louis, C. V. Mosby.

5. Oppe, T. (1960). The emotional aspects of prematurity. *Cerebral Palsy Bull.*, *2*, *4*, 233.

6. Kaplan, D. N., and Mason, E. A. (1960). Maternal reactions to premature birth viewed as an acute emotional disorder. *Am. J. Orthopsychiat.*, *30*, 539.

7. Richards, M. P. M. (1978). Possible effects of early separation on later development in children. In *Early Separation and Special Care Baby Units*,

F. S. W. Brimblecombe, M. P. M. Richards and N. R. C. Roberton (eds), Clinics in Developmental Medicine. London, SIMP/Heinemann Medical Books.

8. Minde, K. K. (1980). Bonding of mothers to premature infants: theory and practice. In *Parent-Infant Relationships*, P. M. Taylor (ed.). New York, Grune and Stratton.

9. Goldberg, S. (1978). Prematurity: effects on parent-infant interaction. *Pediat. Psychol., 3*, 137.

10. Rosenfeld, A. G. (1980). Visiting in the intensive care nursery. *Child Devel., 81*, 939.

11. Frodi, A., Lamb, M., Leavitt, L., Donovan, W., Neff, C., and Sherry, D. (1978). Fathers' and mothers' responses to the faces and cries of normal and premature infants. *Devel. Psychol., 14*, 490.

12. Gray, J. D., Cutler, C. A., Dean, J. G., and Kempe, C. H. (1980). Prediction and prevention of child abuse. In *Parent-Infant Relationships*, P. M. Taylor (ed.). New York, Grune and Stratton.

13. Jacques, N. C. S. (1978). *The Role of Early Mother-infant Contact in the Developing Mother-child Relationship*. Unpublished MSc thesis, University of Cambridge.

14. Jeffcoate, J. A. (1979). Improving communication in a special care baby unit. *Early Hum. Dev., 3*, 341.

15. Jeffcoate, J. A. (1980). Looking at the need for support for families of low birth-weight babies. *Health Trends, 12*, 29.

16. Leiderman, P. H., and Seashore, M. J. (1975). Mother-infant neonatal separation: some delayed consequences. In *Parent-infant Interaction*, Ciba Foundation Symp., No. 33 (New series). Amsterdam, Elsevier.

17. Douglas, J. W. B., and Gear, R. (1976). Children of low birth weight in the 1946 national cohort. *Arch Dis. Child., 51*, 820.

18. Harper, R. C.. Sia, C., Sokal, S., and Sokal, M. (1976). Observations and unrestricted parental contact with infants in the neonatal intensive care unit. *Pediatrics, 89*, 441.

19. Blake, A., Stewart, A., and Turcan, D. (1975). Parents of babies of very low birth weight: long-term follow-up. In *Parent-infant Interaction*, Ciba Foundation Symp., No. 33. Amsterdam, Elsevier.

20. Winnicott, D. W. (1964). *The Child, the Family and the Outside World*. London, Pelican Books.

21. Hawthorne, J. T., Richards, M. P. M., and Callon, M. (1978). A Study of parental visiting of babies in a special care unit. In *Separation and Special Care Baby Units*, F. S. W. Brimblecombe, M. P. M. Richards and N. R. C. Roberton (eds), London, SIMP/Heinemann Medical Books.

22. Jeffcoate, J. (1977). *A Study of the Need for Care and Support for Families of Low Birthweight Babies*. Dissertation, University of London.

23. Mason, E. A. (1963). A method of predicting crisis outcome for mothers of premature babies. *Public Health Report, 78*, 1031.

24. Blake, A., Stewart, A., and Turcan, D. (1975). Parents of babies of very low birth weight: long-term follow-up. In *Parent-infant Interaction*, Ciba Foundation Symp., No. 33. Amsterdam, Elsevier.

25. Seashore, M. H., Leifer, A. D., Barnett, C. R., and Leiderman, P. H. (1973). The effects of denial of early mother-infant interaction on maternal self-confidence. *J. Pers. Soc. Psychol., 26*, 369.

26. Crosse, V. M. (1971). *The Pre-term Baby and Other Babies with Low Birth Weight*. Edinburgh, Churchill Livingstone.

27. Baum, J. D., and Howat, P. (1978). The family and neonatal intensive care. In *The Place of Birth*, S. Kitzinger and J. A. Davis (eds). Oxford, Oxford University Press.

28. Fanaroff, A. A., Kennell, J. H., and Klaus, M. H. (1972). Follow-up of low birth weight infants – the predictive value of maternal visiting patterns. *Pediatrics*, *49*, 288.

29. Hunter, R. S., Kilstrom, N., Kaybill, E. N., and Loda, F. (1978). Antecedents of child abuse and neglect in premature infants: a prospective study in a newborn intensive care unit. *Pediatrics*, *61*, 629.

30. Hawthorne Amick, J. T. (1981). *The Effect of Different Routines in a Special Care Baby Unit on the Mother-infant Relationship: An Intervention Study*. Unpublished PhD dissertation, University of Cambridge.

31. Rosenfield, A. G. (1980). Visiting in the intensive care nursery. *Child Devel.*, *51*, 939.

32. Paludetto, R., Faggiano-Perfetto, M., Asprea, A. M., De Curtis, M., and Margara-Paludetto, P. (1981). Reactions of sixty parents allowed unrestricted contact with infants in a neonatal intensive care unit. *Early Hum. Devel.*, *5*, 401.

33. Klaus, M. H., and Kennell, J. H. (1976). *Maternal-infant Bonding*. St Louis, C. V. Mosby.

34. Taylor, P. M., and Hall, B. L. (1980). Parent-infant bonding: problems and opportunities in a prenatal center. In *Parent-Infant Relationships*, P. M. Taylor (ed.). New York, Grune and Stratton.

35. Minde, K., Shosenberg, N., Marton, P., Thompson, J., Ripley, J., and Burn, S. (1980). Self-help groups in a premature nursery – a controlled evaluation. *J. Pediatrics*, *96*, 933.

36. Kellman, N. (1980). Risks in the design of the modern neonatal intensive care unit. *Birth and the Family Journal*, *7*, 243-8.

37. Lewandowski, L. A., and Kramer, M. (1980). Role transformation of special care unit nurses – a comparative study. *Nursing Research*, *29*, 170.

38. Brown, J. V., La Rossa, M. M., Aylward, G. P., Davis, D. J., Rutherford, P. K., and Bakeman, R. (1980). Nursery-based intervention with prematurely born babies and their mothers: are there effects? *J. Pediatrics*, *97*, 487.

39. Hack, M., De Monterice, D., Merkatz, I. R., Jones, P., and Fanaroff, A. A. (1981). Rehospitalization of the very low birthweight babies. *Amer. J. Dis. Child*, *135*, 263.

40. Campbell, D. M. (1982). *The Evaluation of Aspects of Neonatal Paediatric Services*. Unpublished PhD thesis, University of Cambridge.

41. Smeriglio, V. L. (ed.) (1981). *Newborns and Parents. Parent-Infant Contact and Newborn Sensory Stimulation*. Hillsdale, New Jersey, Lawrence Erlbaum.

42. Masi, W. (1979). Supplemental stimulation for the premature infant. In *Infants Born at Risk*, T. M. Field (ed.). New York, SP Medical and Scientific Books.

43. Scott, S., and Richards, M. P. M. (1979). Nursing low birth weight babies on lambswool. *Lancet*, *i*, 1028.

44. Richards, M. P. M. Unpublished observations.

8 THE ROLE OF THE NURSE IN MOTHER-BABY INTERACTION

Jean Boxall and Chris Whitby

Introduction

The nurse has a central role to play in facilitating mother-baby attachment. Many neonatal nurses may not realise just how important this is, but major contributions can be made which not only improve care of parents and families but give enormous job satisfaction.

Antenatal Period

The senior neonatal unit (NNU) nurses should be involved in preparing parents for the birth of a premature baby. With 'at risk' patients who spend weeks on the antenatal ward, parents should be seen at some stage during the admission. In many other cases (Table 8.1) the mother

Table 8.1: Conditions for which Mothers May Be Admitted Antenatally and Benefit from Visits by Neonatal Nursing Staff.

Pre-term labour
Premature rupture of membranes
Twins or higher multiples
Haemolytic disease of the newborn
Maternal diabetes
Severe pre-eclampsia
Recurrent ante-partum haemorrhage
Poor fetal growth
Assorted medical complications

may be a patient in the maternity hospital for assessment pre-delivery for long enough to allow one or two visits from the nursing staff. The nurses should also attempt to visit any anxious parents who have had a previous stillbirth, neonatal death or pre-term delivery.

These visits from the neonatal nursing staff are usually welcomed by both the parents and midwifery staff. Problems and anxieties can be discussed, both parents can be invited to visit the NNU and if necessary arrangements can be made for them to discuss their problems with a paediatrician. Some of the more common questions asked by parents in this situation are 'Will my baby be alright?', 'What are his chances?', 'What sort of problems may he have?', 'Can I see him?', 'And how often?', 'Who else can see him?', 'Will I be able to breast feed?', 'How long will he be in hospital?'

The experienced nurse, who has seen many happy outcomes from difficult pregnancies, can answer these questions in a very positive way. She can use photographs of previous successful cases to reassure the anxious parents, giving optimistic predictions so that both parents embark on labour and delivery with clear information and hopeful anticipation. The discussion also gives her a chance to outline the routines in the NNU, such as the visiting arrangements for parents, siblings and other relatives, as well as describing standard procedures such as Dextrostix in babies of diabetic mothers, phototherapy and exchange transfusion for rhesus babies and the techniques for ventilatory support and pO_2 monitoring in infants likely to be very pre-term and at risk from respiratory disease.

Perinatal Period

The labour ward midwife present at delivery is the key person initiating the family-baby contact. During her training she is taught to foster this contact by:

(1) encouraging fathers to be present throughout labour and at the birth;
(2) delivering the baby onto the mother's abdomen, and/or allowing her to lift the baby out;
(3) encouraging early skin and eye contact between mother and baby;
(4) putting the baby to the breast as soon as possible.

When delivery is likely to produce a baby requiring NNU admission, in addition to having a labour ward midwife present to carry out these routines, it is helpful to have a neonatal nurse present with the paediatrician, not only to help with the resuscitation, but also to help with the care of the parents who must be kept well informed about what is happening to their baby. This nurse may need to reinforce information given by the paediatrician, or supply that information herself if the paediatrician is preoccupied with the medical care of the baby.

If the baby needs to go to the NNU, the parents should be allowed to see him if it is at all possible before he leaves the labour ward, and the nurse or the paediatrician should explain to the them the transport incubator and any other equipment being used; they must emphasise, even at that stage, that parents will always be very welcome on the NNU. Although some fathers will wish to stay with their wives for some time in this situation, others may wish to, and should be allowed to, accompany their baby and the paediatric team to the NNU.

Babies Born Elsewhere (See also Chapter 10)

It is important to remember that most parents require an explanation of why their baby cannot be cared for in the local unit, and we have found that antenatal parentcraft evenings are a good opportunity to mention that some babies who become very sick after delivery will need to be transferred to the regional centre.

While waiting for the flying squad to arrive the local nurse should:

(1) let the parents see the baby;
(2) ask the mother if she wishes to breast-feed, and explain the breast milk banking procedures;
(3) get relevant notes ready;
(4) take blood from the mother, and get a consent form signed in case operation is required after transfer;
(5) take a photograph of the baby for the mother to keep, and give her a parents' booklet if one is produced by the regional centre;
(6) arrange christening if necessary.

Good communication between nurses and the local unit and the regional centre is essential. One way of doing this in the UK is for some of the local nurses to be seconded to the centre for a day visit, a refresher course, or a Joint Board of Clinical Nursing Studies neonatal course.

The Management of Parent-baby Attachment in the Unit

Cross-infection

Most of the arguments for the trappings of 'preventing infection', such as visiting restricted to parents only and the use of gowns, overshoes and masks, are ill-founded. The nursing staff should appreciate that the mother is the cleanest person handling her baby provided she washes her hands carefully. Grandparents and the baby's siblings are not a hazard, again providing they wash their hands, and they are in fact important components for sealing the new baby into the family unit.

Parents, relatives, or other visitors with infections should not handle the baby. Any information booklet given to parents should state clearly that people with colds, coughs, stomach upsets, infected lesions, or temperatures should not visit the unit.

Receiving the New Father into the Unit

The nurse welcoming a new father should remember that he will be apprehensive yet excited, hoping that all will be well. The visit should not be rushed, and if the baby is needing urgent medical attention when the father arrives he should be asked to wait outside and offered a cup of tea or coffee. However, if the baby is not seriously ill, the father can be allowed in straightaway, and he may feel more involved if he can help with such things as completing the cot card after the baby is weighed.

The father needs a very careful introduction to this alien environment. A friendly positive approach is most important as he will be influenced by the attitude of the staff. Encouraging comments such as 'Many babies of his weight do well', or 'He is doing quite well considering he is so small', or 'We expect he will respond to the treatment', can be made. Phrases such as 'We are very worried about him', or 'Your baby is very poorly', or 'He needs a lot of oxygen', should be avoided as a greeting, and questions about prognosis should normally be left to the paediatrician.

If the nurses and doctors are negative and gloomy about a baby, then the father will be also. An upset father may display great anger and neeed extra understanding to overcome this with a few moments of privacy and someone to talk to. He may become over-protective towards his wife, advising her not to visit because she might 'get fond of him'. Both parents may then emotionally turn away from their baby to protect themselves from painful involvement. This goes against the basic normal emotions, those of wanting to love and care for their child no matter what may happen.

When taking the father into the unit, the importance of hand-washing should be explained, and he should be warned that, if the baby is in intensive care, it will be hot, and that the baby will be connected to various tubes and monitors. These should all be explained to him when he is beside his baby's incubator. The father, like the mother when she comes to the unit, should be encouraged to touch and stroke his baby; he should also be asked about the choice of name for the baby. Finally, he should be given a photograph of the baby, and in our unit a copy of the neonatal unit booklet for parents (see Appendix) for him and his wife to keep.

Mother's First Visit

Every effort should be made to get the mother and baby together as soon as possible. If mother is seriously ill and cannot be moved to the NNU, but the baby is well enough, he should be taken to see his mother. More commonly, the mother, despite premature delivery, is well enough to be taken to the NNU – in a wheelchair if necessary – and this should always be done irrespective of whether the baby is in intensive care or not. However, many mothers need a lot of encouragement to make their first visit. Often, a woman is afraid of what she might see or hear or even of being sick or fainting, though this rarely happens. She may feel that she cannot face this first visit alone and if her husband is not present she may elect to stay away from her baby until he comes back several hours or even a day later.

In this situation a senior nurse from the NNU should visit the mother on her ward and should always volunteer to accompany her to the NNU. Positive encouragement is often helpful; there are always good things to say about the baby, describing his face, eyes and hair, using the photograph given to the father earlier. Further encouragement, such as saying 'It's important for you to see him – he will know you are there' or 'He needs you', may be needed. Most women give in to this gentle persuasion, and with the support from the nursing staff which they subsequently receive, never regret their decision to visit the baby.

When the mother does come to the unit, it is valuable to introduce her to the sister in charge and also to the nurse looking after her baby, the attitude of these people should always be positive and as encouraging as possible. The mother should be shown how to wash her hands, but if she cannot get out of a wheelchair a hand rub can be used. She should be taken to her baby's incubator and with care a wheelchair can be manoeuvred close enough to the incubator for her to be able to reach in and touch her baby. She should be given as much access to him as possible by opening up portholes, removing the baby's gloves and bootees, and by removing cling film or radiant heat shields. The nurse may need to show the mother what to do, without making her feel self-concious, by gently stroking the baby's arm or leg and talking to him at the same time.

The single or separated mother is very vulnerable at this time. She may need to bring her own mother or other members of her family when she visits, or she may want the baby's father or current boyfriend to visit with her and support her; this should always be allowed. Grandparents and siblings should be greeted in the unit in the same way, and the support they give to parents recognised and appreciated. A few toys provided in the unit waiting room for siblings to play with, reassures the parents that children are really welcome, and not 'a nuisance', 'in the way', or 'noisy'.

Subsequent Management of Both Parents

The management of lactation in these parents is described in detail in Chapter 12. As the baby improves, the parents will depend on the nurses to show them the other caretaking activities they can perform for their baby. The nurse's role will become that of someone who befriends, teaches and guides, and allows both parents to feel fully involved in the care of their child. Whilst the baby is on the ventilator the parents can do many things such as:

(1) Soothing, stroking and comforting him when he cries (despite the fact that he is on a ventilator) after painful procedures such as blood-taking or oral suction.
(2) Helping the nurse to make him comfortable, change his nappy, put on his bootees, and smooth or help to change his sheets; they are usually happier to leave his hat to the nursing staff, since they are often afraid of dislodging the endotracheal tube or the nasogastric tube.
(3) Tube feeding their baby, if possible with mother's own expressed milk. Once shown how, not only are mothers safe to do this, but they are eager to do so; they soon learn at what time their baby is fed, and appear on the NNU at the appropriate minute.
(4) Washing their baby with water or moisturising antiseptic cream.
(5) Buying their baby a small soft toy to sit in his incubator; this

acts more as a morale booster for mother and the nurses.

(6) Doing their baby's mouth toilet.

(7) Knitting hats, bootees and other items of clothing for the baby.

When the baby is off the ventilator, but still requires oxygen, all the above things can be done, but now the mother, under supervision, can hold her baby. An oxygen mask is placed so that oxygen blows around the baby's face. At first the baby may be out of the incubator for only a few minutes while the sheet is changed, but gradually the time out of the incubator can be increased. A useful aid at this point is the PR10 Apnoea Monitor (Graseby Electronics Ltd.), which is small and moves with the baby, and therefore allows respiration to be monitored even when the baby is in mother's arms.

With a little practice parents learn to hold a baby attached to an apnoea monitor, cardiac monitor, $Tcp0_2$ monitor and an intravenous drip or even an umbilical artery catheter. In this situation they should sit as close to the incubator as possible, and the nurse should place the baby in the parent's arms, ensuring that none of the intravenous lines or monitoring equipment becomes disturbed.

Holding the baby for the first time is one of the most important steps for the parents. Comments such as 'I can't feel him' from mothers holding these very low birthweight babies should be received sympathetically, and they should be reassured that he will soon feel like a normal weighty cuddly baby. For the baby still nursed in an incubator but out of oxygen, mother can get him out of the incubator herself and hold him for a long period of time, and change his sheets as well as do all the things described above. Once the baby is in a cot he will be well enough for the parents to bath him, and they can also help to weigh him. They should be encouraged to provide normal baby clothes, not only to keep him warm, but to make him look like a real baby; special premature size clothing can be obtained (Dollycare; Crosby). Involvement with feeding continues at all stages (see Chapter 12) and the parents should share their involvement with grandparents and their other children.

It is always important that the parents and not the nurses are seen to do first-time things such as the first cuddle. This prevents parents developing feelings of jealousy towards nurses or feeling that the baby is responding more to the nurse than to themselves. When a mother comments that her baby seems to respond more to the nurses she needs reassurance that she – the mother – is the person who loves him, never pricks or hurts him and that she touches him in a different way which he recognises.

Parents of Infants in Long-term Intensive Care

These babies and their parents require a lot more time and help. The nurse's role is particularly important, and is mainly supportive, helping to keep a loving contact between the parents and their baby over long and difficult weeks. The nurse should always be as positive as possible in her attitudes, helping the parents to feel that their baby is special. Parents may tend to withdraw from the situation, but should be encouraged to visit and be with their baby as much as possible.

When such parents are at home, the telephone becomes their extra link, and they should be free to call at any time, several times a day if they want to. First thing in the morning and last thing at night are favourite times. Many parents will think that constant phone calls are a bother unless they are specifically told that they are welcomed by the NNU staff. Some parents may wish to stay in the hospital all day; a sitting room with facilities for them to make snacks should therefore be available on all NNUs.

Care of the Terminally Ill Child

This can be emotionally demanding and draining. Not all nurses are able to cope with this situation but all should understand the effects of grief and the mourning process. It is important to identify those nurses who find this type of work difficult, whilst, at the same time, not putting an unbearable burden on those who have a particular skill in terminal care, by always using them for this task. The nurses should always have a senior person to turn to if they find the strain of terminal care too much. Open discussion between them and the medical staff will identify problems in this area, such as ethical issues, so that in-service training can be given as necessary.

There are practical aspects to terminal care which should always be considered. Are the chairs comfortable for the nurses and parents to sit in and cuddle the baby? A rocking chair is very soothing. Is there an area which can be screened so that nurses and parents can hide their tears? Are the chaplain and social worker supportive? Is there a special viewing cot in the mortuary? Always offer to arrange for the baby to be christened or to arrange a similar religious observance which can be a great comfort to the parents and nurses at these times. Parents who want to stay with their dying baby can use the unit mother-and-baby room. Nurses should also be able to give correct information on registering the death and on burial and cremation (see Chapter 14).

The Congenitally Abnormal Child

When a child is born with a congenital abnormality, the role of the nurse is that of supporter, comforter, listener and source of information (see also Chapter 13). Maintaining contact between the parents and their baby is essential. Congenitally malformed infants should not be taken away and hidden in the neonatal unit, never to be seen again. Facing up to what is wrong with the baby is best done immediately, not several hours later when the parents have wondered, worried and hoped during the agonising intervening hours before they are told the worst.

Babies with Spina Bifida

These babies rarely have respiratory problems and can be shown to the parents in the labour ward, allowing them to have some time with their baby who will probably need to be admitted to the NNU for assessment. As in other situations the father should be invited to come to the unit with the baby, though he may prefer to wait with his wife.

Parents of infants with open spina bifida for whom no immediate surgical intervention is planned may need a few days to decide whether they will take their baby home. In our experience, most parents, after a week or so, elect to do so. This decision is, nevertheless, very difficult for parents, and they should never be rushed or pressurised, just encouraged to visit frequently and to be as involved in feeding and caring for their baby as other parents. If the parents do take the baby home, the community staff need to be involved in the shared care of the baby and in the support of the parents, and should therefore meet them prior to discharge.

Babies Born with Down's Syndrome

These babies, unless they are ill, should not be separated from their parents, and should stay with the mother on the postnatal ward (Chapter 13). When to tell them the diagnosis should be decided on an individual basis and should usually be done by the paediatrician before the baby leaves the maternity hospital.

Babies with Other Malformations

If the baby's medical condition allows it, he should always stay with the parents on the postnatal ward, though babies likely to require urgent surgery or needing added oxygen will need to be in the NNU. The same sort of support as that given to the parents of infants with spina bifida is appropriate, and in addition the nurse should be aware of the voluntary organisations available for many types of handicap, and in addition should know the names of the local representatives.

9 THE ROLE OF SOCIAL WORKERS IN THE NEONATAL INTENSIVE CARE UNIT – VIEWS OF A NEONATOLOGIST

Sheldon B. Korones

Total intensive care of sick neonates requires a major commitment from physicians, nurses and social workers whose respective activities aim to satisfy the broadly based needs of infants and their families. The importance of physicians who are appropriately trained for neonatal intensive care has never been difficult to propagate, even if one is occasionally not convinced of it. In the case of nurses, a change from the role of physician's handmaiden to the physician's colleague began in the late sixties. However, appreciation of the important role that can be played by social workers has yet to become general, judging from the large number of neonatal intensive care units (NNICUs) that have too few or none on their full-time staff.

Protracted intensive care has meant survival of an increased number of very small infants and has, in turn, imposed severe stresses on their parents. The need for social and emotional support for parents is an essential part of total neonatal care. Temperamentally and professionally, no one is better equipped for this task than the neonatal (or perinatal) social worker.

Should not physicians be the primary source of emotional support? In years past the physician's responsibilities and activities on behalf of patients were total, but the only contemporary expressions of this historic role in the United States are family practitioners and general paediatricians. An inverse relationship between the degree of specialisation and the capacity for ongoing emotional support of patients has developed. Depersonalisation of medical care during the past decades has been largely due to the increasing use of technology and scientific knowledge and a degree of specialisation that has become narrower and deeper as a consequence. Neonatologists are subject to this process, and preoccupation with the physiological condition of their patients may preclude the thoughtful, expert and time-consuming effort that is inherent to emotional support of parents. This does not exonerate neonatologists of a need for compassion, nor an obligation to communicate openly and sincerely with parents. However, it does exclude them from the protracted periods of time that must be devoted to psychosocial needs of parents.

If physicians cannot provide the necessary parental support, why cannot this be done by nurses? Exceptions notwithstanding, the nurse in the intensive care unit is not a social worker, either by education or by commitment to the task that confronts her. Assuredly, there is an orientation to social work in all of us – physicians and nurses alike. This is one of several personal attributes that significantly influence us in the choice of a career in neonatal intensive care. But beyond this consideration, we are plainly inadequate for the psychosocial task. In contrast to medical and nursing staff, the social worker is free to communicate, contact and mingle with parents beyond the bedside – in the office, in the follow-up clinic, during home visits and during frequent phone conversations. Furthermore, social worker training is steeped in psychosocial matters, and their effectiveness in this area is enhanced with accumulating experience.

The roles of physicians, nurses and social workers often overlap. However, we consider these overlaps to be an advantage rather than a difficulty since separate disciplines, utilising their primary responsibilities as a focal point of parental contact, reinforce each other in the total effort. The social worker is primarily responsible for co-ordination of the psychosocial care, whereas nurses, who are often the first to encounter parents, brief them about the medical situation, assess their reactions, attempt to comprehend their attitudes and support them during those stressful moments. They function similarly during subsequent visits and vigils, and one can see that during these encounters they have roles that commonly accrue to physicians or social workers. Physicians also play multiple roles. They dwell upon explanations of physiological disorders and on predictions of outcome, but their effectiveness would be very limited if they avoided all emotional and social issues.

The psychosocial concerns of physicians and nurses should tend to reinforce the social worker's principal commitment, and the latter's concern with medical matters is reciprocally constructive. In our unit, therefore, social workers require sufficient knowledge of medical events to relate them to psychosocial difficulties. For example, explanations of medical difficulties by physicians and nurses are often so replete with scientific terms that parental understanding is limited, but the social workers can reduce confusion by offering subsequent explanations that are more easily understood. Parents are less restrained and self-conscious in the presence of a social worker; they more readily acknowledge confusion and ask more questions. The social worker is also an intermediary, relaying to the physician the parental anxieties that arise from a technical explanation of their infant's condition.

These reflections are an attempt to convince those who are sceptical, and to reinforce those who are already convinced, of the need for a special role for social work in neonatal intensive care units.

Development of Social Worker Involvement in Neonatal Care

The urgent need to alleviate emotional crises imposed upon parents by severe illness of their newborn infants became apparent very early in the history of neonatal intensive care. The first social work programmes, for the specific purpose of parental support, were established almost simultaneously, though independently, in the middle 1960s by Ruth Breslin at Yale University, Rose Grobstein at Stanford University and Jean Washington at the University of Colorado, and they demonstrated a need and an effective response to it. Their programmes flourished as a direct consequence of vigorous personal effort.

Our programme in Memphis started in 1968 without knowledge of the previous activities elsewhere. We acquired our first two social workers in 1970, and soon thereafter expanded to our present staff of six individuals. My recognition of the need for social work originated in preceding years of private paediatric practice. In that setting, the paediatrician is a friend who is available to discuss all aspects of childhood care. After several months of fruitless effort, it became obvious that the nature of intensive newborn care and the size of our unit precluded a similar approach. Our social work programme was naively motivated by a simple desire to provide skilful friends for troubled parents of sick neonates.

The Memphis Programme

The Medical Scene

The Newborn Center is probably the largest single neonatal intensive care unit in the United States. It is located in the E. H. Crump Women's Hospital and Perinatal Center, occupying an entire floor of 26,000 sq. ft in this seven-storey building (Figure 9.1). Space for infant care is comprised of a large room of 6,600 sq. ft (Figure 9.2) in which 60 babies can be housed for maximal and intermediate care. An adjacent room of 1,000 sq. ft accommodates 20 additional infants for minimal care. The

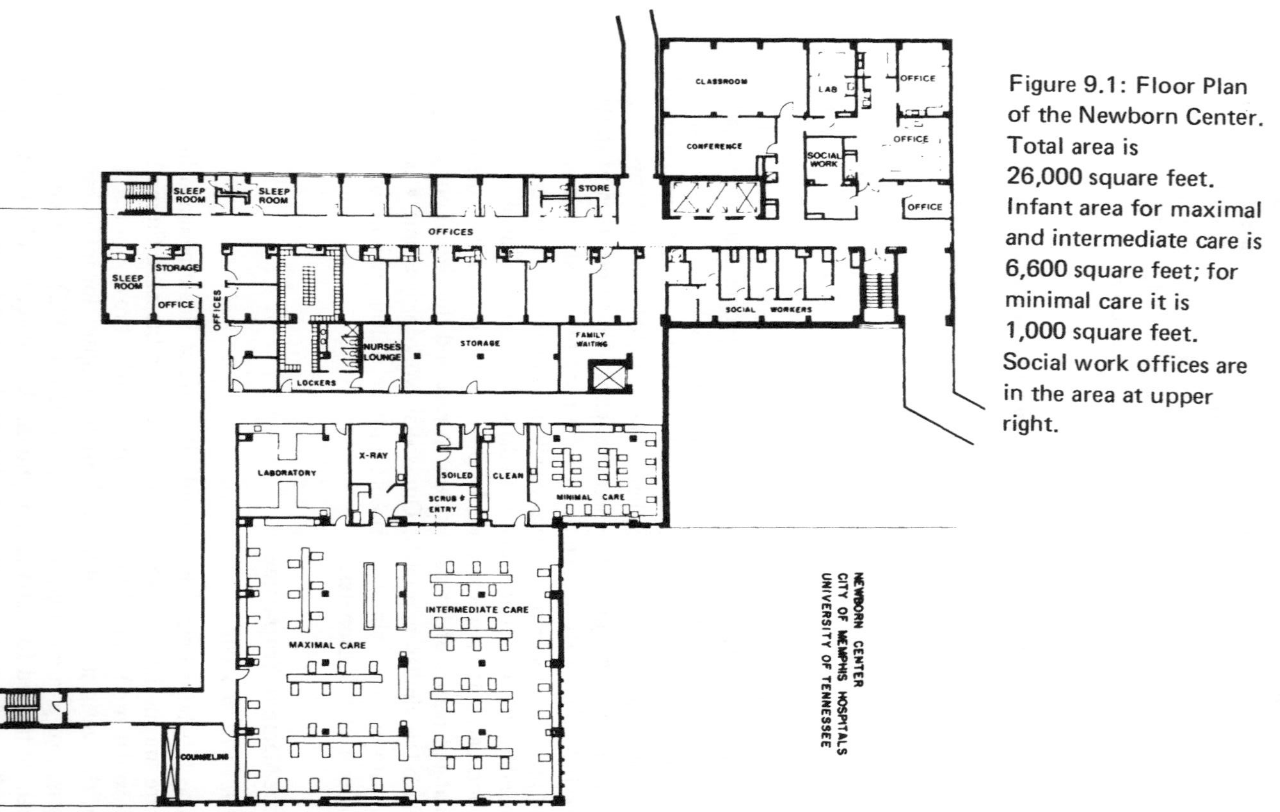

Figure 9.1: Floor Plan of the Newborn Center. Total area is 26,000 square feet. Infant area for maximal and intermediate care is 6,600 square feet; for minimal care it is 1,000 square feet. Social work offices are in the area at upper right.

Figure 9.2: View of a Portion of the Infant Area for Maximal and Intermediate care. One half of this 6,600 square foot room is visible in the picture.

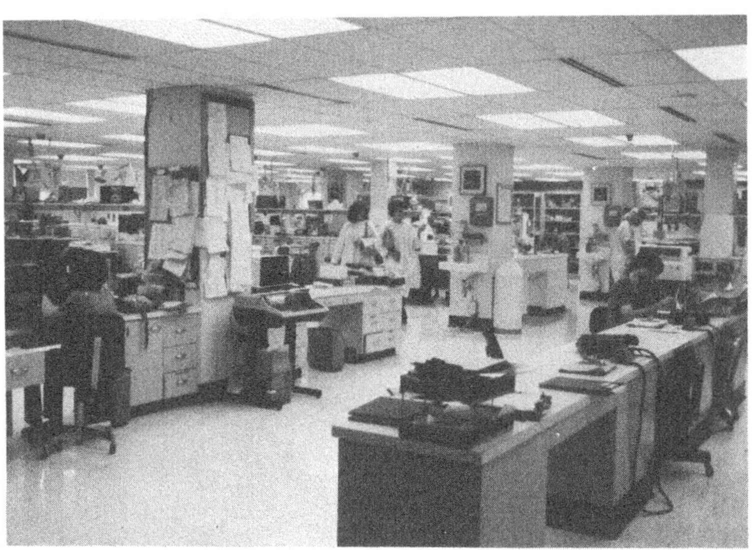

Well Baby Nursery is situated one floor below the Newborn Center. Its daily census ranges from 70 to 110 babies.

Individual offices for the six social workers and the social work secretary is provided on the same floor as the Newborn Center. The presence of all the staff close to the NNU assures frequent informal as well as formal interdisciplinary contacts. Furthermore, the social workers with ready access to the infants in the nursery are not visitors, they are a fixed part of the scene – no less than nurses, physicians or laboratory technicians.

Over 1,200 infants are admitted annually; approximately 250 of them are transferred in our newborn transport van (Figure 9.3) from hospitals situated within 150 miles of Memphis. Many families are of low socio-economic status. The overall incidence of low birthweight is 15 per cent among the babies born in our hospital. Emergencies are common and recurrent. The environment can best be described as one of ordered chaos.

Figure 9.3: Newborn Transport Van is Equipped for all Functions that Transpire in the Nursery Itself. Thirty feet long, it contains two radiant warmers and other devices identical to those in the intensive care nursery.

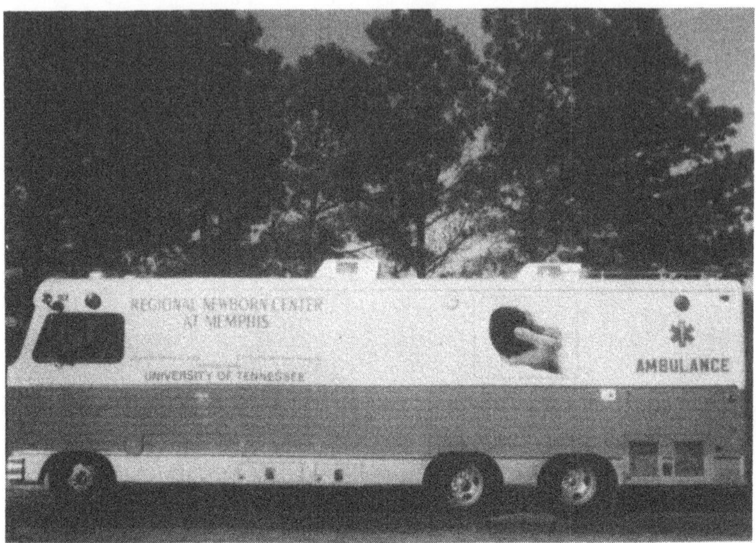

The Social Work Component

Administrative Relationships and Patient Assignments. The six social workers, including their supervisor, work full-time in our NNU. They maintain effective liaison with other hospital social workers, but a clear administrative independence is maintained. Their salaries are provided by the Newborn Center and they are responsible to its director, but matters intrinsic to the social work section are the responsibility of its supervisor. Generally, the director of the Newborn Center restricts administrative decisions to issues that concern the entire facility, particularly as these relate to interdisciplinary relationships.

Patient relationships and their management are the sole concern of the social workers. They make at least one initial contact with every patient admitted to the unit. Files are formally opened on a fraction of all admissions, according to priorities based upon the infant's medical disorder. For example, an attempt is made to follow every infant whose birthweight is less than 1.50 kg. Families are then followed after discharge from the nursery, until the infant's first birthday. Post-discharge contacts largely take place in our Follow-up Clinic, and to some extent during home visits. This system cannot provide in-depth social service to all 1,200 families whose babies are admitted to NNU. Since psychosocial problems pervade the population, we reason that severity of illness distinguishes those families who are most in need of long-term support and priorities are established accordingly. Although social work involvement is not dependent on physical referrals, these occur frequently for families who did not have a file opened after their original contact with the social worker.

Acquisition of Medical Knowledge. The scope of the responsibility of the social workers for their clients is wide. In most instances, psychosocial difficulties are firmly related to the event that threatens an infant's life. The multiple ramifications of the former are within the special expertise of the social workers. However, we have also emphasised the need for familiarity with medical concepts and terminology. In-service sessions have provided an excellent introduction. Fortunately, the turnover of social workers is negligible and repetition of courses has been infrequent. Constant intermingling with physicians and nurses is probably the most important way of learning. The presence of a social worker on each of two teams of physicians during daily teaching rounds has increased the understanding of medical concepts. Recognising the importance of medical knowledge for perinatal social work, the Tennessee Perinatal Care System, sponsored by the State of Tennessee, has published 'Educational Objectives in Medicine for Perinatal Social Workers' (see appendix to this chapter), which sets out to describe the medical information that a perinatal social worker should acquire.

Service to Parents. In essence, the social worker is a compassionate activist. The list of his functions is lengthy and the scope of non-medical support is broad. The social worker is a parent advocate to the nursery staff, an interpreter of medical jargon and concepts to parents, a procurer of tangible necessities for parents, a co-ordinator of the staff's efforts at emotional support, a counsellor in all forms of grief, a source of information on available community facilities, a facilitator of conferences, an arranger of post-discharge follow-up, an adviser on financial problems, and a vocal conscience in the ethical dilemmas that characteristically recur during neonatal intensive care.

Crisis support is provided during hospitalisation and the parents are repeatedly advised of the anticipated schedule of treatment and ultimate discharge. Help with transport is provided in an effort to encourage frequent visiting. We offer a toll-free telephone line for calls from out-of-town families. In cases of imminent death, the social worker's advice on parental attitudes is essential for appropriate management. The freedom with which parents converse with social workers is an immense advantage in informing us about individual fears of and attitudes toward the death process.

Crises that are associated with the infant's hospitalisation are often demanding. An extreme example of a mother comes to mind, who though innocent, was accused of shooting her former husband. Her social worker arranged for free legal counsel. An enormous number of anecdotes that illustrate diversity of function could be recorded, but they would be more entertaining than instructive. The point to emphasise is that the task is very broad, and we believe that no one but a neonatal social worker could provide this type of service to the parents.

Our follow-up process would suffer seriously without co-ordination by social workers. The system that provides medical attention to the poor is complex and often incomprehensible to those for whom it was designed. Return visits to our clinic are easily arranged. However, many of our infants require simultaneous attention in several clinics besides our own, such as neurology, neurosurgery, pulmonary medicine, cardiology, or gastroenterology. Assistance to parents often involves the making of appointments and going with them to the clinic, particularly in an emergency. The social worker interprets, advises and supervises compliance with physicians' instructions.

Staff-directed Functions. Of the three disciplines that provide neonatal care, social work is the only one which also directly serves the nursery staff. The most frequent contacts are with nurses. With depth of knowledge and adeptness at counselling, the social worker is effective in calming frustrations which may arise when a nurse is angry at neglectful or unconcerned parental attitudes, or is uncomfortable or disturbed about the ethics of a decision to continue or end treatment of a baby. Similarly, the problems of physician trainees are often brought to the social worker's attention. The ethical rationale of decisions, unacceptable parental attitudes and controversies with nurses are probably the most frequent problems.

Conclusions

Neonatal intensive care is an interdisciplinary effort that must involve physicians, nurses and social workers. Assignment of a token, part-time social worker to the intensive care nursery is self-defeating. The care of parents during and after their infant's hospitalisation is a full-time job. Although the contributions of nurses and physicians are essential, continuous support also requires a commitment that is precluded by their schedules. Parental support requires the expertise of individuals who are educated to understand the emotional ramifications of perinatal crises and are otherwise unencumbered with medical responsibilities. Their education, temperamental inclination and eagerness to expend vigorous efforts, singularly qualify social workers to provide the psychosocial support that many parents are forced to depend upon. Neonatal (perinatal) social work relates biological disorders to parental psychosocial stress; this is the core of its unique expertise. As such, it is indispensable to the totality of neonatal intensive care.

APPENDIX

To provide a training programme for the social workers employed in the way outlined in the preceding chapter, a task force of social workers in the Regional Perinatal Centers in Tennessee produced these 'Educational Objectives in Medicine for Perinatal Social Workers'. We felt that they give the best outline we have seen of the core of knowledge which should be acquired by all non-medical personnel involved in the care of both sick and healthy newborn babies and their families. We have therefore reproduced it in its entirety.

Educational Objectives in Medicine for Perinatal Social Workers

Introduction

The unique medical and psychosocial problems of the high-risk mother and baby require a rapidly expanding technology and specialised expertise among all disciplines in the perinatal setting. The psychosocial and emotional costs that are intrinsic to the high-risk mother and her family are complicated further by the recent technical advances in our setting. Thus, the social worker must acquire special knowlege in order to assist these families.

The demands of social work practice in a Level III Perinatal Center require special training beyond the basic knowlege and skills of social work.

Areas of essential knowledge include:

A. Prenatal care and nutritional requirements during pregnancy.
B. Course of pregnancy, including high-risk factors, complications and fetal demise.
C. Care of newborns, including high-risk infants.
D. Continuation of care of mother and infant through the first year of life.
E. Knowledge of medical setting, environmental and familial factors affecting parent-child relationships.
F. Appropriate and maladaptive responses to situations occurring in the Level III Perinatal Center.

Areas of essential skills include:

A. Assessment and evaluation of the patient's adaptation to the pregnancy, including high-risk pregnancy.
B. Assessment and evaluation of the patient's family and/or significant others in relation to the patient's pregnancy.
C. Interpretation and clarification of physiological, psychosocial, nutritional, and medical issues during the course of pregnancy and post-partum care.
D. Interpretation and clarification of physiological, psychosocial, nutritional

and medical issues due to the birth of the high-risk infant; evaluation of the parental relationship with the infant to encourage attachment and healthy interaction.

E. Assessment of the family network regarding the understanding of, and adaptation to, the high-risk infant's condition.

F. Supportive services to families, including crisis intervention, therapeutic counselling, patient advocacy in the health care system and special resource identification/utilisation.

I. Pregnancy

A. Rationale. From a psychosocial point of view, pregnancy has been defined as a developmental crisis. There are obvious physiological changes taking place which are accompanied by psychological adjustments. A basic understanding of these adjustments and the stresses that affect pregnancy is essential for assessment of the maternal response and that of her family as well.

B. Terminal Objectives. The social worker will be able to describe the physical and psychological stages of pregnancy, evaluate the familial stresses that have significant impact on pregnancy, and identify unusual or abnormal reactions to pregnancy.

C. Behavioural Objectives. Upon completion of this unit, the social worker will be able to:

(1) Define the following terms and effectively explain their meaning to parents:
   a. Gravida
   b. Para
   c. Gestational age
   d. Rho GAM
   e. Amniotic fluid
   f. Placenta
   g. Trimester
   h. Bag of water
   i. Urinalysis
   j. Gestational diabetes
   k. Caesarean section
   l. Anaemia
   m. Fundal height
   n. Bed rest
   o. Fetus
   p. Uterus
   q. Cervix
   r. Braxton-Hicks contractions.

(2) Outline the physiological changes in the mother and the fetus during each trimester of pregnancy.

(3) Describe the three stages of psychological and emotional adjustment to pregnancy experienced by both the mother and the father.

(4) List unusual pressures or stresses in family circumstances which may

affect the mother's perception of the infant and her ability to relate to the infant.

(5) List changes in role and lifestyle as a result of pregnancy.
(6) List symptoms of a poor adjustment to pregnancy.
(7) Describe typical behaviours indicating planning and preparation for the coming infant.
(8) List available birth control methods and discuss the advantages and disadvantages of each.
(9) List community resources available to the pregnant woman.
(10) Describe the physiological and emotional changes experienced by the post-partum mother.
(11) Describe the various types of labour/delivery and anaesthetics in current use.

II. The High-risk Pregnancy

A. Rationale. The high-risk pregnancy contributes additional anxieties to the already existing stresses of pregnancy. In addition to medical treatment required for the mother, special considerations are pertinent if both parent(s) are to adapt optimally to the high-risk pregnancy.

B. Terminal Objectives. The social worker will be able to recognise the emotional impact of a complicated pregnancy and be able to provide services to the parents.

C. Behavioural Objectives. Upon completion of this unit, the social worker will be able to:

(1) Define the following terms and explain their meaning in simple terms to parents:
   a. Hypertension
   b. Eclampsia
   c. Pre-eclampsia, toxemia, and pregnancy-induced hypertension
   d. Gestational diabetes/diabetes
   e. Placenta previa
   f. Abruptio placenta
   g. Ultrasound
   h. Amniocentesis/genetic amniocentesis
   i. Fetal monitoring
   j. Proteinuria
   k. Sickle cell trait/anaemia
   l. Erythroblastosis
   m. Oxytocin challenge test
   n. L/S ratio
   o. Intrauterine growth retardation (IUGR)
   p. Fetal demise
   q. Premature rupture of membranes (PROM)
   r. Incompetent cervix
(2) Define in lay terms the evaluative medical techniques used in the management of the pregnancy.
(3) Identify environmental factors that contribute to high-risk pregnancy.

(4) List special needs of the mother requiring long-term hospitalisation.
(5) Discuss the effect of high-risk pregnancy on the parents' self-perceptions.
(6) Define the elements of anticipatory grief and their purpose.
(7) Discuss adolescent development in relation to teenage pregnancy.
(8) List community resources available to the high-risk pregnant woman.
(9) Describe the physiological and emotional changes experienced by the high-risk post-partum mother.
(10) Describe the effect of a Caesarean section on the mother's body image and self-perception.
(11) Discuss the effects of substance abuse on pregnancy outcome.
(12) Describe the course of complicated labour/delivery and anaesthetics currently in use.

III. The High-risk Newborn

A. Rationale. An important function of the social worker in the Level III Newborn Intensive Care Unit (NICU) is liaison between parent and medical personnel. A clear understanding of the disease and treatment of diseases of the newborn is essential in fulfilling this role.

B. Terminal Objectives. The social worker will be able to interpret accurately, to reinforce medical information given to the parents by the medical staff, and to assess the family's understanding of the infant's condition.

C. Behavioural Objectives. Upon completion of this unit, the social worker will be able to:

(1) Define gestational age in relation to the high-risk infant.
(2) Identify physical characteristics of pre-term infants at varying gestational ages.
(3) Define the terms SGA, AGA and LGA and relate them to immediate medical/psychosocial expectations.
(4) Define the following terms and explain their meaning to parents:
    a. Apgar/Dubowitz scores
    b. Cold stress
    c. Pneumothorax/pneumomediastinum/interstitial emphesema
    d. Hyaline membrane disease/respiratory distress syndrome/respiratory insufficiency of prematurity
    e. Retained fetal lung fluid
    f. Meconium/meconium staining/meconium aspiration
    g. Congenital pneumonia/bronchopulmonary dysplasia
    h. Cerebral edema
    i. Seizures
    j. Intracranial haemorrhage/intraventricular haemorrhage
    k. Hydrocephalus
    l. Rh and ABO incompatability
    m. Jaundice/polycythemia/anaemia/kernicterus/thrombocytopenia
    n. Erb's palsy
    o. Bacterial and viral infections
    p. Sepsis

q. Meningitis
r. Necrotising enterocolitis
s. Hypoglycaemia/Hyperglycaemia
t. Congenital heart disease
u. Patent ductus arteriosus

(5) Explain in layman's terms the function of the following:
a. Respirator
b. Continuous positive airway pressure (CPAP)
c. Pancuronium
d. Digitalis
e. Chloral hydrate
f. Exchange transfusion
g. Apnoea and heart rate monitor
h. Hematocrit
i. Diuretic
j. Intravenous fluid
k. Phototherapy
l. Nasogastric feedings
m. Endotrachial tube
n. Umbilical artery catheter
o. Computerised Axial Tomography (CAT) Scan
p. Theophylline/caffeine
q. Ventricular-peritoneal shunt
r. Radiant warmer bed/incubator
s. Transcutaneous oxygen monitor
t. Sector scanner

(6) List developmental, medical and nutritional milestones necessary to case management in a NICU and be able to interpret them in layman's terms.
(7) Define the specific elements of the social work role as an integral part of the multidisciplinary team.
(8) List community resources available to the family of the high-risk infant.

IV. The Parent-infant Relationship

A. Rationale. Assessment of the parent-infant relationship is an important social work function in a non-risk or a high-risk situation. The incidence of abuse and neglect is increased in the medically high-risk population of infants. The need for specialised care at birth can threaten the parent-infant relationship in that the parent's ability to relate to the baby can be seriously affected.

B. Terminal Objectives. The social worker will be able to differentiate healthy and unhealthy parent-child relationships, and support/enhance development of more positive relationships.

C. Behavioural Objectives. Upon completion of this unit, the social worker will be able to:

(1) Describe the common parental reactions to the birth of an infant.
(2) Describe the common parental reactions to a neonate.
(3) Identify the stages of grief.

(4) Describe the effect of grieving on the parents' ability to relate to the infant and the hospital staff.
(5) Identify observable attachment behaviours.
(6) Define what is meant by an attitude of 'optimistic realism' in working with parents.
(7) Identify obstacles in the hospital setting that interfere with the parent-child interaction and discuss ways to minimise them.
(8) Discuss the effect of past losses and other experiences on parents' ability to relate to the infant.
(9) Identify and list family support systems and community support systems.
(10) Discuss patterns of visitation and calling the nursery in relation to parent-child relationships.
(11) List factors that can affect visiting or calling by the family network.
(12) List family dynamics that indicate the parent may have problems relating to the child.
(13) List factors indicating that the situation is beyond the parent's ability to cope, thus necessitating referral to Protective Services and/or other appropriate resources.

V. Infants with Handicapping Conditions

A. Rationale. An infant with handicaps, whether mild or severe, can devastate a family. Often these children are the targets of neglect. Nonetheless, with appropriate management, a positive nurturing relationship can be established.

B. Terminal Objectives. The social worker can help facilitate interaction between the family and infant and apply the knowledge of parent-infant relationships to this high-risk situation.

C. Behavioural Objectives. Upon completion of this unit, the social worker will be able to:

(1) Characterise the grief process in various situations encountered in the perinatal setting.
(2) Explain the significance of early contact between parent and infant and family involvement.
(3) Describe theories of parent-infant attachment as they relate to the handicapped infant.
(4) Describe the characteristics of chronic sorrow.
(5) Identify developmental milestones and potential crisis stages for families with handicapped children in helping them to set realistic goals.
(6) Compile a list of appropriate follow-up resources for families with handicapped children.
(7) Define in layman's terms the following handicapping conditions:
    a. Hydrocephalus
    b. Down's Syndrome
    c. Cleft lip and palate
    d. Spina bifida
    e. Retrolental fibroplasia
    f. Cerebral palsy

g. Microcephaly
h. Failure to thrive
i. Fetal alcohol syndrome
j. Congenital heart disease

VI. Follow-up of the High-risk Infant

A. Rationale. Release from the hospital can present a new crisis and increased anxiety for the parents as caretakers. Once the baby is home, parents should know that the social worker is available for support, advice and referral to appropriate resources.

B. Terminal Objectives. The social worker will be able to assess the family's ability to cope with a high-risk infant at home, recognise appropriate or inappropriate development in the infant, and be familiar with community resources.

C. Behavioural Objectives. Upon completion of this unit, the social worker will be able to:

(1) Discuss parents' need to be prepared for the baby's discharge after a lengthy hospitalisation, and make arrangements for such preparation in the nursery.
(2) Outline gross motor development during the first year of an infant's life.
(3) Adjust developmental expectations for a premature infant according to gestational age.
(4) Recognise patterns of maladaptive parenting.
(5) Discuss ongoing reassessment of the mother-child relationship to identify inappropriate maternal responses.
(6) Discuss the role of the social worker in co-ordination of all follow-up in relation to medical and psychosocial needs.
(7) List causes of failure to comply with medical recommendations.
(8) List available community follow-up resources.

VII. Death of an Infant

A. Rationale. Traditional views hold that parents need not grieve a perinatal death, reasoning that there has been insufficient time for attachment. Actually, suppression of grief can prolong the grieving period, affect the parents' ability to function adequately, and thus interfere with all relationships including those relationships with children at home or with infants yet to be born.

B. Terminal Objectives. The social worker can encourage a healthy expression of grief, inform parents of anticipated symptoms of grief for the infant, and recognise pathological grief symptoms.

C. Behavioural Objectives. Upon completion of this unit, the social worker will be able to:

(1) Define the psychological purposes of grieving.
(2) List the stages of the grief process.
(3) Discuss the uniqueness of a perinatal death in contrast to other deaths.

(4) Discuss ways to initiate a positive grief response by the family in the nursery.
(5) List typical physical and psychological responses of the family to perinatal death.
(6) List signs of pathological grief in a family following perinatal death.
(7) Discuss the social work role in relation to staff's responses to perinatal death.
(8) Discuss parental reactions to funeral arrangements/hospital disposal and/or autopsy of their deceased infant.
(9) Discuss major obstacles within the hospital setting and/or presented by hospital staff that may impede the grief process.

10 MANAGEMENT OF FAMILY PROBLEMS ARISING IN REFERRAL UNITS

Roberta Siegel, Edward Goldson, Perry M. Butterfield and L. Joseph Butterfield

Introduction

In order to address the medical and psychosocial needs of pre-term infants and their families, a Family Care Program has been developed at The Children's Hospital regional referral centre in Denver, Colorado. This chapter will discuss the approaches used to help both the parents and the perinatal health team in the care of outborn premature infants.

We have identified certain phases of the hospitalisation of a sick newborn that both he and his parents will experience. Each phase has its own issues and tasks that must be mastered if the parents are to resolve the crisis precipitated by the birth of their infant. These are:

(1) the stabilisation of the infant in the hospital and then the transport to the neonatal intensive care unit;
(2) adaptation to the intensive care environment and the acute period of the infant's hospitalisation;
(3) convalescence;
(4) discharge; and
(5) post-discharge adaptation.

These are not disjointed processes, but rather a continuum proceeding from sickness to health, during which a number of transitions take place and must be facilitated.

Stabilisation and Transport

At the time of transport and during the acute phase of the infant's hospitalisation, parents are experiencing anticipatory grieving or withdrawal from the relationship with the infant established during pregnancy, feelings of guilt and failure,[1,2] and grief over the loss of the expected, idealised child.[3] Both mother and father may independently focus on events that occurred during the pregnancy which they think may have been related to the premature birth and illness, events such as intercourse, smoking and work demands. While some parents place the responsibility on themselves, others may shift the blame onto others – their spouse, the extended family, nurses, the doctor, or God. Often both parents are concerned with the disappointment that they have caused each other.

The decision to transfer the infant to a regional intensive care unit in itself can initiate a grief reaction,[4] particularly if the events surrounding the labour, delivery and postpartum period have indicated to the parents that the chances for the intact survival of their infant are diminished. If this does occur, parents become involved in anticipatory grieving. For some parents, attaching to a critically ill infant may be too overwhelming and they may withdraw in an effort to protect themselves from their feelings of loss, disappointment and guilt.

All these feelings must be taken into account if stabilisation and transport is to be done successfully.[5] The sensitivity with which the family is handled by the medical team effecting the transport and the manner in which the process of transport is handled is crucial to the developing relationship between the parent(s) and the infant, and between the parent(s) and the hospital staff, since this may be the only contact the parent(s) has with the team during the time the parent(s) is separated from the infant. The management of this situation can significantly influence the dynamic process that is involved in attaching to and coping with a critically ill infant.[6]

During stabilisation and transport we have found that early communication with parents is essential. The statements made are critical because they influence parental perceptions of their infant's condition, which can linger in their minds and may help determine how parents relate to their infants. We have found it best to talk to parents together, and to give prompt, direct explanations in a calm manner. This helps to decrease their misconceptions and distortions, and helps to increase the communication and support between them. Not talking to the parents at this stage only increases their anxiety and adds to their growing fantasies.

Telling parents what measures are or will be done to assist the baby can be helpful and reassuring because this helps psychologically to orientate and organise the parents at a time when they are feeling very vulnerable and out of control. Although it is normal to be guarded, the medical team can comfortably tell the parents the known facts about the baby's condition and what treatment is being provided without making any prognostications about the future. It is extremely helpful and important to discuss with the parents at this time plans to feed their infant. In many situations, it will be possible for mothers to breast-feed a sick infant once he has recovered and, in the interim, for her to express her breast milk which can be frozen, transported and given to her own infant.

Before the infant is transferred, the transport team should give the parents an opportunity to see their infant. This facilitates attachment, decreases exaggerated fantasies, decreases withdrawal from the infant, and enhances parental ability to grasp the reality of the infant's condition, especially if the infant may die or there is likely to be a long period of time until the parents can visit the infant. Touching or holding can provide parents with an emotional experience that is sustaining and reassuring, and helps them through a critical period of separation. Mother and father may differ as to whether they wish to see the infant; their individual preferences should be respected and they should not be forced to see their infant.

To help familiarise and orientate parents to the regional centre, they should be given preparatory information and a description of the intensive care nursery. Providing parents with a booklet that includes basic information and illustrative pictures is extremely useful.

The estimated length of time of the transport should be given. The parents should be contacted after the infant has been admitted to the unit and evaluated, with a personal phone call from the nursery staff (physician, nurse or social worker) giving details about the infant and also an inquiry about their plans for visiting. Parents usually feel more comfortable when they have a specific name to relate to, and the staff can be better prepared to talk to parents when they know when they will arrive.

Adaptation to Intensive Care and the Acute Period

Following the infant's transport to the neonatal intensive care unit, parents have feelings of separation, loss and family disruption. Communication is essential for families that are separated by long distances; telephone communication plays a major role and a routine telephone calling schedule should be established. Sometimes the local or referring physician is asked to contact the family personally in order to supplement telephone communication.

Parents separated by distance can send family pictures, clothing, mobiles, simple toys and even cassette tapes so that the infant can hear their voices. Pictures of the infant can then periodically be sent to the parents. Mothers who are expressing their breasts can send frozen breast milk and even their breast pads to familiarise the infant with their scent.

We continually encourage parents living out of town to visit their infants, and if possible to stay nearby. Because finding accommodation and meals can be overwhelming for the parents at this time, we provide them with a list of inexpensive housing and restaurants located near the hospital. These houses have sleeping and eating facilities, and provide parents with a comfortable home-like atmosphere at a nominal charge. Natural support systems emerge from among the parents staying at these homes. Siblings are also encouraged to visit the infant and are given explanations at that time about their new brother or sister which are commensurate with their emotional and cognitive development.

Perinatal social workers are available to all families to assess and evaluate their psychosocial functioning and provide supportive counselling. The social workers assess the family's relationship to the infant as well as the social and psychological functioning of the family and their adaptation to the birth of the sick infant and subsequent hospitalisation. In addition, they co-ordinate the discharge planning and follow-up care for the infant's medical and developmental needs as well as for the family's emotional needs.

Our programme has developed the position of Family Care Co-ordinator, an experienced neonatal nurse who serves as a liaison between parents and hospital staff. She teaches well and special baby care, and in addition assists out-of-town parents in dealing with their financial and housing needs, provides emotional support to the families, screens the families psychosocially, and refers them to the social workers when necessary. She also participates in the discharge teaching and planning for patients in addition to teaching and assisting mothers with breast feeding and pumping.

Another valuable means of providing emotional support to these parents is the use of 'graduate parents'. These are parents who have had a baby in the intensive care unit and are selected because they have successfully dealt with the crisis of the birth of their sick infant. They provide support to parents by sharing common reactions, feelings and experiences about having a hospitalised infant. We can often locate a 'graduate parent' or couple in the same small or rural community as that in which the parents live. Graduate parents in Denver can also offer considerable practical help to parents who are visiting from out-of-town by offering friendship and personal hospitality. In addition they can visit selected infants whose parents are unable to visit frequently and initiate written correspondence with these parents.

The first visit to the Neonatal Intensive Care Unit is generally the most stressful, since the high technology and chaotic appearance of a high-risk nursery is a frightening experience to parents. The members of the nursery team should be available to welcome the parents, to explain the procedures and equipment, to review the infant's course, to answer questions and give emotional support. Since many parents are unable to express their concerns or even ask questions, the team must help them to do so. Facilitating the parents' relationship with the infant is essential, and can be done by offering them opportunities to touch, stroke, hold, feed, diaper, turn him and put lotion on him even if he is on the respirator. Pointing out some of the unique personal characteristics of the infant is important and helps parents better identify with, and relate to, their baby. Thereafter, regular conferences are held with the family and medical team to give constant medical information and emotional support. To expand this support, classes are offered and group counselling sessions are also made available. The intent of these sessions is to provide specific didactic information and to discuss the parents' concerns and experiences resulting from their infants' hospitalisation, and its effect on their family functioning. The sessions are conducted by a perinatal social worker and other members of the staff (e.g. physician, nurse, chaplain).

Convalescence

During the convalescent period the following goals should be accomplished:

(1) the establishment of convalescent or transitional care;
(2) teaching care-giving skills to the parent;
(3) teaching the parents about the infant's medical, social and developmental needs;
(4) facilitating the infant's highest level of behavioural and physiological organisation; and
(5) facilitating family reorganisation.

To help parents accomplish these goals we have taken two approaches. The first one involves the transfer of the infant to his hospital of birth, or a hospital closer to home in order to facilitate the emerging relationship between the parents and their infant. In such instances, the parents are informed of the impending transfer and a complete summary of the baby's hospital course is prepared for the receiving primary physician.

An alternative approach we have taken is to transfer to the Family Care Center,[7] an eight-bed transitional nursery at our hospital. This nursery is designed to create a less intensive milieu, where fewer invasive, diagnostic and monitoring procedures are used and where parents can initiate their care-giving role. They are encouraged by the medical and nursing staff to assume an increasing role in the infant's daily care, and definite tasks such as feeding, bathing and the administration of medications are assigned to them. Although the parents do not make the final decisions regarding care, they are nevertheless included in the decision-making process.

Child developmentalists, occupational and physical therapists evaluate the child and consult with the parents, alerting them to their infant's specific and general developmental needs. This, as well as the teaching provided by the medical staff, helps the parents develop their own sense of competence as caretakers, and achieve a greater understanding of their infant's distinctive qualities and needs.

Another issue that arises at this time is the parental adjustment to the hospitalisation, including family or marital disruption, and financial concerns which need to be addressed, evaluated and intervention provided when appropriate. Parents may exhibit a variety of negative behaviours including non-visitation, hostility toward the hospital staff, and reluctance to interact or participate in caretaking activities with the infant. The perinatal social worker, who is recognised as someone functioning outside the immediate medical care of the infant, is available to help parents deal with these feelings in addition to helping staff understand the parents' psychosocial functioning and their response to the infant's hospitalisation. In order to facilitate communication amongst the hospital staff, weekly meetings of the entire multidisciplinary team, on all the infants in the Family Care Center, are held during which time the psychosocial care plans are developed.

Discharge

Discharge presents another stressful yet exciting event for parents as they realise their responsibilities. This often exacerbates many of the fears and doubts they have experienced during the hospitalisation.

Appropriate discharge planning is therefore critical to give the parents a sense of competence in the care of their child as well as knowledge of what support systems are available in the community. Basic well-baby care activities are taught to the parents, together with any specialised techniques which may be required for their infants such as gastrostomy feeding, management of a tracheotomy, pumping a ventriculo-perinatal shunt, or the use of apnoea monitors. Basic cardio-respiratory resuscitation is also taught to many parents. Many families are also referred to the visiting nurse service for post-discharge follow-up, and if, at the time of discharge, the child demonstrates any physical or developmental problems he may also be referred directly to an appropriate agency.

Post-discharge

Maintaining contact with, and providing support for, parents after their infant has been discharged from the nursery is necessary. Feelings of relief and joy on going home from the hospital are clouded by feelings of loss and anxiety as the parents withdraw from the expertise and support of the hospital and its staff. Confidence which had been gained within the nursery quickly erodes when the baby continues to sleep through feedings, stiffens and rejects cuddling, vomits when handled and turns blue with a diaper change. It is common to see parents overfeed and over-stimulate the child, whereas other parents may withdraw from the infant and provide little interaction or stimulation. Parents of premature or small-for-gestational age babies report recurring anxieties throughout the first year. Their relationships with their infant, which they describe as 'difficult' or even 'stressful',[8-10] can actually be more detrimental to the development of their infant than the previous perinatal stress.[11-13] This may potentially account for the increased incidence of abuse and neglect among infants discharged from neonatal intensive care units.[14-16]

The hospital offers a programme of education counselling throughout the first year. Monthly visits are made to the home initially, and then the parents and the child come to the hospital developmental playroom. These visits are always followed by a letter which reiterates our observations and includes suggestions encouraging positive interaction between parent and child. A phone call to the parents is made a week later which ensures that we have a continuous contact with the family. This programme was initially conducted as a clinical research project.

Statistically significant differences in maternal confidence and in Bayley Mental Developmental scores have been demonstrated beween these families and a matched control group.[17]

A developmental follow-up clinic also monitors the development of the infants at 3, 9 and 15 months (corrected for gestational age) and at the time of their second birthday. The clinic is staffed by a developmental paediatrician, a paediatric psychologist, audiologist, speech pathologist, social worker and occupation and physical therapists, and provides assessment, diagnosis and recommendations for treatment.

Conclusion

This chapter has described a comprehensive programme designed to meet the medical and psychosocial needs of the outborn premature infant and his parents. It has identified the various phases of the infant's hospitalisation, the particular issues that arise and the interventions that have been developed to help parents and their infants with these problems. This is a broad-based, interdisciplinary programme that is initiated at the time the infant is referred to our intensive care centre and goes through the first two years of life. The Family Care Program has proven to be an effective means of providing support both to the parents and the infants who sustain a premature birth and require intensive care.

Acknowledgement

Supported in part by grants and contracts with the Colorado Department of Health, The March of Dimes Birth Defects Foundation, The American Lung Association of Colorado, The McArthur Family Foundation, an anonymous gift in the memory of Pauline Hoff Carey, and an anonymous gift.

References

1. Kaplan, D. M., and Mason, E. A. (1960). Maternal reactions to premature birth viewed as an acute emotional disorder. *Am. J. Orthopsychiatry*, *30*, 539.

2. Prugh, D. (1953). Emotional problems of the premature infant's parents. *Nurs. Outlook*, *1*, 461.

3. Solnit, A. J., and Stark, M. H. (1961). Mourning and the birth of a defective child. *Psychoanal. Study Child, 16,* 523.

4. Benfield, D. G., Leib, S. A., and Reuter, J. (1976). Grief response of parents after referral of the critically ill newborn to a regional center. *N. Engl. J. Med.*,

294, 975.

5. Siegel, R. (1983). A family-centred program of neonatal intensive care. *Health Soc. Wk.* (in press).

6. Siegel, R., Gardner, S., and Merenstein, G. (1983). Families in crisis: theoretical and practical considerations. In *Handbook of Neonatal Intensive Care*, G. Merenstein and S. Gardner (eds). St Louis, C. V. Mosby Co., to be published.

7. Goldson, E. (1981). The family care center: a model for the transitional care of the sick infant and his family. *Child. Today*, *10*, 15.

8. Broussard, E. R. (1979). Assessment of the adaptive potential of the mother-infant system: the neonatal perception inventory. *Seminars in Perinatology*, *3*, 91.

9. Brown, J. V., and Bakeman, R. (1979). Relationships of human mothers with their infants during the first year of life. In *Maternal Influences and Early Behavior*, R. W. Bell and W. P. Smotherman (eds). New York, Spectrum.

10. Field, T. (1981). Gaze behaviour in normal and high risk infants during early interactions. *J. Amer. Acad. Child Psych.*, *20*, 308.

11. Bell, R. (1979). Parent, child and reciprocal influences. *Amer. Psychologist*, *34*, 821.

12. Sameroff, A. J., and Chandler, M. J. (1975). Reproductive risk and the continuum of caretaking casualty. In *Review of Child Development Research, Vol. 4*, F. D. Horowitz, M. Hetherington, S. Scarr-Salaaptek and G. M. Siegel (eds). Chicago, University of Chicago Press.

13. Sander, L. W. (1975). Infant and the caretaking environment. In *Explorations in Child Psychiatry*, E. J. Anthony (ed.). New York, Plenum Press.

14. Klein, M., and Stern, L. (1971). Low birthweight and battered child syndrome. *Amer. J. Dis. Child.*, *122*, 15.

15. Elmer, E., and Gregg, G. S. (1967). Developmental characteristics of abused children. *Pediat.*, *40*, 596.

16. Goldson, E., Fitch, N. J., Wendall, T. A., and Knapp, G. (1978). Child abuse: its relationship to birthweight, Apgar score and developmental testing. *Amer. J. Dis. Child.*, *132*, 790.

17. Butterfield, P., Harmon, R., Miller, L., and Culp, A. (1982). How to read your baby. Abstract submitted to Developmental Psychology Research Group meeting, June 1982, Estes Park, Colorado.

11 PSYCHOLOGICAL AND PSYCHOTHERAPEUTIC SUPPORT OF STAFF AND PARENTS IN AN INTENSIVE CARE BABY UNIT

Helen Bender and Alison Swan-Parente

Introduction

The clinical work discussed in this chapter was undertaken in the neonatal intensive care unit of a London teaching hospital with a large regional catchment area. Liaison between the Department of Child Psychiatry and the Department of Paediatrics led to a child psychotherapist becoming attached to the unit. Thus parents and families had access to a psychotherapist, and at the same time a staff group was set up both to feed back relevant information to the staff and to give them support and a forum for discussing their own needs and difficulties.

Recognition of the emotional needs of both staff and parents on neonatal intensive care units has been growing. The work of, among others, Klaus and Kennell[1] in the USA and of Macfarlane[2] and Brimblecombe *et al.*[3] in the UK has emphasised the role of the neonatal period in the formation of the relationship between parents and their baby. There can be few postnatal environments less conducive to this process than a NNICU, which can be a strange, frightening, noisy and technologically formidable place. If, however the subtle and complicated two-way process of attachment[4] does not take place, the family may be at a serious psychological risk; thus, for example, several studies suggest that premature babies are over-represented in the population of children abused by their parents.[5]

We believe that a psychotherapist, by focusing on the internal, subjective world of parents, babies and staff, can help to alleviate the anxiety which often permeates a NNICU. We hope that he or she can partly unravel the complex psychological processes which inhibit (a) unit policies intended to alleviate stress, (b) optimal functioning by the staff and (c) attachment between parents and babies, and that the staff can be helped to reinstate parents in their parental role. It is perhaps helpful to both parents and staff to be able to air important emotional issues with a member of the team who is non-medical and therefore not involved with the specialised life-saving work of the unit.

Working with Parents

The parents of pre-term babies often experience emotional states such as anxiety, shock, numbness and agoraphobia which seem to be pathological, but can be looked on as the normal reaction to a traumatic event. These parents are also often 'at risk', however, because a higher proportion of them than in the general population come from lower socio-economic groups and they have suffered deprivations which may have contributed towards their infant's prematurity. When they are additionally emotionally deprived by this crisis they often need and benefit from psychotherapeutic intervention.

We feel that the important contributions of this type of intervention are:

(1) *Observation*. Brazelton[6] maintains that sharing the observable behaviour and reactions of a baby with the parents can become a powerful technique enabling a professional to establish an early working relationship with the family. Psychoanalysts have emphasised the value of attentive observation and reflection as a healing process in itself.

(2) *Assimilation*. The whole experience of childbirth, which culminates in a baby's admission to the NNICU, may remain confused, unresolved and unassimilated in the parents' minds. This needs to be carefully talked over and 'integrated' before the parents can move on and attend to the new demands of being parents. These 'undigested' experiences then become more bearable, and thus in caring for the parents one can, in turn, help them to mobilise their own capacities as caretakers.[7]

(3) *The Airing of Irrational Fears*. Many parents have irrational fears and have questions that require much patient explanation before they are able to take in the real situation. Often, the worse the fear is, the harder it is to ask the direct question and therefore parents need plenty of time and a patient listener. Examples of these questions are: Why did I go into premature labour? Will it happen again? How long will my baby be in here? Will my baby be normal? Will it grow as quickly as a full-term baby? There are many secret worries in each question, e.g. Should I have had sexual intercourse during pregnancy? Was I working too hard? Do all pre-term babies grow up brain-damaged?[8]

There seem to be specific crises at different stages of the baby's hospital stay: the initial traumatic stage when the baby is critically ill; the chronic stage, when parents may be at risk because the drama has receded but feelings of numbness and distance persist, sometimes leading to a dropping off of visiting; and the discharge stage where parents need a great deal of reassurance and support about their ability to cope alone at home.[9]

Working with Medical and Nursing Staff

In order to effect any changes in the routine and procedures of a NNICU, the emotional needs of the medical staff and nursing staff must be considered. Although policies can be introduced which have been formulated to keep abreast of any developments reported in the literature, their success or failure will in turn be related to how these affect the staff on an unconscious level. Unit policies of parental involvement in the caretaking team, for instance, although theoretically acknowledged to be beneficial, may arouse very ambivalent feelings amongst the staff.[10]

Clearly it is not appropriate to separate the practical and the psychological aspects of what constitutes stress on a NNICU. It is a multiplicity of factors which leads to the high rates of a stress-related illness, low morale and absenteeism termed 'burn out', defined as 'loss of motivation for creative involvement – a way of feeling and behaving'.[11]

Amongst these stress factors are: responsibility for the lives of very fragile babies; constant exposure due to the nursery layout necessary for the intensive care of neonates; the need to have understood considerable technological complexities; the need to make quick, unsupported decisions during crises; the expectations of expertise sometimes put on very inexperienced staff; disruptive shifts and rotations; staff shortages; the low status and pay of nursing staff; frequent death and loss of babies; rage, frustration, envy and other very strong feelings as well as the moral and ethical dilemmas of working on such a unit.[12-17]

Suggestions and attempts to alleviate stress have been diverse, but certain features recur as important:

(1) that there is a need for quiet, reflective moments within a setting where action sometimes takes the place of thought;
(2) that there should be a forum for expression – a neutral territory in which everyone can contribute equally irrespective of hierarchical structures; and
(3) that time be given to the interpretation of observations and opportunities be opened to explore and encourage intuitive feelings.[10]

The Staff Group

It was with the above principles in mind that the idea of a medical and nursing staff group was first negotiated five years ago. In the early days, the difficulties in establishing the group seemed innumerable, and despite apparent enthusiasm we encountered many months of setbacks, initially over attendance. The feelings of hopelessness, impotence, isolation and rejection that we experienced at those times offered us the key to understanding the essential problems facing staff in neonatal intensive care. In a series of meetings with senior nursing staff it was recognised that it was important to provide a regular time and place where the continuity of the group could foster and facilitate the exploration of feelings about the babies, the parents and the staff themselves. At the same time it was acknowledged that people's defences needed to be maintained and respected. With these in mind to guide the practice of the group, we hoped to achieve a more satisfying way of working, by helping the group to focus on staff experiences and to enable them to use fully their own expertise.

In the early meetings nurses most often used the group to explore their perceptions of particular babies and families. It seemed very important to confirm that these intuitions were extremely valuable tools and could be as important as their technical skills. The group also functioned as a centre for communications and a vehicle for collating and exchanging information in which the therapist (with the parents' permission) fed back information from her sessions with parents. The following incident highlights the importance of information sharing, and illustrates how changes are part of a cyclical process, and how an intervention may at any point effect a change.

> Mr and Mrs A were referred because the nursing staff observed that Mrs A in particular was expressing some reluctance over handling her premature baby daughter (30 weeks gestation), when opportunities for doing so were offered. In the interview it emerged that the parents had suffered the neonatal death a year earlier of their baby, Elizabeth. Mrs A conceived again quite quickly and, despite her wishes, an unsympathetic GP insisted on booking her in to the same hospital. The new baby, called Lisa, was immediately transferred, with the mother, from that hospital to our unit because of her prematurity and their lack of facilities. Lisa's birthday fell on the first anniversary of her sister's death. Mrs A yearned to hold Lisa, but had been warned by her own mother of the dangers of 'infecting' such a tiny baby, and therefore stifled her longings. Mr and Mrs A made

two requests: (i) that Lisa should remain on the unit and not be returned to the other hospital should her condition improve; they felt safe on the unit and grateful for the good caring; (ii) that Mrs A might be allowed to hold the tube during a feed because, although she was expressing breast milk it was difficult to feel like a mother when she could not see the baby taking it in, and she felt, to quote, 'unconnected'.

I agreed to pass this on to the staff, and when the interview was over I asked if I might be introduced to Lisa. She was indeed a beautiful baby and whilst admiring her I noticed some quite vigorous movements and commented on them to the parents. That afternoon, in the group, I related back much of our interview and the staff felt they now understood the situation better, having been unaware of much of the history. The following week my arrival on the unit was greeted by a delighted Mr and Mrs A, who were holding and cuddling Lisa. Apparently Mrs A had been sitting by the incubator watching Lisa, when she noticed her sucking the corner of the cot sheet. She called over one of the nurses, who confirmed the vigour of the action and suggested quite simply, 'Why don't you try putting her to the breast?' Encouraged and supported by the nurse, mother did so; and at 30½ weeks Lisa gained the distinction of being the youngest baby on our unit to become fully breast fed.

Issues Common to Both Staff and Parents: I, Themes

We have noticed some common themes arising for both staff and parents, and shall characterise them here as rivalry, identification, guilt separation and mourning.

Rivalry

Parents often felt rivalry with staff because they felt that their baby had been 'taken over'. They felt that the staff spent more time with babies, fed them, understood the technology and seemed to be more confident with them. We know how easy it is to undermine any new parent's confidence, and parents of babies on a NNICU are especially vulnerable. Most parents reported that they did not feel that the baby was really theirs until he or she was at home.

In the group, staff quite readily acknowledged feelings of rivalry, anger and hostility, and sometimes said that in a similar situation they would be better mothers and visit unfailingly. They frequently felt irritated by mothers who, for example, had not understood the conversion of imperial into metric units. This was understood in terms of the staff projecting their own feelings of inadequacy into the parents. The difficulty centred around the fact that the staff were constantly feeling the helplessness and pain of not being able to save babies, yet at the same time were needing to contain parental projections of hope, potency and idealisation. It was extremely difficult to be in touch with the parents' envy of them as coping, capable surrogate mothers when, at times, they felt so helpless themselves.

Identification

Parents often identified their own confused, hurt feelings with that of their baby, and in consequence need parenting themselves in order to parent their baby.

> Mrs W, whose baby was very ill with respiratory distress syndrome and heart failure, sat crying with her baby, talking about his pain and wondering aloud how she could have been so selfish that she could want a baby so much that she could put him through this.

When parents are suffering like this they need not only to be able to express their feelings to another, safe person, but to be looked after in small, practical ways.

Student nurses seemed particularly aware of the impact of the NNICU on parents, and could identify with their feelings of inadequacy. One nurse recalled how her rosy fantasies about intensive care nursing being about 'plumping up and nurturing somewhat undersized infants' were shattered by the reality of accepting that 'caring' frequently involved inflicting painful procedures on infants whose future life and development were uncertain. Staff, like parents, were reminded of some of their own babyish distressed feelings by these distressed babies.

Separation/Attachment

The generalised anxiety which any new parents feel when separated from their baby was greatly exacerbated by conditions on the unit. Not only was there separation and a feeling of alienation from the baby whilst the parent was visiting, but fatigue, fear and helplessness made parents long to be away from the unit. Once away, however, there was often a strong anxiety that something might have happened to the baby; this is realistic, but fuelled by unconscious guilt and conflicts about anger and dependency. Some parents described feelings akin to agoraphobia, and others reported a feeling of numbness and being suspended in time, always with a nagging sense of wanting to be somewhere else.

Because of these feelings it is crucial to permit visiting and telephone calls from parents at any time of the day or night.

Separation and attachment were also central preoccupations for the staff. Rotational policies and a shift system often militated against the formation of very close attachments to babies and parents. Some staff saw this policy as a disadvantage and felt the need to augment and cement their attachment by discreetly visiting on off-duty days. Others felt grateful that the system allowed them to maintain a distance, and protected them from the overwhelming pain and acute distress when 'their baby' died.

Mourning/Attachment/Guilt

Parents of a pre-term baby always experience some mourning and grief. The loss of the experience of the last trimester of pregnancy contributes towards making attachment to the baby difficult,[18] as does the loss of the wished for 'normal baby'[19] and the threat of losing this baby.[20] These losses can evoke former unresolved grief and mourning which then becomes overwhelming. This is especially true of parents who have experienced a previous miscarriage or stillbirth.

> Mrs M was causing concern to the staff because of her rejecting statements about her baby after his birth, and then her apparent lack of feeling when he died after 24 hours. A long talk with her revealed that her beloved mother had died of cancer two years previously, and she had been very stoic about this. During several sessions she cried for her mother, and on leaving the hospital said that she felt much better and might really want another baby in the future.

The constant reality of babies dying on the unit made death, and the feelings of tremendous guilt and depression that it aroused, the most difficult thing of all for the staff to deal with. The effects of the sudden death of a long-stay baby would resonate throughout the unit.

> A superhuman effort was made for a particular baby who had spent eight weeks on the unit. Having survived major setbacks he just 'went off' one night. After unsuccessful attempts at intubation he sustained massive brain damage and died despite weeks of care and effort. The entire staff's grief was most acute, and the unit went into a state of mourning. We had seen the parents both prior to, and immediately following, the baby's death. We had also accompanied the parents to the mortuary, where the mother finally felt free to hold the baby, unencumbered by the machinery which had hampered their contact during his lifetime. Afterwards, Mrs S, feeling unable to return to the unit, asked us to please convey her

gratitude to the staff for all the loving care she, her husband and her baby had received – they had all become 'family' to her. In the group, when we described the details of Mrs S's leavetaking of her baby, almost every member broke down and cried freely. It had been the staff's own pain at losing the baby which had led to the hasty dispatch of the body from the ward, and their attempts to dissuade us from supporting the mother's wish to hold and say goodbye to her dead baby.

Issues Common to Both Staff and Parents: II, Defence Mechanisms

We have observed that parents and staff employ various defence mechanisms to help them deal with the psychological stress, pain and conflict thrown up by the birth of a severely ill baby. The most common of these seem to be avoidance and denial, displacement, splitting and projection, manic reparation and magical thinking.[21]

Denial and Avoidance

This takes several forms:

Mrs P reported that on looking at her critically ill baby for the first time she said to herself that there was nothing wrong with him and he would be out of the unit in a few days.

Parents sometimes do not name their babies, avoiding attachment in case of loss. Some parents begin to say that they are too busy to visit their baby (reality factors such as other children at home have to be taken into account when considering this reaction, see Chapter 10), and one 15-year-old mother said that she could not visit because she had to go shopping for clothes so that she could be presentable to the doctors. A common phenomenon is that parents ask questions about their babies and are then unable to hear the answers so that the staff have to be infinitely patient in repeating simple information. If the underlying fantasies are first elicited from parents, staff find it easier to convey the real facts.

Avoidance of the group sessions by medical and nursing staff paralleled this avoidance in the parents. The therapist would arrive for the group meeting, and suddenly doors would close and the staff seemed to disappear. Some staff admitted that this was often the only way they could deal with their anxiety when the parents of a dying baby arrived to visit. Again, for example, there was a nurse who was adamant that unlike in adult intensive care nursing, one could not get involved with babies. Nurses often reported losing interest in a very sick baby who might die, or a feeling of anger towards that baby. Sometimes they requested to be moved on into a different nursery within the unit.

Displacement

Some parents deal with their feelings by displacing them onto other things or events. The focus of those feelings almost always has a basis in reality, but may become emphasised to the exclusion of other feelings about the baby.

> One father, for example, was only able to talk about his baby's life-support equipment, worrying whether the dials were accurate, etc. One mother decided that the baby's room was inadequately decorated and exhausted herself redecorating it.

Projection/Splitting

These are complex defence mechanisms involving blaming other things and people for things for which one unconsciously blames oneself, and splitting feelings into those which are all good and those which are all bad.[22] We often see how obstetricians are blamed for everything which has gone wrong, and how staff on the NNICU are idealised. At other times it is the NNICU that receives *all* the blame, or one particular doctor. Parents can often blame each other.

> Mr H, the father of a child irreversibly brain damaged at birth, pointed out that his wife's uncle was mentally handicapped, and blamed his wife's blood for his son's condition.

Not surprisingly, marital tensions are particularly common among parents whose emotional needs are individually so great, and only very well adjusted relationships survive the stress without difficulties.

Manic Reparation

Parents sometimes deal with the guilt about their own damaging infantile feelings by compensating for them. This is normally quite an adaptive defence as it involves caretaking and such activities as fund raising for the unit. Clearly not all caretaking is defensive, but staff can be aware that when it has a manic quality other, more painful, feelings may be behind it. Following a baby's death, it was not uncommon for staff to console themselves with the thought that the mother would soon be pregnant again.

Magical Thinking and Intuition

This is an area which we as psychotherapists tend to accept rather than to analyse. Icons, lucky toys and prayers have different meanings to different people and are often extremely important. Intuitive feelings are also respected.

> Mrs M, a Ghanaian mother, begged that her child be allowed to stay one more night rather than be transferred to a paediatric ward. Since her concern was so great this was accepted. Her child went into heart failure that night, and was saved by procedures unavailable on the paediatric ward. Another mother, unable to comprehend explanations of her child's condition, knew that he was going to die hours before he actually did, just by touching his skin.

Many practical steps can be taken to facilitate the interaction between parents and babies and, in some measure, to reduce their immediate distress. Doherty[23] described the importance of the initial visit to the unit, and we would add that liaison between the obstetric wards and the NNICU is essential to the success of this introduction. She describes how parents are encouraged to touch and stroke their babies as soon as possible, to look at them and to talk to them. Other ways of fostering parental relationships are stressed in other chapters in this book.

Although these types of steps towards facilitating parent-infant attachment are crucial, their *implementation* is often fraught with difficulty and the outcome of these interventions alone is questionable. We would contend that additional psychotherapeutic help is needed for parents and staff on NNICUs if the grief and pain of the experience is to be confronted and worked through.[24–26]

Hospitals, now efficient at saving lives and usually preventing serious handicap in babies, need to give consideration to other aspects of neonatal care in order to ensure the best possible development of infants within their families. Too much reliance is placed on the dedication and understanding of hard-pressed medical and nursing staff, with no official policy directed towards the psychological aspects of neonatal care. A trained psychotherapist who is in close liaison with the staff is an important member of a caring team where stress is part of the daily caseload. We cannot yet evaluate the long-term effects of these interventions, but can only hope that one important result will be to alleviate anxiety and thus to free the caretakers from distortions of their perceptions, enhancing their ability to confront the infant's illness as realistically as possible.

It is preferable that help be offered *during* the crisis, rather than much later when the traumatic evidence of failure may be a battered or an unthriving child.

References

1. Klaus, M., and Kennell, J. (1975). *Maternal-Infant Bonding*. St Louis, C. V. Mosby.

2. Macfarlane, J.A. (1977). *The Psychology of Childbirth*, London, Fontana.

3. Brimblecombe, F. S. W., Richards, M. P. M., and Roberton, N. R. C. (eds). (1978). *Separation and Special Care Baby Units*, Clinics in Developmental Medicine. London, Spastics International Medical Publications/Heinemann.

4. Freud, W. E. (1981). To be in touch. *Child Psychotherapy*, 7, 141.

5. Lynch, M. A., and Roberts, J. (1977). Predicting child abuse: signs of bonding failure in a maternity hospital. *Brit. Med. J.*, *1*, 624.

6. Brazelton, T.B. (1980). Behavioral competence of the newborn infant. Symposium on Birth, Interaction and Attachment, Cleveland, Ohio, 9-12 November 1980.

7. Bender, H., and Elkan, J. (1980). Unconscious aspects of communication about the birth. Unpublished paper.

8. Breen, D. (1981). *Talking to Mothers*. London, Gill Norman.

9. Swan-Parente, A. (1982). Psychological pressures in a neonatal ITU. *Brit. J. Hosp. Med.* (March), 266.

10. Bender, H. (1981). Experiences in running a nursing staff group in a hospital intensive care unit. *J. Child Psychotherapy*, 7, 152.

11. Marshall, R. E., and Kasmin, C. (1981). Burnout in the NNICU. *Pediatrics*, *65*, 1161.

12. Stepney, R. (1981). The problem of working in ICUs. *World Medicine* (25 July), 25.

13. Walker, C. H. M. (1982). Neonatal intensive care and stress. *Arch. Dis. Childhood*, *57*, 85.

14. Szur, R., and Earnshaw, E. (1979). Experiences with newborn and very young infants. *Nursing Times* (30 August).

15. Astbury, J., and Yu, V. Y. H. (1982). Determinants of stress for staff in a neonatal intensive care unit. *Arch. Dis. Childhood*, *57*, 108.

16. Duff, R. S., and Campbell, A. G. M. (1971). Moral and ethical dilemmas in the special care nursery. *New Eng. J. Med.*, *289*, 890.

17. Stahlman, M. (1979). Ethical dilemmas in perinatal medicine. *J. Paediat.*, *94*, 511.

18. Raphael-Leff, J. (1982). Psychotherapeutic needs of mothers-to-be. *J. Child Psychotherapy*, *8*, 2, 3.

19. Kaplan, D. M., and Mason, E. A. (1960). Maternal reactions to premature birth. *Am. J. Orthopsychiatry*, *30*, 539.

20. Benfield, D. G., Leib, S. A., and Reuter, J. (1976). Grief response of parents after referral of the critically ill newborn to a regional centre. *New Eng. J. Med.*, *294*, 975.

21. Winnicott, D. W. (1975). *Through Paediatrics to Psychoanalysis*. London, Hogarth Press.

22. Klein, M. (1955). *On Identification*. Vol. 3 of Collected Works, *Envy and Gratitude and Other Works* (1946-63). London, Hogarth Press/Institute of Psychoanalysis, 1973.

23. Doherty, C. (1975). The baby in the ICU and the family. *Australian Nurses' Journal*, 7, 31.

24. Brown, J. V., La Rossa, M. M., Aylward, G. P., Davis, D. J., Rutherford, P. K., and Bakeman, R. (1980). Nursery-based intervention with prematurely born babies and their mothers: are there effects? *J. Paediat.*, *97*, 487.

25. Jeffcoate, J. (1980). Looking at the need for support of families of low birthweight babies. *Health Trends, 12*, 29.

26. Siegal, E., Bauman, K. E., Schaefer, E. S., Saunders, M. M., and Ingram, D. D. (1980). Hospital and home support during infancy. Impact on maternal attachment, child abuse and neglect and health care utilization. *Pediatrics*, *66*, 183.

12 BREAST FEEDING FOR VERY LOW BIRTHWEIGHT BABIES

Chloe Fisher and J. D. Baum

A mother's own milk is the ideal food for her own healthy term baby. It remains uncertain however which milk or milk formula is best suited for the very low birthweight baby. Recent studies suggest that human milk and particularly the infant's own mother's milk may be the food of choice for such babies.[1]

In this chapter we discuss first the problems which beset the mother who wishes to supply her own milk for her very low birthweight baby. We then discuss the range of problems which relate to the collection, storage and processing of donated human milk for the feeding of the pre-term infant whose mother's own milk is insufficient or unavailable.

The Practicalities of Establishing Breast Feeding for Very Low Birthweight Babies

A mother who wishes to breast-feed a baby of very low birthweight on a neonatal intensive care unit faces a range of difficulties which do not apply to the mother with a healthy term infant. An intensive care unit is a place of intense activity orientated towards measuring and controlling physiological variables and intervening to deal with recurrent crises. The staff are under continuous stress. Successful breast feeding under these conditions would be difficult *even* for a mother with a healthy responsive term infant. It is therefore important that one member of the staff, preferably a midwife, should take special responsibility for the mother who is attempting to establish lactation and has a very low birthweight baby. She should be carefully taught to express her milk in order to establish and maintain her lactation. She can express at times convenient to the hospital routine, usually 3-5 hourly, except perhaps at night.

Who is Responsible for the Breast Feeding Mother?

There is a danger that the breast feeding mother whose baby is in the intensive care unit may herself be unsupervised. Her bed is in the postnatal ward while the baby is in the neonatal unit. Unless a deliberate attempt is made to identify who is primarily responsible for the mother's care, it is possible for her to fall between the two groups. In most hospitals the primary responsibility for breast feeding practice on both the postnatal ward and the neonatal unit rests with the midwives. However, it is important that other members of staff, especially the resident medical staff, also have a working knowledge of the problems of lactation and the policies for dealing with them as they exist in their hospital. In particular all members of staff should recognise how stray remarks and contradictions can confuse and demoralise the vulnerable mother of a low birthweight baby struggling to establish her lactation.

The First Crisis in Breast Feeding Confidence

Whether the mother is collecting her milk by manual expression or by using a hand-held or electrical pump, a variety of worries and problems may be encountered which need to be recognised by members of the staff. The first crisis in the mother's confidence is likely to arise when she notes the relatively small volumes of milk collected at each pumping session. She needs to be reassured that the amount of milk expressed in the first few days after delivery in no way predicts her long-term ability to breast-feed her baby successfully.

Many weeks elapse after the birth before a very low birthweight baby is ready to feed directly at the breast. For much of this time most mothers will be at home and must be thoroughly familiar with whichever method they have chosen for expressing their milk (see Addendum to this chapter). The expressed milk that the mother collects at home should be placed in sterile containers and stored in the refrigerator if it can be delivered to the neonatal unit daily. If the mother is unable to take the milk to the unit daily, it should be stored in the freezing compartment of the refrigerator or in a deep freeze, where it can be stored for up to two weeks. The fresh refrigerated milk would be used for the mother's own baby on a daily basis. The frozen milk would be used to supplement the baby's needs and any excess added to the pool of donated milk for other babies in the unit.

The Second Crisis in Breast Feeding Confidence

The majority of mothers settle down to the routine expression of their milk. However, it is not uncommon for a mother to become very despondent if her baby has difficulties in fixing and feeding when first put to the breast. This is the second crisis in the establishment of successful breast feeding. The mother may interpret this temporary failure of fixation and sucking to signal rejection of her baby, adding further to her confusion about her role as the caretaker of her own baby. Both parents may become anxious, particularly if the successful establishment of breast feeding is the only factor delaying the baby's homecoming. This is a time for further sensitive encouragement and support for the mother by all members of staff.

The Initiation of Suckling

Time should be set aside for the baby to be in skin-to-skin contact with his mother's breasts. During these periods every effort should be made to ensure privacy for the family group. Although a screen across a cubicle might be adequate as a visual barrier it needs to be respected by members of staff so that the mother is not constantly interrupted for ward nursing and medical routines.

Every effort must be made to provide the ideal physical environment on the neonatal unit for the breast feeding pair. This means a comfortable chair or settee with a supply of pillows to ensure that the optimal position of the baby feeding at the mother's breast can be achieved and varied according to the day-to-day needs. While it is generally understood that a mother needs tranquillity for successful breast feeding, recognition is not given to the importance of the physical alignment of the baby at the breast for the mother's comfort and for the success of an individual feed.

This time of familiarisation for the mother with her baby at her breast is important from another point of view. Up till this stage the baby has been in danger of dying and under the constant care of (and in many ways a possession of) the staff of the neonatal unit; now it appears that the baby is likely to survive and be cared for by the mother herself.

Specific Problems of the Very Low Birthweight Baby at the Breast. Most problems of breast feeding mothers with term infants can be solved by expert assistance from an experienced midwife. These problems tend to occur more commonly on the neonatal intensive care unit when babies make the transition from tube feeding to breast feeding. The baby's mouth is small compared with that of a term infant; as a result the baby may produce nipple traction and trauma, making breast feeding both uncomfortable and ineffectual. These factors may be interpreted to mean that breast feeding is unsuccessful because the baby is immature, weak, or accustomed to tube or bottle feeds. In fact it is really an exaggeration of the problems that a breast feeding mother with a term infant may face in the first few days after birth. The mother needs to be shown by a skilled midwife how to 'tease' the baby to open his mouth wide and adequately fix on the areola each time he suckles.

During this phase of transition when the baby is beginning to suck at the breast, his feeds will initially be completed by tube. There appears to be no scientific evidence to identify whether it is preferable to complete the baby's feeds by complementary tube feeds or by feeding from a teat and bottle. While a lot of anxiety is often concentrated on this issue, it would seem reasonable, in the absence of evidence to the contrary, for staff on different units to approach this problem in different ways.

The Third Crisis in Breast Feeding Confidence

Prior to the parents taking the baby home it is important that the mother should spend 24 hours or more in residence in the hospital taking charge of all aspects of her baby's care. However, at least of equal importance is the provision of professional support specifically related to breast feeding for the first few days after the mother takes her baby home. In every case the person responsible for providing this support, whether community midwife or health visitor, needs to be clearly identified. If this last stage of transition from breast feeding in hospital to breast feeding at home is mismanaged, then the end result will be a hungry baby, sore nipples and a distressed mother. It will then appear to the family doctor that he has little option other than to advise formula feeding.

Donor Breast Milk for Very Low Birthweight Babies

There are times when a mother wishing to breast-feed her infant on a neonatal intensive care unit cannot meet the baby's daily requirements through fluctuations in her own milk supply or difficulties in visiting the baby in hospital. Furthermore, there are many mothers who are unsuccessful in establishing lactation or never wish to do so. In order to feed all very low birthweight infants with human milk, some system of human milk banking must be established.[2] This depends upon adequate and reliable supplies of donated breast milk.

The Collection of Donor Breast Milk

In this section a description is given of one approach to the collection of donor breast milk.[3] The milk collected for the Oxford Human Milk Bank is mostly drip breast milk – that milk which drips spontaneously from the non-feeding breast in about 20 per cent of lactating mothers.[4] Drip milk donors contribute 50-100 ml of milk per 24 hours. Individual mothers may contribute to the bank anything from 100 ml to 40 litres of drip breast milk over a period of time. In addition expressed milk is donated to the bank by some mothers whose babies are on the neonatal unit and who produce in excess of their own babies' needs.

The fat concentration of drip breast milk is substantially lower than that of expressed milk.[5-7] Nevertheless there are two reasons why, despite this, we prefer to collect drip breast milk for the Oxford Human Milk Bank. First, drip breast is a 'waste' product, the collection of which has ecological appeal. Secondly, collecting milk in this way avoids the necessity of donating mothers having to 'pump' their breasts, which many mothers find unattractive as an idea. Furthermore the expression of milk requires a substantial capital investment in breast pumps, and it means that the mother is producing milk over and above the needs of her own baby, which is worrying in terms of possible nutritional consequences for both the mother and her own baby.

The milk is brought to the human milk bank, which in the John Radcliffe Maternity Hospital is situated adjacent to the special care baby unit. The mothers are not paid for their milk, nor are the midwives paid for their additional work. We believe that involvement with giving spare milk to the bank is gratifying for the mothers and in practice leads them, together with the community midwives, to publicise the charitable idea of providing spare human milk for babies who have special need of it. Central to the efficiency of the system is a high rate of breast feeding in the maternity hospital and in the community, so that many mothers may each be donating small volumes of drip breast milk daily, thereby maintaining an adequate flow of milk to our milk bank. Between 50 and 90 mothers are donating drip breast milk at any one time and the volume arriving at the milk bank has varied between 50-100 litres per month (Figure 12.1).

Banking of Donor Breast Milk

In the human milk bank the individual bottles of frozen milk are placed in a reception deep freeze. At a convenient time supplies of this milk are removed and allowed to thaw at room temperature. The milk is then pooled and pasteurised.[4] One bottle of milk is sent for bacteriological analysis, and if no growth is reported (after blood agar plating), the remaining milk is transferred to a third freezer ready fc· use. Orders

Figure 12.1: The Volumes of Donor Breast Milk Arriving at the Oxford Human Milk Bank Analysed on a Month-by-month Basis, Showing that this Varies between 50 and 100 Litres per Month with a Trend in Recent Months for Increasing Volumes of Milk to be Donated.

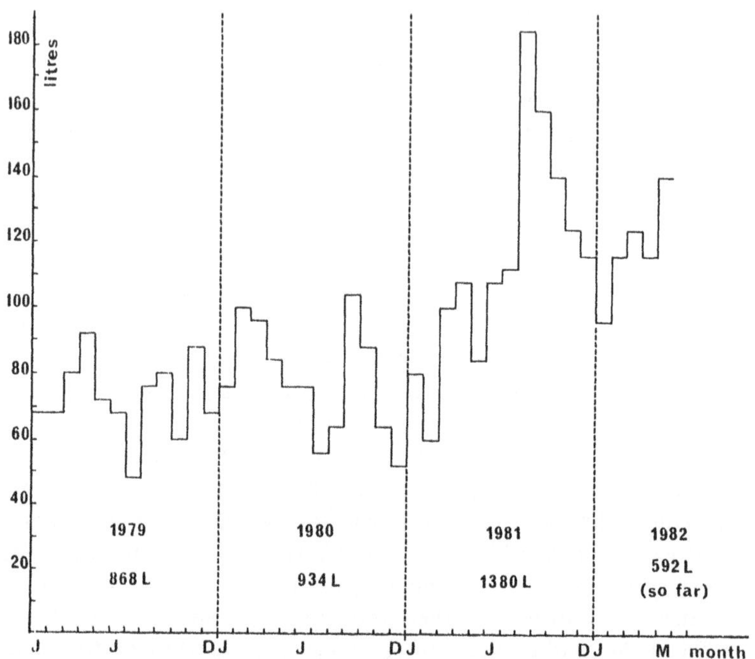

for human milk are placed one day in advance whenever possible. In this way the nursing auxiliary in charge of the milk bank can thaw the necessary volumes of milk early the following morning. It should be noted that the processing of the milk is carried out by one part-time nursing auxiliary.

Donor Breast Milk in the Neonatal Unit

For the very low birthweight baby whose mother is not contributing her own milk, feeding is started with banked human milk and continues until the baby weighs about 1.50 kg. At this stage a change to a proprietary formula milk is considered. The timing of this change is variable depending upon the baby's health, plans for transfer to another hospital or discharge home, the number of babies in the nursery and the amount of milk available in the human milk bank.

The banked milk, which has been thawed, is distributed in the nursery according to the needs of the individual babies. Every effort is made to avoid leaving large volumes of human milk at ambient temperature (25° C) in the neonatal unit because of the risk of bacterial growth. Pasteurised milk is also available for babies of mothers on the postnatal ward who may be undergoing initial difficulties with breast feeding, to babies admitted to the neonatal surgical unit and as an interim measure to babies of mothers in the community who may be undergoing temporary breast feeding problems.

Problems in Quality Control in Human Milk Banking

Nutritional Value. There are many nutritional considerations which come under the heading of quality control. These include the concentration of vitamins, trace minerals, calcium, phosphorus, sodium and potassium, lactose, amino acids, protein and fat. In this discussion we shall refer only to the problems of controlling the fat concentration of human milk since this lends itself to simple monitoring and possible manipulation. Furthermore fats are the main determinant of the energy value of human milk and can be measured simply by the 'creamatocrit' method.[8]

The creamatrocrit has allowed the investigation of the variability of the fat concentration in individual donated human milk samples. This variability would interfere with any attempt to regulate the fat and energy content of banked human milk. The problem is overcome to a large extent by pooling the milk. The composition of pooled drip milk compared with that of mature expressed milk is shown in Table 12.1.

Table 12.1: Composition of Pooled Drip Milk.

		Pooled Drip Milk[a]	Pooled Mature Expressed Milk[b]	
		mean ± SD (N)	mean and range	
Fat	(g/dl)	2.2 ± 0.8 (17)	4.5	(1.3 – 8.3)
Lactose	(g/dl)	6.5 ± 0.1 (9)	6.8	(5.0 – 9.2)
Protein	(g/dl)	1.0 ± 0.2 (9)	1.1	(0.7 – 2.0)
Sodium	(mM/l)	5.5 ± 1.6 (27)	7.4	(2.6 – 19.1)
Potassium	(mM/l)	16.1 ± 1.5 (27)	13.0	(9.5 – 16.4)
Calcium	(mM/l)	6.9 ± 0.8 (22)	8.5	(4.3 – 15.3)
Magnesium	(mM/l)	1.2 ± 0.2 (22)	1.7	(0.8 – 2.5)
pH		6.75 (10) (range 6.58-7.04)	7.01	(6.40 – 7.60)
Osmolality (mOsm/kg water)		285 ± 9 (22)		

Notes: a. 48 hr collections from N donors (Gibbs *et al.*).[4] b. Macy and Kelly.[6]

Monitoring the fat concentration of banked milk does not indicate the fat and energy available to the recipient infants. Some fat may be lost by adherence to the walls of the feeding tube and syringe, particularly if the milk is infused into the baby rather than given as a bolus. Estimates of the fat lost in this way have been as high as 30 per cent.[7] Furthermore, not all the fat reaching the baby's stomach is necessarily absorbed. We believe that there is a variable and sometimes very substantial fat malabsorption in pre-term and low birthweight infants which may play a significant role in their failure to gain weight, particularly when they are seriously unwell. The severity and variability of this steatorrheoa can be monitored in a simple way using the 'steatocrit' test.[9]

Bacteriological Surveillance. For each species of bacteria a thermal death line can be plotted: that is the time/temperature exposure which will effectively reduce a given bacterial count to zero. In order to reproduce this effect and to heat-treat milk precisely under routine milk bank conditions we developed the Oxford Human Milk Pasteuriser (Vickers Medical, Basingstoke, Hants RG24 9NP).[4] In this machine, milk is heated rapidly to 62.5°C, held at that temperature for 30 minutes and then cooled rapidly. In recent experiments we have used a temperature of 56°C and a holding time of 15 minutes and shown that milk samples are rendered sterile with starting counts of 10^7 organisms per ml of *Escherichia coli, Staphylococcus aureus* and group B β-haemolytic streptococci.[10] In addition, the percentage survival of immunoglobulin A, lactoferrin and lysozyme approaches 100 per cent at these settings compared with lower and variable survival using the classical pasteurisation settings of 62.5°C for 30 minutes.[11]

Is Donor Breast Milk Suitable for the Nutrition of the Low Birthweight Infant?

In our nursery the majority of very low birthweight infants, particularly those weighing less than 1 kg at birth, take 2–4 weeks before they regain their birthweight and start to gain weight steadily. This is the result of many influences, including the complications associated with very low birthweight and immaturity, which frequently make it impossible to achieve even modest feeding targets on a regular basis. Furthermore, there is the variable, and often considerable, loss of energy as unabsorbed fat present in the baby's stool.[9] At the same time there are great uncertainties about the ideal food for such low birthweight infants. It may be that part of the explanation for their relatively slow weight gain is that they need a milk with a higher protein and energy content than that which is suitable for the term infant. It was to this end that we developed the concept of separating milk into its component parts to be added to pooled banked milk, with the object of giving low birthweight and sick infants a fortified 'human milk formula' designed to meet their specific nutritional requirements.[11] Recently the methodology for separating milk has been simplified with an improvement in the speed and precision of the process.[12] Table 12.2 gives the results of fortifying pooled milk with human milk fat and protein, indicating the feasibility of the exercise.

Table 12.2: Protein and Fat Concentrations (Mean ± s.e.m.) in Pooled Human Milk and in Human Milk Formula.[11]

	Pooled Breast Milk	Human Milk Formula
Protein, g/100 g (n = 8)	1.44 ± 0.01	2.53 ± 0.04
Fat, g/100 g (n = 8)	2.43 ± 0.08	4.46 ± 0.30

However, some caution is in order here. The history of neonatal intensive care has included a number of clinical catastrophes resulting from the uncontrolled adoption of new and attractive ideas.[13] While it is natural that we should be anxious when low birthweight and sick newborn infants fail to gain weight over days and even weeks, the final arbiter as to whether or not this short period of relative undernutrition is harmful must rest upon follow-up studies. It will require careful long-term evaluation of growth and intellectual function to determine whether the initial patterns of postnatal growth among low birthweight infants have repercussions in later childhood. Preliminary data from the Oxford cerebral palsy study show that in terms of length and head circumference there is no difference between babies less than 1.50 kg (born in Oxford 1978 and 1979 and fed on routine banked drip breast milk) and matched controls born at term, when measured at nine months and 18 months corrected postnatal age – see Table 12.3.[14]

Conclusion

There are many unanswered questions in relation to the ideal approach to feeding the very low birthweight infant. Some mothers will wish to establish and sustain their lactation in order to give their milk as their

Table 12.3: Follow-up Measurements at Nine and 18 Months Corrected Postnatal Age for Babies Born 1.50 kg or over and Matched Control Babies Born Normal Weight at Term. There is no statistical difference between the two groups. The mean ± standard error is shown.[14]

		1.50 kg or over (n = 20)	Term Controls (n = 20)
9 Months	Length (cm)	68.3 ± 3.5	69.9 ± 2.3
	Head Circ. (cm)	45.4 ± 1.2	45.6 ± 1.0
18 Months	Length (cm)	77.3 ± 3.8	78.8 ± 2.6
	Head Circ. (cm)	47.6 ± 1.2	48.2 ± 1.1

contribution to the care of their own infant while he is at his smallest and sickest. Others will wish to go further than this and hope to breast-feed their infant when he comes home from hospital. These mothers require the time and skilled assistance of members of the staff of the neonatal unit if the various crises of breast feeding are to be avoided.

If human milk is considered the ideal food for all very low birth-weight babies, then for those whose mothers do not provide their own milk some safe system of human milk banking must be established. The system which we employ in Oxford is simple to organise and safe in terms of protecting the very low birthweight infant against milk contaminated with large numbers of bacteria. However, a great deal of controlled experimental work is required before it becomes clear which is the best system of banking human milk and indeed whether human milk is, as we suppose, the ideal nutrient for very low birthweight babies.

Addendum

Breast Expression

The choice of method to be used for milk expression will be governed by the equipment available in the area. Most maternity hospitals, or at least their special care units, provide electric pumps for use during the mother's stay, and occasionally after the mother has gone home. All the electric pumps currently available appear to be effective though expensive. A pump hire scheme has been established in the UK.[15] A few mothers may develop an intense dislike for the 'relentless' machine and alternative methods available are manual expression and hand-operated pumps.

Manual expression is the simplest, involving no extra equipment. It is a difficult technique to learn and some mothers never master it. Others find it painful, tiring and time consuming. Advice on the techniques of manual expression is readily available.[16] Hand-operated pumps are the most commonly used for milk expression at the moment. The simple breast reliever has so many disadvantages that it makes it inadvisable for long-term expressing. The vacuum is difficult to control and the hand movement required is tiring. The initiation of lactation by this means is rarely successful; when the milk supply is plentiful the mother has to empty the small reservoir frequently, which is messy and tiring. A more recent model provides a slightly larger reservoir. The other models of hand-operated pumps offer finer control and larger reservoirs for the milk. In these, the vacuum may be created by operating a hand lever or moving the inner of two cylinders like a large syringe.

Useful Points

(1) The breast cup should not be pushed hard against the breast as this makes the breast retract instead of allowing the areola to be drawn into the pump.
(2) Lifting the breast from underneath with one hand may greatly increase the efficacy of expressing.
(3) Milk expression does not necessarily reveal all the milk that is in the breast; it is much less efficient than the suckling baby.
(4) Initially, a small or premature baby may not be capable of sustained suckling; it is therefore advisable that after the feed, the breast should be expressed to maintain the lactation.
(5) Efficient breast expression may increase lactation when it appears to be diminishing.
(6) Where there is choice in the size of breast cup, the mother should try all of them because one may enable her to express very effectively while another may make it almost impossible to do so.
(7) The mother should aim to express five or six times in 24 hours.

References

1. Baum, J. D. (1980). Preterm milk. *Early Human Development*, *4*, 1.

2. DHSS (1981). *The Collection and Storage of Human Milk*. Report on Health and Social Subjects, 22. London, HMSO.

3. Baum, J. D., Fisher, C., and Smith, M. A. (1980). *Guide to Human Milk Banking*. Basingstoke, Vickers Medical Publications.

4. Gibbs, J. A. H., Fisher, C., Bhattacharya, S., Goddard, P., and Baum, J. D. (1977). Drip breast milk: its composition, collection and pasteurisation. *Early Human Developm.*, *1*, 227.

5. Davies, D. P., Carroll, L. and Derbyshire, F. (1980). Collecting and banking human milk. *Brit. Med. J.*, *281*, 1350.

6. Macy, I. G., and Kelly, H. J. (1961). Human milk and cow's milk in infant nutrition. In *Milk: The Mammary Gland and its Secretion, Vol. 2*, S. K. Kon and A. T. Cowie (eds). New York, Academic Press, 265-304.

7. Spencer, S. A., and Hull, D. (1981). Fat content of expressed breast milk: a case for quality control. *Brit. Med. J.*, *282*, 99.

8. Lucas, A., Gibbs, J. A. H., Lyster, R. L., and Baum, J. D. (1978). Creamatocrit: simple clinical technique for estimating fat concentration and energy value of human milk. *Brit. Med. J.*, *279*, 1018.

9. Phuapradit, P., Narang, A., Mendonca, P., Harris, D. A., and Baum, J. D. (1981). The steatocrit: A simple method for estimating stool fat content in newborn infants. *Arch. Dis. Child.*, *59*, 725.

10. Wills, M. E., Han, V. E. M., Harris, D. A., and Baum, J. D. (1982). Short-time low-temperature pasteurisation of human milk. *Early Human Developm.*, *8*, 71.

11. Lucas, A., Lucas, P. J., Chavin, S. J., Lyster, R. L. J., and Baum, J. D. (1980). A human milk formula. *Early Human Development*, 4, 15.

12. Williams, A., and Baum, J. D. A system for the separation of human milk IgA. In preparation.

13. Baum, J. D., Macfarlane, A., and Tizard, J. P. M. (1977). The hazards of neonatal intensive care. In *The Benefits and Hazards of the New Obstetrics*, T. Chard and M. Richards (eds). London, Spastics International Medical Publications/Heinemann.

14. Macfarlane, A. (1982). Personal communication (study in progress).

15. Helsing, E., and Savage King, F. (1982). *Breast Feeding Practice*. Oxford, Oxford University Press.

16. Leibhaber, M., Lewiston, N. J., Asquith, M. T., and Sunshine, P. (1978). Comparison of bacterial contamination with two methods of human milk collection. *J. Pediat.*, *92*, 236.

13 CARE FOR THE FAMILY OF AN INFANT WITH A CONGENITAL MALFORMATION

Marshall Klaus and John Kennell

The birth of an infant with a congenital malformation presents complex challenges to those who care for the affected child and family. A major malformation occurs in two of every 100 births. Thus almost every nurse or physician will have a part in the care of these babies. Yet despite the relatively large number of infants with anomalies, understanding of the development of parental ties to a malformed infant remains incomplete. Investigators agree that the child's birth often precipitates a major crisis.

The early recorded history of human society indicates that malformed infants have been treated in widely differing ways and have evoked a broad range of emotional reactions: 'Sculptures, carvings, and drawings of abnormal births by ancient peoples antedate the arts of reading and writing. During times when human deities were worshipped, it was the unusual human being who assume divine status.'[1]

The parental reactions are turbulent, and the usual pathways for the development of close parent-infant bonds are disrupted. The goal is best described by Bettelheim: 'Children can learn to live with a disability. But they cannot live well without the conviction that their parents find them utterably loveable... If the parents, knowing about his (the child's) defect, love him now, he can believe that others will love him in the future. With this conviction, he can live well today and have faith about the years to come.'[2]

During the course of a normal pregnancy, the mother and father develop a mental picture of their baby. Although the degree of concreteness varies, each has an idea about the sex, complexion, colouring, and so forth. One of the early tasks of parenting is to resolve the discrepancy between this idealised image of the infant and the actual appearance of the real infant. The dreamed-about baby is a composite of impressions and desires derived from the parents' own experience. If the parents have different racial backgrounds, the task of reconciling the image to the reality is more complicated. However, the discrepancy is much greater if the baby is born with a malformation (Figure 13.1).[3]

The reactions of the parents and the degree of their future attach-

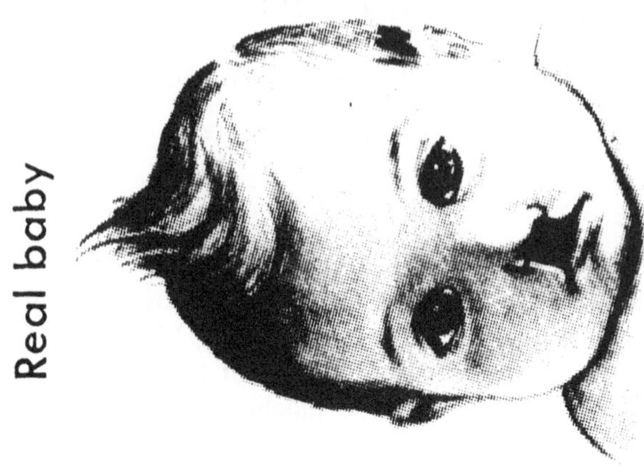

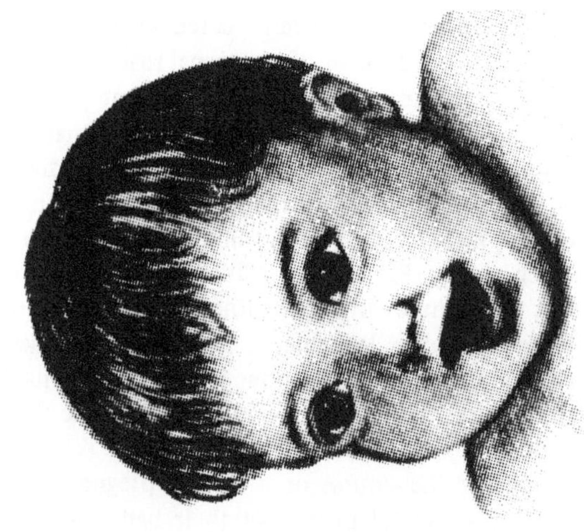

Figure 13.1: Image and Reality.

ment difficulties depend, in part, on the properties of the malformation: Is it completely correctable or is it noncorrectable? Is it visible or invisible? Is it familial? Is it life-threatening? Does it affect the central nervous system? Does it affect the genitalia? Is it a single or multiple malformation? A number of investigators have noted that the more visible the defects are the more immediate will be the concern and embarrassment. Even a minor abnormality of the head and neck results in greater anxiety about future development than an impairment of another part of the body.[4]

In several studies parents have reported that when they saw their infants for the first time, the malformations seemed less alarming than they had imagined. Seeing the children allayed some of their anxiety. The information that something was wrong with the baby was often far more disturbing than the sight of the child. Both the mothers and the fathers were greatly relieved when they actually saw their children.[4-6]

Some parents were reluctant to see their babies at first, expressing a need to temper the intensity of the experience. When these parents did see their babies, it seemed to mark a turning point, and caretaking feelings began to be elicited. Roskies[7] studied the mothers of children with phocomelia due to thalidomide. She describes four mothers who were debating whether or not to institutionalise their children. The issue was settled when they saw their infants and found aspects they could 'cherish'. From our clinical experience the parents of children with visible anomalies had a shorter period of shock and disbelief than did the parents of a child with a hidden defect. The shock of producing a baby with a visible defect is stunning and overwhelming.

Two-thirds of the mothers of babies with spina bifida preferred to be told about the diagnosis as early as possible.[8] Any delay tended to heighten their anxiety. They objected to being given an unnecessarily gloomy picture at first on the one hand and on the other hand they objected to having the seriousness of the condition minimised at first. The parents attached great importance to the approach and general attitude of the medical and nursing staff. They often did not recall the words of the nurse, obstetrician, or pediatrician but did remember their attitude. Mothers who were hurt by an apparent lack of sympathy tended to attribute the abruptness to a lack of feeling in the informant. Most mothers were impressed by the kindness and sympathy extended to them by the nursing and medical staff. Small acts of kindness were clearly remembered for years: 'The initial counselling of the mothers of malformed infants can make a lasting impression.'[8]

The original creative work of Solnit and Stark[3] has become the foundation of most therapeutic approaches to the parents of the malformed infant. Their seminal work concluded that:

(1) The infant is a distortion of the dreamed-of or planned-for infant (Figure 13.1).
(2) The parents must mourn the loss of this infant before they can become fully attached to the living defective infant.
(3) Along with this proces of mourning there is a large component of guilt that takes many forms and requires great patience of the caregiver, since the parents may repeat the same questions and problems many times.
(4) There is resentment and anger, which nurses, paediatricians and obstetricians must understand, since it is sometimes directed towards them.
(5) The physician, nurse and social worker should not interpret to the parents that the grief they are feeling is due to the loss of the expected perfect child, nor should they compare the mourning response with any others the parents might have experienced, since it may rob the mother of the full strength and depth of her own grief by intellectualising it.
(6) The task of becoming attached to the malformed child and providing for his ongoing physical care can be overwhelming to parents at the time around birth, when they are physiologically and psychologically depleted.
(7) The mourning cannot be as effective when the damaged child survives. The daily impact of this child on the mother is unrelenting and makes heavy demands on her time and energy.

Our studies[5] confirmed the work of Solnit and Stark[3]. Despite the wide variations among the children's malformations and parental backgrounds, a number of surprisingly similar themes emerged from the parents' discussion of their reactions. Generally they went through identifiable stages of emotional reactions, as shown in Figure 13.2, which is a generalisation of the complex reactions of individual parents.[5] Although the amount of time that a parent needed to deal with the issues of a specific stage varied, the sequence of stages reflected the course of most parents' reactions to their malformed infant.

The first stage was shock. Most parents' initial response to the news of their child's anomaly was overwhelming shock. All but two of the parents reported reactions and sensations indicating an abrupt disruption

Figure 13.2: Stages of Emotional Reactions of Parents.

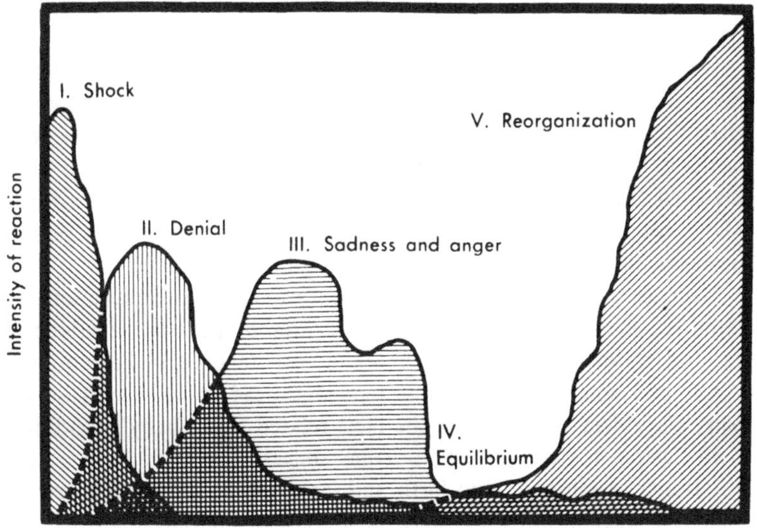

of their usual states of feeling. One of the fathers explained, 'It was as if the world had come to an end.' Many parents noted that this early period involved irrational behaviour, characterised by much crying, feelings of helplessness and occasionally an urge to flee.

In the second stage, denial, each parent reported that he or she wished either to be free from the situation or deny its impact. Many parents tried to avoid admitting that their child had an anomaly. Some parents mentioned that the news of the baby's birth did not make sense. Although every parent reported disbelief, the intensity of the denial varied considerably.

In the third stage, the most common emotional reaction was sadness. One mother reported, 'I couldn't stop crying. Even after a long while I cried about it.' A smaller number of parents reported angry feelings. A mother reported that she was angry and 'hated him (the baby) or hated myself'. In most instances, mothers were hesitant about becoming attached to their babies.

In the fourth stage, equilbrium, parents reported a gradual lessening of both their intense emotional reactions and anxiety. As their feelings of emotional upset lessened, they noted increased comfort with their situation and confidence in their ability to care for the baby. Some parents reached equilibrium within a few weeks after the birth, whereas others took many months. Even at best, this adaptation continues to be incomplete. One parent reported, 'Tears come even yet, years after the baby's birth.'

In the final stage, reorganisation, parents begin actively to deal with responsibility for their children's problems. Some mothers reported that they had to reassure themselves that the baby's problems were nothing they had done. Positive long-term acceptance of the child involved the parents' mutual support throughout the time after birth. Many couples relied heavily on one another during the early period; however, the crisis of the birth separated some parents.

The parents progressed through the various stages of reaction differently, despite the important similarities in parental reactions to various malformations. Some parents did not report initial reactions of shock and emotional upset but tended instead to intellectualise the baby's problem and focus on the facts related to the baby's condition. Some parents were unable to cope successfully with their strong emotional reactions to the birth and, as a result, did not achieve an adequate adaptation; they were in a state of continous sorrow that lasted long after the birth.

A lack of opportunity to discuss the infant's diagnosis can create a situation in which the parents feel overwhlemed and unable to gauge the reality of their child's abnormality. If the mourning process becomes fixed as a sustained atmosphere of the family, the image of the desired, expected, healthy child continues to interfere with the family's adaptation. It is remarkable that parents who cope with the intense emotional experience engendered by the birth of an infant can assimilate the child into the family and begin responding to his needs as readily as they do.

It is necessary to consider just what characteristics constitute optimal adaptation. If sorrow, depression and anger are natural responses to the birth, and if the infant evoking these feelings continues to live, what is the right balance between mourning and acceptance? Olshansky[9] coined the term 'chronic sorrow' to describe some of the enduring aspects of parental reactions in adapting to a retarded child. Chronic sorrow at some level may be constantly present in parents, especially if the child will always be dependent on them, as in some cases of retardation. To expect the disappearance of the painful impact of this child on the family, under the guise that these feelings must be 'resolved', can only force parents to deny their real feelings to professionals who may want to help. Professionals might consider the rewards of shepherding a child with problems to a more successful level of functioning along with the need to come to grips with the malformation in the first place.

Many parents also struggle with these issues and search for some explanation of why this has happened to them. Sometimes these struggles include much concern over the exact cause of the problem, which can be frustrating if a cause cannot be determined. When there is no acceptable medical explanation for the child's birth defect, the parents' genetic competence is called into question. They may try very hard to find a specific non-genetic cause for the anomaly in order to rid themselves of guilty feelings. Parents of children who develop mental retardation due to an illness, such as meningitis subsequent to birth, for example, seem to adjust much better than parents with a baby retarded from birth.

It is disturbing for parents to encounter a discrepancy between their own intense emotional turmoil and what they believe is a lack of feeling on the part of professionals. The physician's objective professional manner may sometimes be mistaken for a lack of sympathy and may be met by outrage on the part of the parents. Many physicians are able to compromise, maintaining their own standards of correct professional behaviour and at the same time fulfilling some of the parents' needs for support. The baby can be presented to the parents in such a way that his attributes and normal features are highlighted. It is desirable to do this shortly after birth in the presence of both parents. This demonstrates to the parents that the hospital staff consider the baby an acceptable substitute for the wished-for baby and not a 'piece of damaged goods'.[10]

Involving the parents in the care and planning for their infant allows them to enjoy satisfying feedback from him. It is also at this early stage that the groundwork is laid for an effective alliance of parents and professionals concerning treatment.

Nurses and physicians can facilitate the attachment of parents to their malformed infant in the neonatal period and as the child grows. Knowledge about the usual course of parental reactions helps the physician to take this into account in planning interventions. For example, a physician who knows about the disorganisation which parents experience during the stages of shock and denial will realise that information about the child's condition and progress may have to be repeated many times.

The crisis of the baby's birth has the potential for bringing the parents closer, as a result of the mutual support and the communication required for adaptation. On the other hand, in many of the families we have studied, the baby's birth estranged the parents. The ongoing demands of the baby's care increased the isolation between some parents, particularly if they did not share the responsibility. We have used the term 'asynchronous' to describe parents who progress through the different stages of adaptation at different speeds[11] (Figure 13.2). These parents usually do not share their feelings with each other and seem to have particular difficulty in their relationships. Asynchrony often results in a temporary emotional separation of the parents and appears to be a significant factor in the high divorce rate after a major family crisis.

The availability of the paediatrician throughout the child's early years puts him or her in a position to help with the family's adaptation. The paediatrician can be sensitive to the relationship between the parents, can determine which stage of adaptation each parent has reached, can check how aware each partner is of the other's progress, and may be alert to evidence of asynchrony. Parents have told of the importance of identifying the normal features of their child, which become increasingly evident as he grows. The paediatrician has an excellent opportunity to nurture this.

As a physician, nurse, or social worker follows the progress of the parents, each will be struck by the step-by-step nature of adjustment to a stressful situation such as this. There will be a tentative and perhaps ever-changing view of the child's potential. If reality indicates a less hopeful prognosis, the professional can present the news so that the parents can adapt to it in small amounts without losing confidence in themselves. Many parents describe that the most effective way they have found to deal with the challenge is to take things day by day. They try not to worry excessively about the uncertainties in the future or to dwell on the traumatic events of the past. Unless the daily care and planning for the child is affected, this type of reaction seems to serve to protect parents from unbearable pain.

Recommendations for Care

(1) We consider it of high priority to bring a baby to the mother as soon as possible so that both parents can see him and observe his normal features as well as his abnormality. Any period of delay during which the parents suspect or know that their baby may have a problem,

but are unable to see him, heightens their anxiety tremendously and allows their imaginations to run wild. They may jump to the conclusion that the baby is dead or dying while he is actually doing well and the problem is a cleft lip. The longer the period before they see the baby the more distorted and fixed their concept of the baby's condition may become. The parents' mental images of their infant's anomaly are almost invariably much more grotesque than the actual problem. Whatever is said to the parents initially is usually indelibly imprinted on their minds. This places a sobering responsibility on the shoulders of everyone caring for the mother and baby because the words used in discussing the baby with the mother may affect her initial attachment process.

(2) Positive emphasis. When first showing the infant with a visible problem, it is important to show all the normal parts as well and to emphasise positive features such as the baby's strength, activity and alertness. It is surprising that malformations that appear obvious, striking and bizarre to the physician sometimes do not seem to the parents as frightening or disfiguring.

(3) Special caretaking. Most maternity units are designed for the care of normal mothers and babies. Therefore, when a baby is born with a problem such as a congenital malformation, the mother's mood and needs are out of step with the routines of the unit. We find that it is usually best to assign a specific nurse to the mother of a baby with a congenital anomaly. This nurse should have the ability to sit for long periods with the mother and just listen to her cry and tell about the powerful reactions, which are often disturbingly critical and negative. Not everyone on a unit will find this an easy task, so it should be given to someone who feels prepared to assist the parents of an infant with an anomaly.

(4) Parents should not be given tranquillisers, which tend to blunt their responses and slow their adaptation to the problem. However, a sedative at night is sometimes helpful.

(5) Parents who are adapting reasonably well often ask many questions and indeed at times appear to be almost overinvolved in clinical care. We are pleased by this and are more concerned about the parents who ask few questions and who appear stunned or overwhelmed by the problem. Parents who become involved in trying to find out what the best procedures are, and who ask many questions about care, are sometimes annoying, but often make the best adaptation in the end.

(6) Many anomalies are very frustrating to the physicians and nurses

as well. There is a temptation for the physician to withdraw from the parents who ask many questions and then appear to forget and ask the same questions over and over.

(7) Visiting. It is wise to extend the visiting hours in the maternity unit to allow the father to spend prolonged periods with his wife so that they can share their feelings and start working through their sequence of reactions as synchronously as possible.

(8) We have found it best to move at the parents' pace. If we move too quickly, we run the risk of losing the parents along the way. It is beneficial to ask the parents how they view their infant at the beginning of each discussion period.

(9) Possible retardation. We strongly believe that if there is a chance of the infant being retarded, we should not discuss it with the parent unless we know with almost absolute certainty that the infant is damaged. This controversial recommendation stems from the many cases in which excellent physicians expressed this suspicion, but later found that this was incorrect and then discovered that they could not convince the parents that the child was normal even years later. Many of these youngsters have subsequently experienced major developmental disturbances.

(10) Each parent may move through the process of shock, denial, anger, guilt and adaptation at a different pace. If they are unable to talk with each other about the baby, their own relationship may be disrupted. Therefore, we use the process of early crisis intervention and meet several times with the parents. During these discussions, we ask the mother how she is doing, how she feels her husband is doing, and how he feels about the infant. We then reverse the question and ask the father how he is doing and how he thinks his wife is progressing. The hope is that not only will they think about their own reactions but will also begin to consider each other's as well.

References

1. Warkany, J. (1971). *Congenital Malformations: Notes and Comments.* Chicago, Year Book Medical Publishers.

2. Bettelheim, B. (1972). How do you help a child who has a physical handicap? *Ladies Home J.*, *89*, 34.

3. Solnit, A. J., and Stark, M. H. (1961). Mourning and the birth of a defective child. *Psychoanal. Study Child*, *16*, 523.

4. Johns, N. (1971). Family reactions to the birth of a child with a congenital abnormality. *Med. J. Aust.*, *1*, 277.

5. Drotar, D., Baskiewicz, A., Irvin, N., Kennell, J. H., and Klaus, M. H.

(1975). The adaptation of parents to the birth of an infant with a congenital malformation: a hypothetical model. *Pediat.*, *56,* 710.

6. Daniels, L. L., and Berg, G. M. (1968). The crisis of birth and adaptive patterns of amputee children. *Clin. Proc. Child. Hosp. D.C.*, *24*, 108.

7. Roskies, E. (1972). *Abnormalities and Normalities: The Mothering of Thalidomide Children*. New York, Cornell University Press.

8. D'Arcy, E. (1968). Congenital defects: mothers' reactions to first information. *Brit. Med. J.*, *3*, 796.

9. Olshansky, S. (1962). Chronic sorrow: a response to having a mentally defective child. *Soc. Casework*, *73*, 190.

10. Carr, E. F., and Oppe, J. E. (1971). The birth of an abnormal child: telling the parents. *Lancet*, *2*, 1075.

11. Klaus, M., and Kennell, J. (1982). *Parent-Infant Bonding*. St. Louis, The C. V. Mosby Co.

14 MOURNING PERINATAL DEATH

Gillian C. Forrest

In England and Wales over 8,000[1] babies die each year in the perinatal period. In spite of the relative frequency of this tragic event, there has been little systematic research into the effects of the loss of a newborn baby on the family and the best ways of helping parents to cope. Giles[2] published one of the first reports in 1970, when he studied 40 women after their newborn baby died. Other accounts have followed, and it is now established that most women experience grief reactions similar to those following the loss of any loved person as described by Lindemann[3] and Parkes[4]. This is characterised by an initial period of numbness or disbelief, followed within a few hours or days by tearfulness, sadness, lethargy, insomnia, physical manifestations of anxiety (palpitations, choking feelings in the throat, etc.), irritability and social withdrawal. Searching for a cause of the baby's death, guilt and angry feelings are usual in the early stages. These symptoms tend to intensify in bouts – the 'pangs of grief'.

However, from anecdotal accounts of many authors, it is clear that typical grief reactions do occur, particularly after stillbirth. Lewis[5] has described unresolved grief reactions lasting ten years or more, with severe disruption of family relationships and personal functioning during this time. He attributes these abnormal reactions to the 'painful emptiness' and 'unreality' of a stillbirth, which may be enhanced by the management of the event in the maternity unit and later at home. The baby may be removed quickly, before the mother sees it, and the mother then be rapidly discharged. Funeral arrangements may be carried out by the hospital, with no parental involvement, and the baby then buried in a common, unmarked grave. Follow-up arrangements may be haphazard, with little or no opportunity for parents to discuss what went wrong or whether to plan future pregnancies. Professionals, friends and neighbours may all maintain a 'conspiracy of silence', concealing their own distress under aloofness or unavailability. This all contributes to the baby failing to have an identity, and without there being a real object to mourn, the bereavement process is hampered (as happens with relatives of persons 'missing, believed dead').

As an awareness of the plight of these parents has grown, recommendations for improving the management of a perinatal death have been made by obstetricians, paediatricians, psychiatrists and midwives. In the United States, Kennell and Klaus[6] have published guidelines, and in Britain, the National Stillbirth Study Group has produced a leaflet 'The Loss of Your Baby'[7] for parents and staff. These recommendations include encouraging parents to see, hold and name their baby, hold a funeral and have a marked grave, make opportunities for discussions with the medical staff involved, and obtain obstetric and genetic counselling.

To illustrate this approach, the management of a stillbirth or early neonatal death in the John Radcliffe Maternity Unit, Oxford, will be described. The management plan was set up in 1978 as part of a study evaluating the effectiveness of a programme of support and counselling for parents after perinatal death. Fifty families were recruited to the study, and follow-up was continued for 14 months. The detailed results of the study have been reported elsewhere.[8]

A Stillborn Baby

Like other workers in this field, we found that women whose baby had died *in utero* were very fearful of the labour and delivery, and had many unpleasant fantasies about what was happening to their dead baby. One woman wondered how it would be possible to give birth to a dead baby at all; another was tormented by the thought of delivering a 'decomposed, shapeless lump of cells'. If they expressed these uncertainties and fears, they were sometimes called 'morbid' or 'ghoulish' by the staff.

We aim to help parents prepare for the delivery by giving accurate information about any abnormalities known to be present, including the skin changes to be expected and reassuring them about the normal process of birth and pain relief. Husbands are encouraged to remain with their wives during labour. After the baby has been delivered, the midwife or the obstetrician suggests that the parents see and hold their baby and bring him to them. If any abnormalities are present, these are described first and then shown to the parents along with all the baby's normal parts. (In describing this 6 and 14 months later, the parents of deformed babies all focused on these normally-formed parts and none had found the experience of seeing their deformed baby horrifying or distressing.) If the parents do not wish to see the baby at all, a photograph is taken and kept in the notes for possible use later. Many of the parents who refuse, do, in fact, regret their decision weeks or even months later, and are then glad to have the photograph. They are all encouraged to name the baby. Afterwards, some parents like to be left alone together, to share their grief in private.

If a mother has been heavily sedated during labour, or had a Caesarian section, we offer her the opportunity of seeing her baby later when she has recovered sufficiently. One of the midwives may bring the baby to her room, or she and her husband may be taken down to the chapel where the baby is laid out.

A Baby Dying in the Special Care Unit

When a woman is in premature labour, or where there is known to be fetal distress, the paediatrician will try to see the parents before delivery, to prepare them and describe the special care unit. The parents usually see their baby at delivery, before he is taken to the special care unit, but often this is very rushed because of the baby's poor condition. A photograph of the baby is taken as soon as possible for the mother to keep at her bedside. Both parents are encouraged to visit the unit in order to see and touch their baby, and the staff try to keep them closely informed of the baby's progress. When the baby's condition is known to be deteriorating, the parents are told, so that they can be with him when he dies. A minister of religion is called in if they wish. If at all possible, the parents and baby are placed in a separate single room with the minimum of equipment present. They are encouraged to hold him as he dies, and afterwards, if the mother wishes, she can help with the laying out.

Where a baby has suffered irreparable damage during delivery or afterwards, the parents have to adjust from a position of hope of recovery to one of accepting that their baby will inevitably die. This is a most painful transition for them to make, and will produce shock and numbness, followed sooner or later by intense feelings of grief and protest (anger). We try, whenever possible, to break this news to parents in private so that they can release feelings without inhibition. At this time, or later, they will have many questions to ask about what has gone wrong and the information may have to be repeated many times over before they can grasp it. In our experience, parents in these circumstances are seeking explanations and expressions of sympathy from the staff and a chance to ventilate their own feelings. Only when these are absent do they seek legal redress.

The Post-mortem Examination

The information provided by a careful post-mortem examination or necropsy can clearly be important in establishing the cause of the baby's death and in identifying congenital abnormalities and any genetic implications. However, many parents, distraught at losing their baby, find giving consent for this examination very difficult. One mother put it like this: 'She's been through enough. Must she be cut up now as well?' Parents can be helped to overcome this instinctual reluctance to consent by their doctor explaining to them that the examination is necessary to clarify what has gone wrong and if it is likely to happen again. Even so, there will be some parents who refuse. In these circumstances, it is important to assess the likelihood of the necropsy yielding vital information in each individual case, before pressurising the parents to agree. Pressure will make parents feel torn between their protective feelings for their baby, even though he is dead, and their desire to comply with their doctor's wishes. For some of them the only way to resolve this conflict may be to leave the hospital altogether and withdraw from any further contact, thus increasing the likelihood of unresolved grief reactions. It follows from this discussion that the results of the post-mortem examination will be very important to parents, and it is essential that they are given an opportunity later on to receive these. (See section on 'follow-up arrangements' below.)

Afterwards. The parents will be in a state of shock and numbness for a few hours or days before they can accept the reality of their baby's death. One woman, describing her reaction to her stillborn baby, said, 'We looked at her in our arms, and I thought, she's asleep. Why doesn't she just wake up now?' Another said, 'His mouth came open as we held him, and I thought, he's coming alive!' Although medical staff do give explanations to the parents at this stage of what seems to have gone wrong, it is likely that these will have to be repeated later, perhaps several times. It may not be until the follow-up appointment several weeks later that parents are able to take in the information.

Wherever possible, the mother is given the choice of a single room on the isolation floor or in the postnatal ward, or a return to her own (four-bedded) ward. It is perhaps surprising that some women prefer to return to their own ward, for the support of the friends they may have there. A few certainly wish to have contact with other babies straight away, 'I've got to face up to it, and I'd rather do it now than postpone it.'

The parents are given a copy of the 'Loss of Your Baby' leaflet and the telephone number of the local member of the Stillbirth and Perinatal Death Association. The midwives try to help parents express their feelings, and are urged not to hurry away if they come in and find the woman, or her husband, in tears. Lactation is discussed – many women assume that they will not lactate if the baby has died – and help is offered with the necessary registration and funeral arrangements (see below). Discharge is not hurried, to allow time for contact with the hospital social worker, who offers support while mourning is being established and assesses the couple's supportive network at home. The results of the Oxford study and that of Raphael's [9] work in Australia suggest that unsupported bereaved persons are more at risk of atypical reactions, so extra community support is mobilised for any couples in this situation, from ministers, health visitors, the local Stillbirth and Perinatal Death Association, etc. The community midwife and the general practitioner are informed of all babies' deaths as soon as possible, so that they can arrange to visit the parents in the maternity unit before discharge. The couples we interviewed welcomed contact with familiar figures in these early stages, and it greatly increased their sense of being supported if these visits were made.

Registration and Funeral Arrangements

For most young couples, this will be their first experience of bereavement, and they are bewildered by the complicated administrative procedure of registering the baby's death or stillbirth and arranging a funeral. We believe that, by helping parents with these arrangements, some of their distress can be relieved. These have been described in detail elsewhere[10] but a short account is given here.

Registration

In the United Kingdom, all neonatal deaths and stillbirths (i.e. babies born dead after 28 weeks gestation) have to be registered by the Registrar of Births, Marriages and Deaths. Such babies then have to be properly buried or cremated. In some places, a branch of the Registrar's office is attached to the hospital, but in others (including Oxford), parents have to travel to the central office in the town. They take the Medical Certificate of Cause of Death or Stillbirth provided by a doctor to the Registrar's office and he then supplies a Certificate of Burial or Cremation which is required by the undertaker (see Figure 14.1).

Figure 14.1: Registration and Funeral Arrangements.

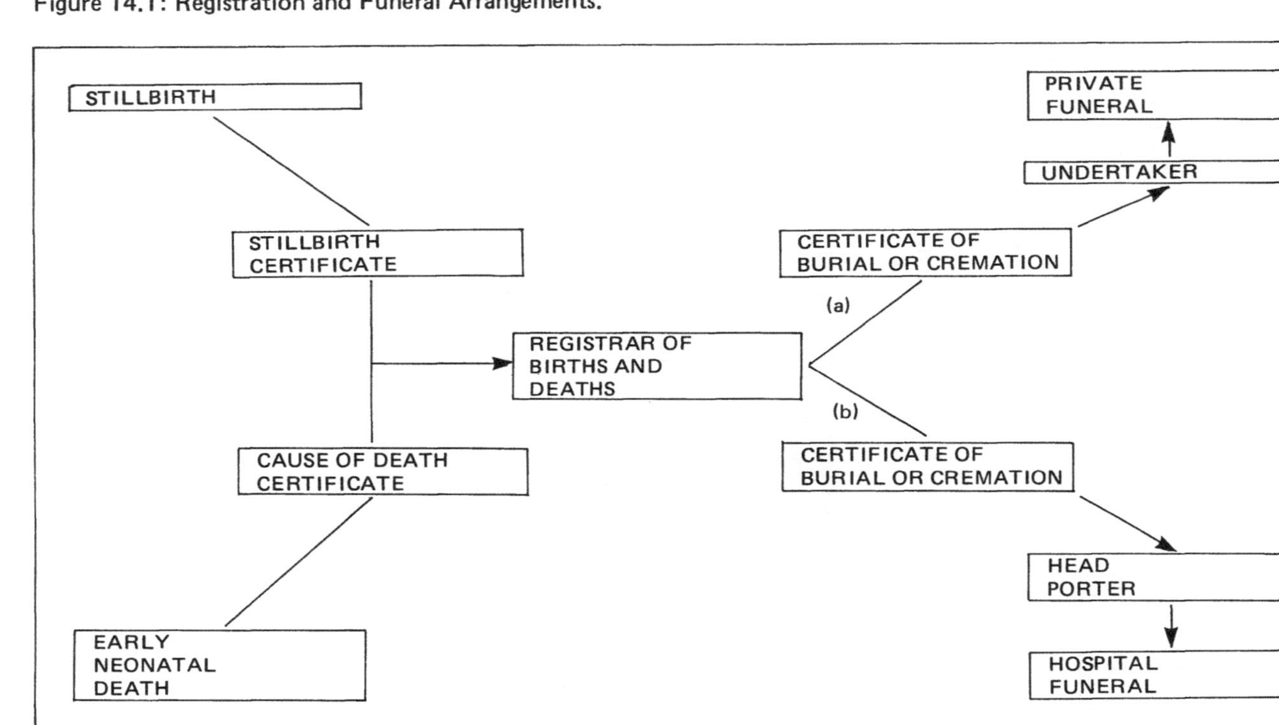

Parents of stillborn babies are often shocked to discover that they cannot register a first name for their baby. Efforts are being made by the National Stillbirth Study Group and others to get the law changed on this point. Meanwhile, in Oxford, we try to overcome this by recording the baby's names in a special register for the parents.

Sometimes – and increasingly – parents of babies under 28 weeks gestation who are born dead ask if they can hold a funeral. This is not a legal requirement, but there is nothing to prevent parents doing so.[11] The undertaker will require a note from the attending doctor stating the gestation of the baby and the (presumed) cause of death, and authorising the undertaker to proceed with burial or cremation.

Funeral Arrangements. The funeral can be arranged either by the hospital (with a contracted firm of undertakers), or privately. The DHSS has directed hospital administrators to meet the costs of any stillborn baby's funeral, unless the parents wish to pay for this themselves. Parents of neonatal deaths may claim the death grant (currently £9) to 'offset' the cost of the funeral.

The advantages of the hospital-arranged funeral are that parents are relieved of the burden of making the arrangements and the costs are minimal. The main disadvantage is that it prevents parents from being involved in this important part of the mourning rituals. In some cases, parents are told that they cannot attend the funeral; they often have great difficulty locating the site of the grave later; and they usually find that they cannot mark the grave. In addition, there are frequently many myths and misconceptions about the hospital-arranged funeral – e.g. that the babies are, in fact, disposed of in the hospital incinerator; that they are buried in mass graves without coffins or ceremony; or that the funeral may be delayed for weeks or months. In Oxford, some of these 'myths' were found to be based on fact – before 1978, babies in our area were sometimes not buried for up to ten weeks and the undertakers strongly discouraged parents from attending the funeral.

To improve the care of bereaved parents, it is clearly important for staff to be able to give them accurate information about the funeral arrangements applying locally, and discuss with them their needs and wishes. Our hospital-arranged funeral provides a white coffin and a grave in the local cemetery which has a total capacity (over the years) of seven babies. Parents can attend and the hospital chaplain is always prepared to offer his services. It is possible for parents to mark the grave by purchasing an exclusive grave for an extra fee. It has also proved possible to overcome the difficulties of finding the grave later by arranging with the cemetery clerk at the local Town Hall for it to be flagged temporarily when parents visit the cemetery. A Bereaved Persons' Welfare Officer has now been appointed, to help parents with these arrangements. She also teaches the maternity staff about these complicated adminstrative procedures.

Follow-up Arrangements

These are planned to ensure that the parents receive obstetric counselling, genetic counselling (where appropriate) and an opportunity to discuss the baby with his paediatrician. As has already been discussed, the post-mortem results are particularly important for parents as they frequently find it so difficult to give consent for the post-mortem. A senior obstetrician (for a stillborn baby) or senior paediatrician (for a neonatal death) include these results in their discussions. We have found that asking general practitioners to do this is unsatisfactory as on the whole they do not have the specialist knowledge to discuss the results and their implications with parents. These follow-up interviews are arranged between three and six weeks after the baby's death or stillbirth – allowing time for the post-mortem results to be available and for the parents to have recovered from the initial numbing impact of the baby's loss. Although parents are usually willing to return to the hospital for the interview it tends to be distressing for them if they are given a routine appointment in the postnatal or paediatric clinic, particularly as this increases the possibility that some member of staff will not realise that their baby died.

The Course of Mourning a Newborn Baby

Grief is usually intense and constant initially, and then gradually the 'pangs of grief' described earlier occur with lessening frequency. They tend to be preciptated by reminders of the dead baby – e.g.: the funeral; the expected date of delivery, if he was premature; the onset of the first period; the first Christmas or anniversary of his death; as well as by less specific things – baby clothes, a piece of unfinished knitting, the baby counter in the chemist's shop.

Insomnia is very common, but is best left to resolve spontaneously over the first few weeks. Ideas of guilt and self-blame may take over from the early searching for extraneous causes of the baby's death and intense guilt feelings may be experienced by women who have had a previous termination of pregnancy. (One woman was convinced that the angry jealous spirit of her terminated baby had taken his revenge on this much loved and wanted baby. She eventually 'appeased' the spirit by buying a set of baby clothes for him and placing them in the coffin.) Many couples experience difficulties relating with their friends and neighbours in the early weeks. They find themselves avoided by those who know that the baby died, and dread being asked about the 'new' baby by those who have not yet heard. Friends may not know that bereaved people need to rehearse the events around the death for a long time, and try to cheer the parents up by switching the conversation to a neutral topic. The parents then feel they are being 'boring' and may withdraw socially for many months until the need passes. Many bereaved mothers experience destructive feelings towards other babies for a time; these are frightening and upsetting and may lead them to withdraw from any contact with children. They are often reassured to find that these feelings occur very commonly and pass with time.

Fathers tend to cope by plunging themselves back into work activities as soon as possible. They appear to have shorter bereavement reactions than the mothers – in our study, 86 per cent of the fathers had recovered from the psychological symptoms of bereavement by six months, compared with only 50 per cent of the mothers. For some couples this disparity in their grief reactions strains their relationship; for others it seems that the man readily takes on the supportive role, and they are drawn closer. Parents with other children at home often describe difficulties handling their questions about the baby, e.g. a four-year-old: 'Why can't you go back to the hospital, Mummy, and fetch her when she's not dead any more?' A three-year-old: 'What did I do? Hurt the baby so it went away?' The children's own grief reactions appear to be relatively brief, except when their parents, usually mother, remain severely depressed, lethargic and withdrawn for several months. Then, naughtiness at home or school, or withdrawal, sadness and preoccupation with death, coffins, etc., may be seen.

Twins

A particularly difficult set of circumstances arises if one twin dies and the other survives. It is quite common for the parents and the staff to rejoice in the survival of the one baby and not mourn the other's death, even to the point of denying his or her existence at all. However, there have been many accounts of subsequent relationship problems between mothers and their surviving twin. He may have to take on the identity of his dead sibling as well as his own, which may be very onerous, or his mother may desperately overprotect him. In other cases the mother may idealise the dead twin and make constant unfavourable comparisons between the survivor and him. These problems can be avoided if time and opportunity are given to the parents to grieve for their dead twin and we aim to do this by encouraging parents to name him, attend the funeral and have a marked grave.

The Next Pregnancy

For many women, recovery is marked by embarking on another pregnancy. However, anxieties have been expressed that women may seek another 'replacement' baby[12] before they have sufficiently mourned the dead baby. It appears that pregnancy inhibits grieving and mourning[13] and so it seems important that women wait long enough to mourn one baby before conceiving again. In any case, they need to feel able to cope with the inevitable anxiety of the next pregnancy and delivery. The Stillbirth and Perinatal Death Association suggest that this may take nine months or more. It is likely to vary a great deal for the individual woman, but the more strongly the identity of the dead baby has been established and the more completely he has been mourned, the less likely it is that the 'replacement baby syndrome' will occur.

Training

To help parents cope with the loss of their baby, staff need some training in the psychological, as well as the technical, aspects of care. Without acquiring some skills in this area, junior medical and nursing staff will tend to withdraw from a situation which is painful and difficult. Apart from lectures, some units have found that discussion groups are helpful, enabling staff to discuss their own, and their patients', attitudes to death and dying. In Oxford, a member of the child psychiatry department regularly attends ward rounds in the maternity unit and special care baby unit, and close liaison has been established with the department of medical social work.

Conclusion

The death of a newborn baby is a tragic event, particularly now that our expectations of the safe delivery of a healthy baby are so high. Mourning can be difficult, but the practical management outlined in this chapter will help reduce the distress of parents and facilitate the recovery of the family from its loss.

References

1. Office of Population Censuses and Surveys (1980). Monitor DH 3 81/3. London, HMSO.

2. Giles, P. (1970). Reactions of women to perinatal death. *Aust. N. Z. J. Obstet. Gynaecol.*, *10*, 207.

3. Lindemann, E. (1944). Symptomatology and management of acute grief. *Am. J. Psychiatry*, *101*, 141.

4. Parkes, C. M. (1964). The effects of bereavement on physical and mental health. *Br. Med. J.*, *2*, 274.

5. Lewis, E., and Page, A. (1978). Failure to mourn a stillbirth – an overlooked catastrophe. *Br. J. Med. Psychol.*, *51*, 237.

6. Klaus, M. H., and Kennell, J. H. (1976). *Maternal-Infant Bonding*. St Louis, C. V. Mosby.

7. 'The Loss of Your Baby'. Booklet produced by the Health Education Council, London, in conjunction with the National Association for Mental Health and the National Stillbirth Study Group.

8. Forrest, G. C., Standish, E., and Baum, J. D. (1982). Support after perinatal death. *Br. Med. J.*, *285*, 1475.

9. Raphael, B. (1977). Preventative intervention with the recently bereaved. *Arch. Gen. Psychiatry*, *34*, 1450.

10. Forrest, G. C., Claridge, R., and Baum, J. D. (1981). The practical management of perinatal death. *Br. Med. J.*, *282*, 31.

11. Jolly, H. (1976). Family reactions to child bereavement. *Proc. Roy. Soc. Med.*, *69*, 835.

12. Cain, A. C., and Cain, B. S. (1964). On replacing a child. *J. Am. Acad. Child Psychiatry*, *3*, 443.

13. Lewis, E. (1979). Inhibition of mourning by pregnancy: psychopathology and management. *Br. Med. J.*, *2*, 27.

15 DISCHARGING PRE-TERM BABIES FROM NEONATAL UNITS

D. P. Davies and F. M. Derbyshire

Until 1978 very low birthweight babies (birthweight below 1.5 kg) who were looked after on the neonatal unit of the Leicester Royal Infirmary Maternity Hospital were required to reach a weight of 2.20 kg before being discharged home. This rather rigid policy was in keeping with traditional practices in Britain of delaying discharge of these babies until they reached a predetermined weight, usually in the range of 2.20-2.50 kg. Our practice changed radically, however, when the results of a randomised control trial conducted on our neonatal unit revealed that these babies could be sent home whatever their weight so long as they were clinically well and had passed the nadir of postnatal weight loss, provided of course that home conditions were satisfactory.[1] These findings confirmed earlier observations from studies undertaken in the USA,[2,3] Jamaica,[4] Zimbabwe[5] and Ethiopia[6].

With so much attention now being given to preventing unnecessary and prolonged separation of mother and baby after birth and with great pressures on cot occupancy in neonatal units, it is a constant source of surprise to us to discover that in Britain weight criteria are still widely used to determine the time to send preterm babies home. In this chapter we present our experiences in sending home preterm babies from our neonatal unit implementing the findings of our earlier research.

Clinical Methods

From January 1978 to June 1980, 103 babies of 32 weeks gestation and under or weighing less than 1.5 kg at birth were discharged home from the neonatal unit of Leicester Royal Infirmary Maternity Hospital when they were clinically well, had passed the nadir of postnatal weight loss and were feeding satisfactorily (three or four hourly on demand). A key to the success of this practice is the early and thereafter regular involvement of mothers and fathers with their baby, in order to help them form the bond which would otherwise have developed had physical separation not been enforced by premature delivery. This begins as soon as the baby is admitted to the neonatal unit when a photograph is taken for the mother to keep at her bedside.

Mother is visited regularly on the postnatal ward by neonatal unit nursing and medical staff if she is unable to visit the baby. As soon as she is well enough, frequent visiting is encouraged. The baby's progress is openly discussed with the parents and all the complicated technological equipment carefully explained in order to lessen the often frightening image of a space-age neonatal laboratory. The neonatal unit then becomes, hopefully, less intimidating. Brothers and sisters are encouraged to visit and toys are provided for them. Two years ago the routine wearing of gowns for staff and parents was abandoned in order to help create a less clinical environment. There has been no increase in the incidence of infection recorded: indeed a saving of several thousands of pounds per year has been made!

The aim of creating as relaxed an atmosphere as possible on the neonatal unit is to help the parents look after their baby as soon and as completely as possible. In the intensive care area this involvement includes gently touching the baby, cleaning the baby's mouth, changing napkins and tube feeding even if the baby is being ventilated. As the baby then progresses from the intensive care area through high dependency to special care, parents are encouraged to spend as much time as possible with their baby – bathing, feeding, making-up feeds and choosing clothes for the day. The attitudes of the nursing staff to feeding are crucial at this stage, as we encourage the babies to pass as quickly as possible through the various phases of tube feeding to breast/ bottle feeding.

Regardless of gestation, weight or age, a small feed of about 5 ml, or for a mother wishing to breast-feed, a short period of sucking at the breast, is offered once a baby ceases to need oxygen and is free of episodes of apnoea and bradycardia. If little interest is shown then this type of feed is offered only once a day. If the baby sucks well, these are increased to twice a day, and a few days later to thrice daily. At this stage the baby would still be having hourly tube feeds. He would then be changed to two-hourly tube feeds and when these were well tolerated to three-hourly. As the suck becomes stronger, a bottle or a breast feed is offered in a ratio of two tube feeds to one bottle or breast feed. Thereafter, and dictated by the baby's behaviour, the baby will be gradually weaned completely from the tube feeding. We have come to recognise that even the smallest of pre-term infants can feed normally at a much earlier age than many give them credit. This is obviously of great importance as we try to get them home sooner.

When the baby is asymptomatic, weather permitting, parents are encouraged to take him for a walk outside the hospital in prams which we provide. This gives the parents precious time to be with their own child, to make them feel they do have a real baby, and above all, to feel they are parents.

Home conditions are assessed by the general practitioner's health visitor when the time is approaching for the baby to go home, and assuming that the parents are happy and in agreement with the early discharge. A check that there are adequate and safe sources of heating (not necessarily central heating) is part of the initial home assessment antenatally by the community midwife and later by the family health visitor. If there are any problems such as damp in the home or lack of heating, this hopefully would be dealt with long before delivery or most certainly before discharge of the baby. The social worker will often be involved in helping to remedy the problem. Once the baby is home the mother is advised to heat the house no differently from normal, but what is emphasised is that during winter months the baby wears a vest constantly and is wrapped in a flannelette wrap under the blankets, that a bonnet is worn during the night and that the baby is roomed in with the parents: their bedroom will usually be warmer during the night than other rooms in the house. We sometimes wonder whether this last recommendation might diminish the chances of 'cot death'. With the baby sleeping at night in the same room as the parents, breathing disturbances would stand a better chance of being heard by the parents, making resuscitative attempts more possible.

Finally, before discharge the mother is encouraged to stay for a couple of nights and to have complete charge of the baby in her room but with the support of staff near at hand for any queries that might arise. After hospital discharge the babies are seen regularly in our follow-up clinic. The babies are seen initially around the time of their expected date of delivery. If at this age they are showing adequate weight gain, subsequent visits are at three-monthly intervals for a further twelve months. More frequent visits will be needed if particular problems develop. All babies will have a detailed neurodevelopmental assessment at eighteen months. The only supplement they receive is a standard vitamin supplement. Iron is not routinely prescribed and haemoglobin levels are not routinely checked.

Results

In this study we present information on the babies up to six months beyond their corrected age of term. Figure 15.1 shows the distribution

Figure 15.1: Individual Weights and Ages at Hospital Discharge.

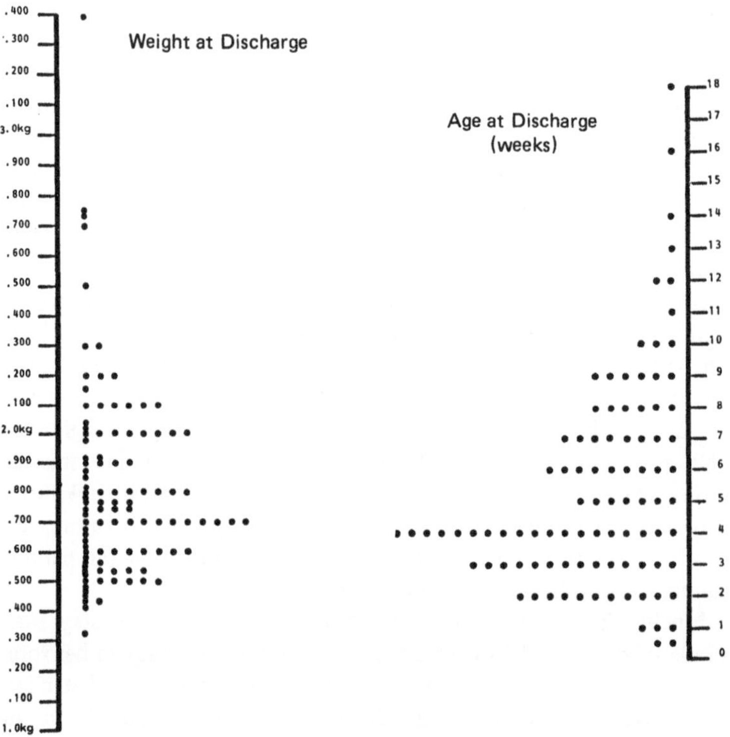

of the weight and age of each baby at discharge. These range from 1.3 kg to 3.4 kg with a mean of 1.83 kg. The average stay in hospital was five weeks, with a range of 3-7 weeks. Eighty-eight (86 per cent) of the babies were home before they had reached 2.2 kg, our previous 'traditional' weight for discharge. Eighteen (17 per cent) were discharged weighing 1.5 kg or less; about half of these were 'light-for-dates'. Social problems were largely responsible for delaying discharge beyond a weight of 2 kg. Examples of these include one mother who was educationally subnormal and needed to stay a long time in hospital before taking her baby home and another mother who was in hospital with ulcerative colitis and wished to see her baby every day. Eleven babies were admitted to hospital during the follow-up period. It is our practice to re-admit to the neonatal unit up to one month after discharge, beyond this time admissions being to a paediatric ward in the main hospital. Only one baby weighed less than 2.2 kg on admission, the indication being a 'top-up' transfusion for anaemia of prematurity. Other than one baby who was admitted with failure to thrive, all gained weight satisfactorily. None of the other babies would have avoided re-admission had they remained in hospital awaiting a discharge weight of 2.2 kg. Reasons for re-admission to hospital were unrelated to the decision when to send the baby home.

Discussion

Our experience over the last 2½ years confirms our earlier findings that there is little to justify the still widespread practice of delaying discharge of small babies from neonatal units until they reach a certain arbitrary weight. Health and progress of the baby along with the home situation are the essential determinants for sending babies home.

The early involvement of parents with their baby and the continuing practical care they are encouraged to give is critical to the success of an early discharge policy. By the time our discharge criteria are fulfilled, the parents are already looking after their baby and the fact that the baby is still often very small seems no longer important. Going home then becomes a logical sequel, irrespective of the age or weight of the baby. However, all these prerequisites are worthless without there being good liaison between hospital and community services, especially the home health visitor. We have a liaison health visitor who visits the neonatal unit daily and notifies the baby's own health visitor of admission, progress and estimated time of discharge. In return, the liaison health visitor notifies the neonatal unit of home conditions, social problems, etc. The family doctor and health visitor will hopefully visit the family at home prior to the baby's discharge to establish an early relationship, thereby smoothing transition from hospital to home care. In Leicester, and in contrast to some other parts of Britain, there is no special community care service for babies discharged from the neonatal unit. Responsibility for supervising the care of these babies at home falls to the general practice health visitor. However, this seems not to significantly increase her workload as babies discharged are scattered throughout the city and at any one time it is unlikely that one health visitor will have more than one small baby. Furthermore, since the babies are healthy, albeit small, there is no real reason why more time should be spent with them than with any other baby. However, we do emphasise that the door is always open to babies who are discharged. Parents are encouraged to phone if they have any queries or problems and to visit at any time. The follow-up clinic is an integral part of this support system since it is organised entirely by the neonatal nursing and medical staff. Parents find it helpful and relaxing to see people whom they know well. Should admission to hospital be necessary in the early weeks after discharge, babies will (with few exceptions) be re-admitted to the neonatal unit and to maintain relationships care will be organised by the same staff that had previously looked after the baby. This can in most instances be assured, as cots are not full of babies waiting to achieve a predetermined weight.

Conclusion

Three possible complications of sending babies home early – feeding problems, maternal anxiety and increased community workload – have not materialised (Figure 15.2). An early discharge policy means fewer nursing hours spent on small but otherwise healthy babies, thereby affording more time for the care of those who are sick. Indeed we have estimated a saving of something in the order of 5,000 nursing hours per year, the amount of time taken to give routine care to babies staying in hospital until reaching a weight of 2.2 kg.

If early separation of babies from their mothers is unavoidable due to premature delivery, at least early re-uniting with the family is possible. The family will also save money on travel and the not inconsiderable inconvenience which so often arises in visiting babies in hospital. Prolonged and unnecessary separation after birth might also be potentially harmful for the psychological well-being of parents[7] and baby. It might also contribute to the risks of non-accidental injury, a problem to which preterm infants who are admitted to a neonatal unit are especially vulnerable.[8] A more critical appraisal of discharge policies might go some way to minimising these hazards.

Figure 15.2: The Balance of Early Discharge.

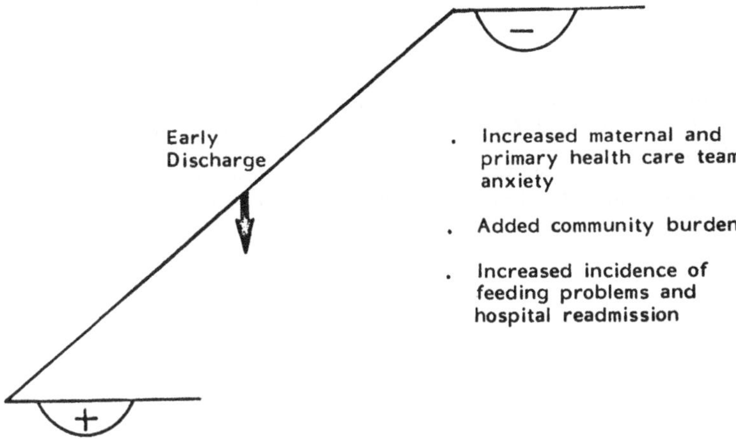
–
Early Discharge
. Increased maternal and primary health care team anxiety
. Added community burden
. Increased incidence of feeding problems and hospital readmission
+

- Saving of money (travel) and family inconvenience
- less interference with early mother-baby attachment
- More efficient use of nursing time on neonatal unit
- Less risk of hospital infection

Acknowledgements

We would like to thank the many nurses and doctors of the neonatal unit of the Leicester Royal Infirmary Maternity Hospital whose constant support and encouragement of parents have made it possible for small babies to be re-united at home with their families at the earliest possible time.

References

1. Davies, D. P., Haxby, V., Herbert, S., and McNeish, A. S. (1979). When should preterm babies be sent home from neonatal units? *Lancet*, *i*, 914.

2. Berg, R. B., and Salisbury, A. J. (1973). Discharging infants of low birth-weight. *Am. J. Dis. Child.*, *122*, 414.

3. Dillard, R. G., and Korones, S. B. (1973). Lower discharge weight and shortened nursery stay for low birthweight infants. *New Eng. J. Med.*, *288*, 131.

4. Lowry, F. M., Jones, M. R., and Shanahan, M. D. (1978). Discharging of small babies from hospital. *Arch. Dis. Child.*, *53*, 522.

5. Singer, B., and Wolfsdorf, J. (1975). Early discharge of infants of low birthweight: a prospective study. *Brit. Med. J.*, *i*, 362.

6. Tafari, N., and Sterky, C. J. (1974). Early discharge of low birthweight infants in a developing country. *Trop. Paediat.*, *20*, 73.

7. Editorial (1979). Separation and special care baby units. *Lancet*, *i*, 590-1.

8. Murphy, J. F., Jenkins, J., Newcombe, R. G., and Sibert, J. M. (1981). Objective birth data and the prediction of child abuse. *Arch. Dis. Child.*, *56*, 295.

Part Three

CASE STUDIES OF ROUTINES USED IN NEONATAL UNITS

INTRODUCTION

J. A. Davis, M.P.M. Richards and N.R.C. Roberton

So much for the theory. In the next six chapters there are descriptions of how paediatricians in Scandinavia, Africa, North and South America, and two hospitals in England, one a teaching hospital and the other a district general hospital, try to put it all into practice.

Each of the units, quite clearly, still has deficiencies in the way it works. For example, in Sweden, so often held up as the paradigm of perfect perinatal practice, 20 per cent of all babies born in the Karolinska are still admitted to the neonatal unit, albeit transiently. However, the author shows quite clearly how one particular group of high-risk infants, those born to diabetic mothers, can, particularly with first class antenatal management of the maternal diabetes, avoid neonatal unit admission. It would be nice if babies in Santiago could be spared a short routine early period of separation from their mothers, and perhaps fewer babies could be exposed to the physical risks of neonatal unit admission in High Wycombe as well as in Stockholm. Yet, none of the other units matches up to the High Wycombe one in the provision of mother-baby rooms. Given the patterns of postnatal ward care in Baragwanath and Santiago, and the weights at which infants are discharged from these units into torrid slum surroundings, it would seem that Cambridge and Montreal are hanging onto their 2.00 kg babies too long, particularly in the light of what is reported by Davies and Derbyshire (Chapter 15).

However, three messages come over loud and perfectly clear from all these chapters.

(1) As well as in 'sophisticated' Montreal or Cambridge, in areas with frightful socio-economic problems like Soweto and Santiago, infants can be safely discharged home when they weigh 2.00 kg or even slightly less.
(2) Mothers, no matter what their educational background, can cope with the immediate post-partum care of healthy infants weighing 1.80-2.00 kg or more.
(3) Extended parental involvement with sick very low birthweight infants is completely possible, as is the establishment of breast

feeding in such infants, and both can be achieved in many different ways given the enthusiastic co-operation of medical and nursing staff.

These three simple aspects of neonatal care are still sadly lacking in many neonatal units across North America and Western Europe. It is clear that they can be done safely and satisfactorily on units not only in socio-economically privileged communities, but can be done equally safely and just as successfully in the third world. Therein lies an important message for us all.

16 SPECIAL CARE WITHOUT SEPARATION: HIGH WYCOMBE, ENGLAND

Donald H. Garrow

Introduction

The special care baby unit (SCBU) at the Wycombe General Hospital has one feature which makes it unusual if not unique: there are enough rooms in the unit to enable most mothers to be admitted with their babies. The unit was planned between 1964 and 1966, and opened ten years later in June 1976. Paediatric and obstetric departments should always be as close as possible to each other, and these two departments at High Wycombe are sited in the same block. The children's ward and labour rooms and theatres are on the ground floor, the postnatal wards on the floor above.

The population of the district served is around 250,000 with about 3,000 deliveries a year and a yearly admission rate to the SCBU of some 250 babies and 200 mothers (see Table 16.1 for 1981 statistics). Though part of a district general hospital, and not a 'regional centre', limited intensive care is practised and two cots are designated for this. Babies who seem likely to require more than a few days of assisted ventilation are transferred to the regional centre, The John Radcliffe Hospital in Oxford.

The generous facilities for mothers in the Wycombe unit were requested not as a result of the work that was being done in the United States on the importance of early contact between mother and baby, but as a natural extension to the practice started 30 years ago by Dr Dermod MacCarthy and his colleagues, of admitting mothers to children's wards and involving them as fully as possible in the care of their own children: an application of the insight into the needs of the mothers of sick infants of Sir James Spence who founded the Babies Hospital in Newcastle-upon-Tyne in 1926.[1,2]

The admission of mothers to hospital with their children is now widely practised throughout Britain, though black spots remain, such as the wards of some surgical specialities. The attitude of paediatricians towards a premature baby has, until recently, been similar to that of such surgeons and dominated by a dread of cross-infection and the

Table 16.1: Wycombe General Hospital Special Care Baby Unit, Patient Statistics, January-December 1981.

Babies admitted to Special Care Baby Unit	293
Mothers admitted to Special Care Baby Unit	187
Number of deliveries in District	3,039
Number in Wycombe General Hospital	2,387
G. P. Maternity Home, Amersham General Hospital	175
G. P. Maternity Home, High Wycombe	476
Delivery at home	1
Babies transferred from other hospitals	16
Babies transferred to other hospitals	27
Number of babies pre-term	164
Number of babies small-for-dates	53
Number of babies low birthweight	142
Number of babies requiring intubation after delivery	59
RDS	46
Umbilical artery catheterised	27
Ventilated	16
Neonatal deaths	16
Hypothermia	16
Hypoglycaemia	6
Jaundice requring phototherapy	98
Infections	41
Blood in stools (all in first six months of year)	24

belief that newborn babies do not mind who looks after them as long as they are fed and kept warm. Whatever the baby may feel, mothers are often upset if their babies are taken away from them, and the common practice in European and North American hospitals of taking babies away from their mothers certainly makes many mothers unhappy and ill at ease. While following premature infants I became concerned at the frequency with which mothers reported feeling remote from their babies. They would say, for instance, 'I felt he wasn't really mine until I got him home.' Sometimes this feeling of the baby not really belonging lasted for weeks or months. Occasionally love seemed not to have been felt at all, but to have been buried under repeated anxieties and demands. It seems possible that some of the later disturbances of mother-child relatonship that every paediatrician sees might be due to neonatal separation interfering with the natural development of maternal feelings.[34] Whether this is true or not, the accumulation of individual anecdotes convinced me that it was at least as wrong and unnecessary to take a newborn baby away from a mother as to separate a toddler or older child admitted to hospital.

The High Wycombe Neonatal Unit

This unit has rooms for nine mothers (rooms 1-9, Figure 16.1). Each mother's room opens on one side to a common corridor through folding panel doors. This corridor provides ready access for her visitors and her obstetrician who looks after her as though she were on a postnatal ward. When the panel doors are closed there is still a gap above, which provides adequate ventilation but defective sound-proofing. The mothers' rooms corridor has direct access to a patio and grass-covered banks. The outside wall is south-facing and consists of fine sheets of glass (12 × 1½ ft), separated by vertical black supporting strips. During the summer, as might have been anticipated, the green-house effect from this arrangement results in intolerable overheating and has necessitated the installation of electrically operated silver coloured blinds. The mothers' rooms open on the other side into the nurseries. Five of the rooms have small intermediate cubicles (1c-6c, Figure 16.1). The nursing areas can, therefore, be approached from the mothers' rooms as well as from a working corridor off which is the nurses' station. As far as possible a mother will be given a room which leads directly into the appropriate nursery. The door between her room and the nursery has an observation panel, and is not felt to be a barrier between her and her baby to whom she is allowed free access at all times.

The number of babies in the unit at any one time has ranged from 5 to 18. On a number of occasions mothers have been unable to accompany their babies because all nine rooms were occupied. Our experience suggests that ten mothers' rooms for 15 cots would be a proper ratio. Our nursing establishment at present is 24 whole-time equivalents, 16 by day and eight by night:

3 sisters	6½ nursery nurses
5½ staff midwives	2½ staff nurses
4 state enrolled nurses	2½ nursing auxiliaries

It might be thought that having mothers continuously around would lighten nursing duties, but this is not so, provision for extra nursing staff being necessary to cope, not so much with the physical requirements of the mothers, as with their natural and inevitable anxieties and questions.

When the unit first opened there were unexpected difficulties. The obstetric and midwifery staff were reluctant to 'discharge' their patients

Figure 16.1: Wycombe General Hospital Special Care Baby Unit.

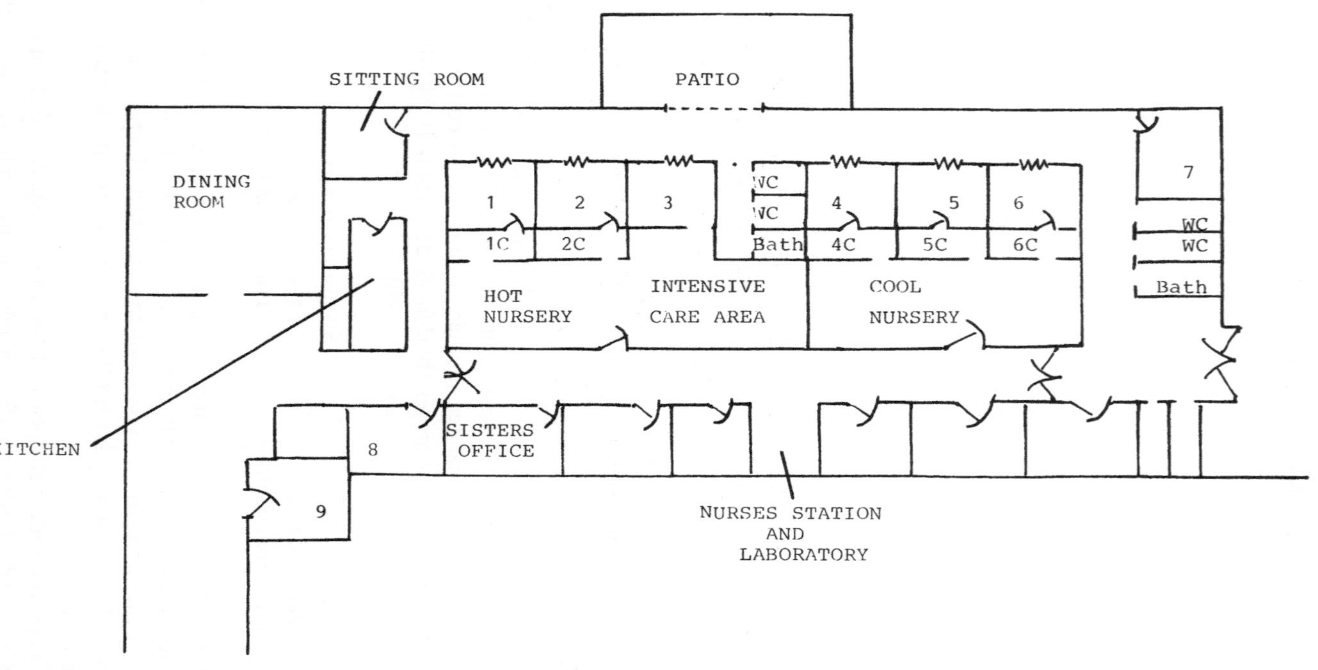

immediately after delivery because of the danger of postpartum haemorrhage. For the first six months that the SCBU was fully functional there was an average delay of 33 hours before mothers could join their infants. This impasse was overcome, not by persuading those in charge that anyone could be quickly trained to recognise the signs of a postpartum haemorrhage, but by employing fully trained midwives to look after the babies *and* their mothers. This simple solution forced on us by interdepartmental protectionism has been, in the long run, of inestimable value. The same nurse looks after mother and baby. This is, of course, how it should be, and to have nurses of different disciplines looking after each is absurd.

Criteria for Admission

Provided she is not ill, the mother accompanies her baby to the unit from the labour ward. Some 80 per cent of the babies admitted have their mothers with them for the first few hours of life. Premature babies, plus all those needing intensive observation or therapy, are admitted to the 'hot' nursery, graduating to the cooler nursery or their mother's room before discharge. We try to keep the number of admissions down (below 10 per cent of the deliveries in the district) and, since the mother comes in with her baby, we hope an admission which turns out to have been unnecessary, will have done no harm.

A number of babies are admitted with comparatively trivial conditions (see Table 16.1). If their mothers had not been able to be admitted with them, they would probably have been managed on the postnatal ward. Since admission to our unit does not entail separation from their mothers we believe that, for instance, phototherapy for hyperbilirubinaemia is better given in the unit. We give phototherapy to full-term babies when their plasma bilirubin reaches 280 mmol/l, and have been impressed by the amount of anxiety caused by this procedure. Having the mothers resident underlines how surprisingly great the anxiety can be – how parents seldom really understand the physiology, and how much patient explanation and re-explanation may be necessary.

Maternal Involvement in Care

A mother's involvement in the care of her baby may include being present and helping with practical procedures such as tube feeding, and sometimes holding her baby for the taking of diagnostic blood samples or lumbar punctures or watching an exchange transfusion. If a baby is on a respirator, the machine and the significance of the monitoring leads are explained as fully as possible. It might seem that to allow a mother to sit by the side of her intensively-cared-for premature infant would be to subject her to an intolerable strain. Physically all she may be able to do is to hold a hand or foot or stroke some small area of her baby not covered by monitoring equipment; but this is something. We believe that the more she can be involved in understanding the problems that arise the better able she will be to cope with her anxieties. By her presence she demonstrates to herself and to the staff that 'this is my baby'.

When she is in her room she knows her baby is 'through there' and that she can, without asking permission, go in at any time and see how things are. Her ordeal and inevitable anxieties enlist everyone's sympathy and understanding. In a sudden emergency she will not be excluded. When the diagnosis is clear, as it may be for instance in the case of a pneumothorax, she will be told what has happened and what needs to be done. When there is uncertainty this is frankly admitted and the purpose of further investigations explained. A mother's involvement is encouraged but of course not insisted upon, and she may need and choose to go home to her husband for a few nights, or have him stay the night with her. We have z-beds for this purpose which can be put up in the mother's rooms, but so far we have no double beds.

Family Involvement

Visiting by fathers, siblings and grandparents is, of course, encouraged. It is a joy for staff to be able to share with the whole family the progress and recovery of any baby, especially when the illness has been severe and there has been much anxiety. The availability of an area which can be used as a common dining room is a great asset; it helps mothers to support each other and feel that they are to some extent 'in the same boat'.

Herding newborn babies together in a SCBU increases the risk of cross-infection. It has been a worry that having families together, as we have, might increase this hazard. We have been particularly sensitive to this possibility, but we have found no evidence that relatives or siblings do in fact bring infection into the unit. In our only outbreak of cross-infection in the unit – rectal bleeding in association with *Clostridium paraputrificum* in stool culture – the organism was probably introduced to the unit by a member of staff.

Procedure on Ward Rounds

On a ward round the baby's case is presented. If the parents are there, they are included in the discussion. If the baby is on a ventilator, both parents will probably be there, eager for the most up-to-date news. If they are not already conversant with the functions of the various leads, the respirator settings, the flow chart for blood gases, and other recordings, they are told about these in appropriate detail. Parents may, of course, have considerable expertise and be helpful in sorting out the problem of record keeping and the breakdown of recording equipment. The mothers are then visited in their rooms. The structure of the unit makes it easy for everyone to observe good manners. Thus, the consultant will knock at the mother's room door, apologise for disturbing her, and with a 'May we sit down?' does so. A discussion takes place, the mother tells what problems there have been with her baby, how they are being tackled and expresses any anxieties that she may have. She may be asked for suggestions for improvements, either to the structure or function of the unit. One mother may find the lack of privacy and inadequate soundproofing a little irksome, another will welcome the arrangement, enjoying the facility of being able to talk to a neighbour as in a dormitory. We have learned that a common dining room is much appreciated, as is the friendliness and support of the other mothers and staff. We have learned how important privacy is and how good it is for a mother to have some time entirely alone with her baby, away from nursing staff whose eyes, however friendly, are inevitably observing and apparently critical.

Care of the Dying Baby

Sometimes every active effort fails and it becomes clear that a baby is dying. After the news has been broken to the parents the baby is taken off the respirator and placed in a cot with its mother in her cubicle, to be watched over and touched and taken, if she wishes, into her arms to die. In the almost open living arrangements of a unit such as ours a death cannot be covered up or denied. Nor should it be so. Though sad, such a death is both graceful and dignified.

Care of the Malformed Baby

The management of a baby with severe congenital abnormalities caused us initial anxieties. The policy that we adopt when a severely abnormal baby is born is as follows: if at birth resuscitation is thought to be required, it is given, since it is usually impossible to judge the severity of the abnormalities in the time available. The news is broken to the parents as early as possible and if possible they are told together. Who does the telling will vary with the circumstances. Also we have to remember that little can be taken in at a first interview, that a mother's initial reaction may not be her considered opinion, and that she will need support on many subsequent occasions. If an operation is possible the choice of its advisability has to be made, but who should decide? Should it be the parents, the family doctor or paediatrician, the grandparents, a panel of experts or a pressure group, religious sect or legal experts? It is very clear to me that it is for the parents to decide with all the help and information they can be given and in my experience they are very good at doing so. It may help to give an example of the way such problems are handled. A baby is recognised within a few hours of birth to be an example of Down's syndrome with duodenal atresia and an operation is required to save life. Parental consent is required for the operation. The parents, in coming to their decision, must be given as much information about the prognosis after the operation as they are capable of grasping; the good as well as the bad. The effects of a handicapped child on other members of the family must be pointed out. Some will feel that they can accept a mongol baby with their other children and others will feel that they cannot. They are told of the help and support that they will receive from parents' groups and from their family doctor, social services and the hospital. The presence of a fatal complication in a baby with Down's syndrome may be regarded as a merciful deliverance and I wholeheartedly support a decision not to operate in these circumstances and give such drugs as may be necessary to prevent discomfort and suffering until the baby dies. The parents will be seen afterwards in order to help them in their grief and to understand the guilt which, however, in my experience is no greater than parents always feel when they lose a child.

The problems of a baby with severe congenital abnormalities such as spina bifida are discussed and re-discussed on ward rounds. It must not be forgotten that other parents on the unit will know something of what has happened and what is being done. They may be upset and need an explanation and support. Parents' wishes must always be respected, but they cannot always be complied with. For instance, if the doctor is asked to kill a baby, he must explain that he must act within the law. I draw a clear distinction between killing and allowing to die. However much everyone may hope for a speedy death, drugs must only be given for pain and discomfort. In following the difficult but consistent course of non-intervention, one can ensure that a child does not suffer, but has full nursing care and the comfort of physical contact. To allow death to come in such a way to a severely handicapped baby may be a seemly and loving thing to do.

Discussion

How important is it to provide rooms for mothers in a SCBU? Might it not be better to allow free access for parents to come and go as they please, looking after their babies during the day and then going home? I have worked in units with both facilities and the difference is very striking. The room that a mother has in High Wycombe is *her* room as well as part of the unit. The nursing staff and mothers get to know each other well and are on first name terms. It is not 'they' who know, telling 'us' who do not know what to do, but women sharing a common task. A nurse will encourage a mother to grin and bear it if she is 'sore down below' following the repair of an episiotomy in the first day or so and will help her to struggle the few necessary paces to see her baby rather than lie back with an analgesic and 'get some rest'. The presence of resident mothers influences the behaviour of medical staff as well as nurses. For example, when working in the unit, medical staff must never forget that there will almost always be mothers within earshot.

Is it really important for mothers to be so much involved with their sick or premature newborn babies? The difficulties in demonstrating objectively that neonatal separation in the long run makes differences at all have been outlined in Chapter 1. That so many families survive neonatal care is merely an indication of how resilient human beings are.

Resilient they may be, but many who have experienced both separation from, and involvement with, their newborn babies feel that it helps to be there. Neonatology, like other branches of medicine, is concerned with humanity as well as science.

References

1. MacCarthy, D. (1957). Mothers in a children's ward. *Public Health*, *71*, 264.

2. MacCarthy, D., Lindsay, M., and Morris, I. (1962). Children in hospital with mothers, *Lancet*, *i*, 603.

3. Garrow, D. H., and Smith, D. M. (1976). The modern practice of separating a newborn baby from its mother. *Proc. Roy. Soc. Med.*, 69, 22.

4. Garrow, D. H., and Smith, D. M. (1978). Relationship between mother and neonate. In *The Place of Birth*, S. Kitzinger and J. A. Davis (eds). Oxford, Oxford Medical Publications, 191.

17 NEONATAL CARE IN THE CAMBRIDGE UNIT

C. Whitby, C. M. de Cates and N. R. C. Roberton

The Cambridge neonatal unit (NNU) has 24 cots and serves three purposes:

(1) It provides all the neonatal services for approximately 4,000 infants delivered per annum in the Cambridge Maternity Hospital (CMH).
(2) It provides neonatal special care for four small neighbouring maternity units (in Ely, Royston, Huntingdon and Newmarket) which together deliver approximately 2,000 babies per annum (Table 17.1).
(3) It is the designated intensive care unit for the East Anglian RHA (Counties of Norfolk, Suffolk and Cambridgeshire), and also provides intensive care for maternity hospitals in the counties of Essex, Hertfordshire and Bedfordshire, thus serving a population of approximately 2.5 million. This regional commitment in the unit comprises about half of all neonates who require intensive care each year, and of these babies about a half are transferred to the CMH *in utero*.

Table 17.1: Catchment Area of Cambridge Maternity Hospital (CMH) Neonatal Unit – Number of Infants Delivered.

	Mill Road (CMH)	Surrounding Maternity Units: Ely, Newmarket, Huntingdon & Royston	Total
1981	4,185	1,818	6,003
1980	4,251	1,850	6,101
1979	4,133	1,815	5,948
1978	3,903	1,764	5,667
1977	3,352	1,846	5,198
1976	3,324	2,061	5,385

From what is written in other chapters in this book, it is clearly important to avoid mother-infant separation in the neonatal period, and in this chapter, we will concentrate on the three aspects of neonatal care in our unit specifically designed to minimise the effect of this separation when a neonate *has* to be admitted to our unit because he is ill or low birthweight. These are:

(1) Strict admission criteria for admission and discharge from the NNU.
(2) Procedures for supporting the families of infants who have to be on the NNU.
(3) Transitional care.

Criteria for Admission to, and Discharge from the NNU

For the reasons given in Chapter 5 we have only two criteria for admission to our unit: (1) a birthweight of less than 1.80-2.00 kg and (2) signs of illness in an infant of any birthweight. In Chapter 5 we have discussed in detail the effects of this policy, and it is clear that it is very rare for infants on postnatal wards to have fits or apnoeic attacks, become hypoglycaemic or seriously jaundiced, or develop late onset respiratory disease, and if they do, they do not come to any harm as a result. In an analysis of over 16,000 babies transferred to the postnatal wards with their mothers over several years our admission policy has been found to be safe.

Early Discharge of Infants from the NNU

With infants for whom there is no alternative but neonatal unit admission one important way of minimising mother-infant separation is to discharge the baby as soon as it is safe to do so. This can be done in three ways:

(1) Infants born to mothers resident outside Cambridge are transferred back to their local hospital with their mothers once they have recovered from their illness.
(2) Infants can join their mothers on the postnatal ward.
(3) Healthy infants whose mothers have been discharged can themselves be discharged as soon as possible.

Infants Discharged to Referring Hospital

Most of the hospitals in our catchment area which refer women antenatally with high-risk pregnancies, or which refer infants postnatally for intensive care, have consultant paediatric services which are fully capable of looking after low birthweight infants requiring only routine neonatal care. It has, therefore, been our policy to discharge to these units infants who no longer require intensive care. Table 17.2 shows that we have become more confident in this practice and have tended to transfer the infants back sooner and at lower birthweights.

Table 17.2: Infants Discharged to Referring Hospital, Age and Weight on Discharge.

	Birthweight below 1.50 kg			Birthweight 1.50-1.99 kg		
	Age on Transfer Back (Days)	Wt on Transfer	No.	Age on Transfer Back (Days)	Wt on Transfer	No.
1977	26	1.35	14	12	1.75	10
1978	26	1.35	19	8	1.66	14
1979	24	1.28	28	9	1.58	26
1980	22	1.34	23	7	1.59	21

Infants Discharged to the Postnatal Wards

Once an infant has recovered from his illness, he is reunited with his mother on the postnatal ward if she is still in hospital, or if the infant still needs some hospital supervision she is encouraged to stay on the PNW with him. Table 17.3 shows that this routine of uniting mothers and babies has been used for an increasing number of babies weighing between 1.50 and 2.00 kg during the last four years. For infants

Table 17.3: Age (Days) and Weight of Infants Transferred to Postnatal Wards after Initial NNU Admission.

	Birthweight 1.50-1.99 kg			Birthweight 2.0-2.49 kg		
	Age on Transfer	Wt on Transfer	No.	Age on Transfer	Wt on Transfer	No.
1977	4.6	1.98	8	2.1	2.21	31
1978	5.1	1.95	8	2.5	2.14	23
1979	6.0	1.82	24	3.8	2.13	30
1980	4.7	1.78	25	2.3	2.14	31

weighing more than 2.50 kg who are admitted to the neonatal unit, early discharge to the postnatal ward is the rule rather than the exception. About 80 per cent of such infants are transferred to their mothers' care after an average stay of only two days on the neonatal unit

(Table 17.4); only a small number of these larger infants are discharged home after a long stay on the NNU.

Table 17.4: Average Duration of Stay (Days) on NNU of Infants with Birthweight over 2.50 kg.

	Discharged to PNW		Discharged Home	
	Average Stay	No.	Average Stay	No.
1977	1.7	71	9.3	25
1978	2.4	49	12.8	13
1979	2.7	53	11.6	13
1980	2.4	76	10.5	12
Total		249		63

Discharge Home

There is no set weight for discharge. Once an infant on the NNU is feeding well three-hourly, and we are satisfied that the home conditions are satisfactory, and that his mother can cope, the infant is sent home. The mean discharge weights of low birthweight infants from our unit is given in Table 17.5.

Table 17.5: Average Discharge Weight and Age of All Infants Discharged Home from NNU, 1977-80.

Birthweight (kg)	Discharge (kg)	Age (Days)	No.
Below 1.50	2.09	48	87
1.50 – 1.99	2.08	26	150
2.00 – 2.49	2.21	15	48

Maintenance of Mother-baby Contact on the NNU

The management of this subject is covered in detail in many other chapters of this book, and the routines followed in our unit are modelled on various practices described in earlier chapters. Those aspects that we would like to emphasise are:

(1) When the infant has to be admitted immediately after birth, if it is at all possible we let the parents see their baby for a short

time on the labour ward, explaining to them why their baby is being admitted.

(2) We allow unrestricted access to the unit for parents.

(3) We allow parental access without gowning or masking, but give careful instruction about hand washing. Parents are encouraged to touch, stroke and talk to their critically ill baby even if he is receiving IPPV, and to get involved by cuddling, feeding and changing older infants even though they may still require oxygen.

(4) We allow unrestricted access for grandparents and siblings, and have a liberal approach to visiting by other family members.

(5) The mother is given a photograph of her infant, particularly if she is unlikely to be able to get to see the baby either because she is in another hospital, or because she is too ill to come from another part of the Cambridge Maternity Hospital to our unit.

(6) We give all parents a unit handbook (see appendix at the end of this book).

(7) We encourage the mother to provide EBM for her own baby with instructions on how to express her breasts and we have electrical breast pumps available for mothers' use (Chapter 12).

(8) Mothers of infants transferred after birth to our unit are also transferred and admitted to the postnatal wards.

(9) Parents are allowed to stay and hold dying infants and to take infants with inoperable malformations home for terminal care.

Transitional Care

When we first set out to use the two criteria for admission to the neonatal unit given earlier, we found that there were no problems with infants weighing more than 2.50 kg admitted to the postnatal wards with their mothers. However, considerable anxieties were expressed about the care of infants weighing less than 2.50 kg. For these reasons we arranged for all babies weighing 1.80-2.50 kg who were asymptomatic and could be kept with their mothers to be admitted to a postnatal ward adjacent to the NNU.

Although this section is entitled 'transitional care' perhaps it should not be given such a grandiose label. No extra facilities or staff are allotted to the ward, and mothers with infants of 2.50 kg or less birthweight are in a minority on the ward. The use of this unit has recently been described in detail elsewhere.[1]

The Ward

Our present postnatal ward has 14 beds; when the new Cambridge Maternity Hospital is completed in 1983 we will use a 26-bed ward next door to the neonatal unit for the same purpose. We have made no architectural adaptations in the present ward; we keep oxygen cylinders and a Matburn suction unit in the nursery, but there is no piped air, oxygen or suction. In the new hospital the nursery on this postnatal ward will be larger than that on the other wards and will have piped air, oxygen and suction; this is, however, because it will be the back-up intensive care unit in the event of an outbreak of severe infection in the main neonatal unit. We would emphasise, therefore, that infants requiring 'transitional care' can be nursed safely on a routine postnatal ward, as we do at present, without the provision of any special or additional care.

Staffing

The nursing staff on this ward rotate through the other departments in the maternity hospital. The daytime establishment at present is one sister, three staff midwives, one SEN, one nursery nurse and nursing auxiliary, plus one or two pupil midwives. The sister stays on the ward for six months and the staff midwives for four months; the nursery nurse, the SEN and the nursing auxiliary are permanent. The nursing establishment for the ward at night is one staff midwife and one nursing auxiliary, but the night rota has been arranged to ensure that there is always a trained nurse in charge of the ward. This nursing establishment was *not* increased when the ward started to admit infants weighing 2.50 kg or less.

The nurses are expected to be able to cope with routine Dextrostix measurements on infants of diabetic mothers and small-for-dates infants, tube feeds, to supervise phototherapy, and to give intramuscular drugs when infants, now well enough to be on the postnatal ward with their mothers, need to complete a course of therapy started while they were still in the NNU. No infants on this ward receive intravenous therapy, oxygen, or are nursed in incubators.

We have found it very advantageous for the neonatal unit nursing officer to be responsible for this ward. She is available for day-to-day advice on the management of small babies, and supervises the in-service orientation of nursing staff joining the ward (who always overlap for one week with those about to leave). No extra medical staff are necessary; SHO and consultant advice is always available from the paediatric staff in the maternity hospital.

Well infants weighing 1.80-2.50 kg, including twins or higher multiples, are admitted to this ward after delivery. Infants of this birthweight or above who needed to be admitted to the NNU at birth, but have recovered from their neonatal illness, are transferred to this ward to be looked after by their mothers, as are infants with malformations which are not life-threatening such as hare lip and cleft palate, and cases of Down's Syndrome (Tables 17.4 and 17.5). All these babies are 'cot nursed' and 'room-in' with their mothers.

Results

The records of 269 infants weighing between 1.80 and 2.50 kg delivered in the Cambridge Maternity Hospital between March 1979 and March 1980, who were candidates for admission to this ward, have been analysed in detail.[1] It proved to be easy, immediately after delivery, to identify with a high level of accuracy those requiring neonatal unit care and those who could go to the postnatal wards with their mothers; only six of 181 infants admitted to the postnatal ward subsequently needed to be transferred to the NNU (Table 17.6 and Figure 17.1). Of 88 infants admitted to the neonatal unit at birth, three died and six were transferred to other hospitals. Sixty-one of the remaining 79 were transferred to the postnatal wards with their mothers and only three cases were subsequently readmitted to the NNU (Table 17.6 and Figure 17.1).

The clinical details of the procedures carried out on the infants in the study are given in Table 17.7, which excludes the nine babies who oscillated to and fro between the postnatal ward and the neonatal unit. It can be seen that these infants were cared for very successfully and safely on the postnatal ward with their mothers providing most of the care. As a result of this unit, 237 (91 per cent) of the 260 infants between 1.80 and 2.50 kg birthweight who survived and stayed in Cambridge went home with their mothers, and a further five (2 per cent) spent some time with their mothers (Table 17.7). Thus only 18 infants of this birthweight did not spend a considerable part of the puerperium with their mothers. That 50 per cent of these infants were breast feeding on discharge is, we believe, yet another vindication of this type of care.

Conclusion

In this chapter, we have discussed a system of providing neonatal care which minimises parent-baby separation in a busy teaching hospital

Table 17.6: (i) Infants Admitted to Postnatal Ward and Subsequently Requiring Admission to SCBU.

Birthweight	Gestational Age	Diagnosis	Age on Admission	Subsequent Course
2.08	34	TTN[a]	4 hours	Transferred back to PNW 2 days. Discharged. Bottle fed. Day 10. Thriving.
2.29	34	TTN	90 mins	Transferred back to PNW 2 days. Discharged. Bottle fed. Day 6. Thriving.
2.47	36	GBS[b] sepsis	6 hours	Transferred back to PNW 6 days. Discharged. Breast fed. Day 12. Thriving.
2.44	37	Feeding problem	24 hours	Transferred back to PNW 2 days. Discharged. Bottle fed. Day 4. Thriving.
2.24	33	TTN	20 hours	Home from SCBU 18 days. Bottle fed. Thriving.
2.24	38	NEC[c]	6 days	Transferred for surgery after 24 hours on SCBU. Necrotic section resected. Home breast fed. 24 days. Thriving.

(ii) Infants Transferred from SCBU to Postnatal Ward and Subsequently Readmitted.

Birthweight	Gestational Age	Admission Diagnosis	Age Transferred to PNW	Age Back to SCBU	Diagnosis	Subsequent Course
2.34	33	RDS[d]	3 days	9 days	Poor feeding	Discharged home. Day 11. Breast fed. Thriving.
1.86	33	Mild birth asphyxia	6 days	11 days	Poor feeding Mum depressed	Discharged home. Day 17. Bottle fed. Thriving.
1.81	35	Mild birth asphyxia	4 days	9 days	Poor feeding Mum depressed	Discharged home. Day 16. Bottle fed. Thriving.

Notes:
a. TTN — Transient tachypnoea of the newborn.
b. GBS — Group B streptococcus.
c. NEC — Necrotising enterocolitis.
d. RDS — Respiratory distress syndrome.

Table 17.7: Data of Infants 1.80-2.50 kg Born in Cambridge Maternity Hospital, March 1979-March 1980.

	Never Admitted to SCBU	Admitted at Birth to SCBU then Transferred to the Postnatal Ward	Always on SCBU
Number	175	58	27
Mean birthweight (kg)	2.27	2.12	1.97
Mean gestation	36.5	35	32.4
Diagnosis on SCBU:			
RDS		14	10
Transient tachypnoea		12	8
Normal prem		17	4
Mild birth asphyxia		5	–
Normal small for dates		4	–
Malformation		1	3(2)[a]
Others		5	2(1)[a]
Transfer to PNW			
Weight (kg)		2.05	
Age (days)		3.4	
Problems on PNW:			
Tube feeding	33	33	
Jaundice	39	12	
(Phototherapy)	(16)	9	
Dextrostix	167	7	
Low values	(5)	–	
Conjuncitivitis	16	–	
Skin infections	2		
Transient tachypnoea	2		
Malformations	6	1	
Antiobiotic (IM, oral or topical)	6	3	
Duration of stay on PNW (days)	8.7	9	
Discharge from hospital:			
Mean age (days)	8.3	13.7	22.7
Mean weight (kg)	2.28	2.18	2.16
Feeding:[b]			
Breast	96	19	10
Bottle	75	35	8
Readmissions:	15	15	2
	3 bronchiolitis 2 hernias 2 pyloric stenosis 2 fracture femur 2 bronchiolitis (1 ? NAI) 1 D & V	4 bronchiolitis 1 failure to thrive (4x) 2 hernias 1 squint 1 pyloric stenosis bronchiolitis (2 admissions)	1 bronchiolitis URT I (2 admissions). 1 apnoea with feed

Table 17.7 (continued)

	Never Admitted to SCBU	Admitted at Birth to SCBU then Transferred to the Postnatal Ward	Always on SCBU
Readmissions:	1 adenovirus pneumonia (died) 1 B4 myocarditis (died) 1 congenital rubella with patent ductus and heart failure	1 disseminated BCG-osis 3 D & V 1 balanitis, skull fracture (2 admissions) 1 dislocated hip	
Cot deaths	1[c]		

Notes:
a. Figures in brackets = deaths.
b. The numbers do not add up to the total since in a few cases the method of feeding at discharge was not recorded.
c. This was the infant with congenital rubella who died 1/52 after being discharged from the children's ward where her heart failure had been controlled.

Figure 17.1: Outcome of Infants 1.8-2.50 kg Born in Cambridge, March 1979-March 1980 Inclusive. Of 260 'Cambridge Babies' who survived, 237 (91 per cent) went home with their mothers and of these 128 (55 per cent) were making some attempt to breast-feed. The figures in brackets refer to the number of babies breast feeding on discharge.

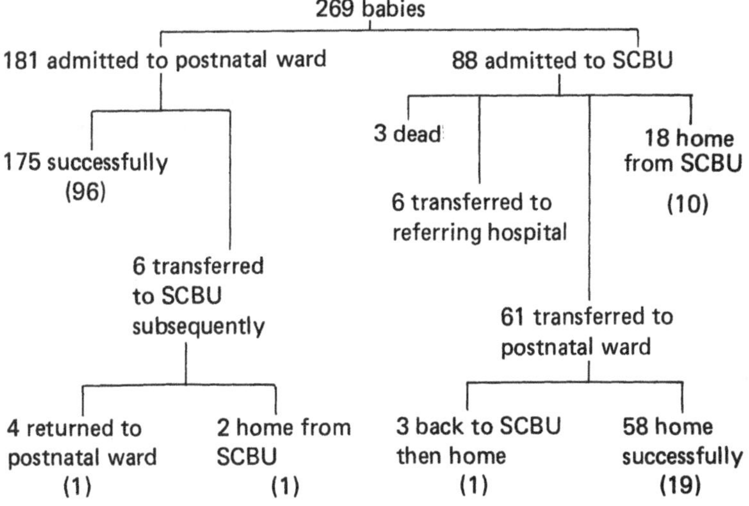

maternity unit responsible for the neonatal care of 6,000 deliveries per annum (Table 17.1) and providing a regional neonatal intensive care service. With this system only 6 per cent of all infants delivered in the Cambridge maternity unit need admission to a neonatal unit (Table 17.8), a figure similar to the number of admissions to NNUs in England and Wales in the early 1960s. Of this 6 per cent many can be transferred to the postnatal wards with their mother after only a short

Table 17.8: Inborn Admissions to Cambridge SCBU, 1979-1980.

Birthweight (kg)	Number Delivered	Number Admitted	Per cent
Below 1.50	120	120	100
1.5 – 2.0	171	136	80
2.0 – 2.5	380	85	22
Over 2.5	7,695	163	2.1
Total	8,366	504	6

stay on the NNU (Tables 17.3 and 17.4). This system of neonatal care gives the maximum opportunity for mothers and babies to stay together, and it is not only entirely safe, but may well be safer than patterns of neonatal care which expose many infants to the hazards of nosocomial infection in an NNU, and compromise mother-infant attachment, increasing the likelihood of serious non-accidental injury in later infancy.

Reference

1. Whitby, C., de Cates, C. R., and Roberton, N. R. C. (1982). Infants weighing 1.8-2.5 kg: do they need neonatal unit or postnatal ward care? *Lancet*, *i*, 322.

18 THE SOTERO DEL RIO HOSPITAL, SANTIAGO, CHILE

Jorge Torres Pereyra

General Factors Involved in Perinatal Risk in Chile

In Chile, where 90 per cent of all births take place in hospital, most neonatal deaths occur during the first week of life, and 57 per cent of infant deaths in the first months (Table 18.1). The outcome of perinatal illnesses depends to a large extent upon the medical care available and, moreover, may be affected by adequate medical planning since it has been suggested that the importance of living conditions as a factor in mortality is less in the perinatal period than subsequently. In Chile the neonatal mortality rate (NNMR) has declined little (Figure 18.1) over the past decade, in spite of the fact that the resources given over to neonatal medical attention have increased.

Table 18.1: Perinatal and Infant Death in Chile, 1980.

	Rate per 1000 Live Births
Perinatal mortality	21.91
Late fetal mortality (stillbirths)	11.34
Early neonatal mortality	10.57
Late neonatal mortality	1.53
Total neonatal mortality	12.10
Total infant mortality (early + late neonatal + deaths 28 days-1 year)	21.2

Demography of South-east Santiago (the Area Served by Sotero del Rio Hospital)

This is one of the seven health districts of Santiago, with a population of nearly 600,000. It has a young, newly urbanised population, with substandard living conditions; only 60 per cent of the dwellings have drinking water, and only 56 per cent have mains drainage. Fifteen per cent of adults are illiterate, 25 per cent of the working population is unemployed and alcoholism and miscarriage are important community

Figure 18.1: Neonatal and Infantile Mortality in Chile and South-east Area of Santiago, 1966-79.

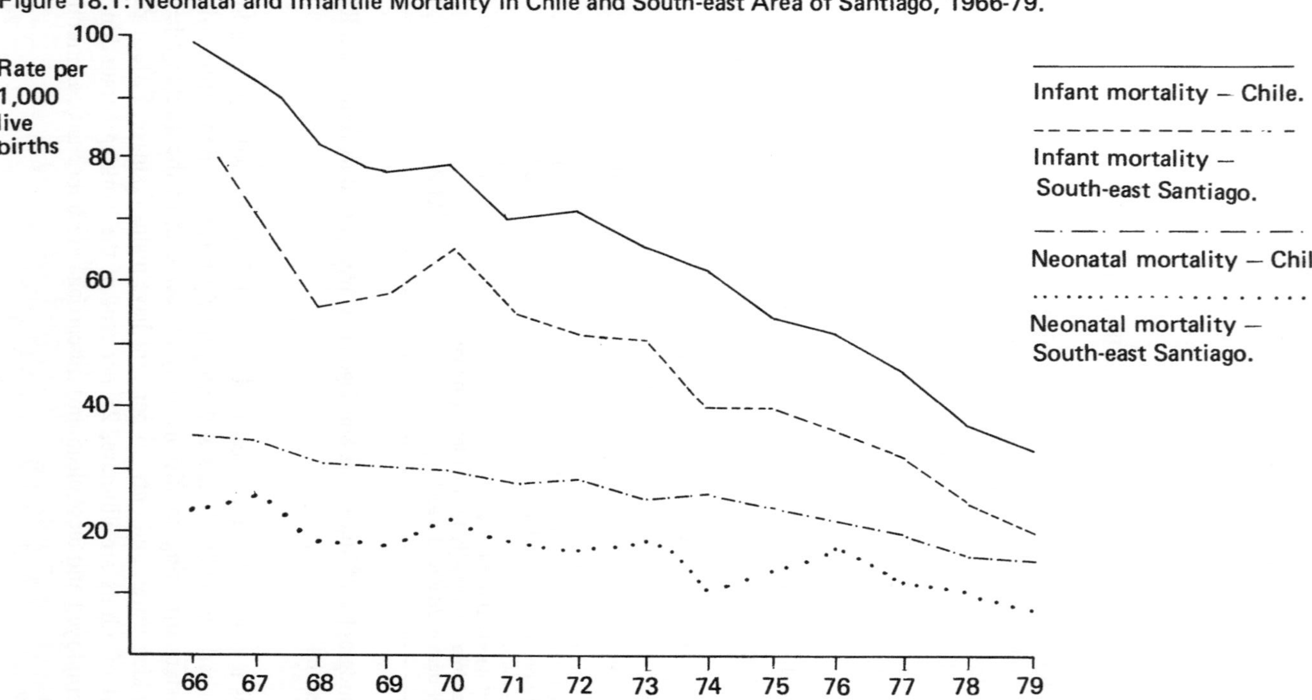

health problems. Family groups are large and often unstable.

Perinatal Medical Care in South-east Santiago

The neonatal unit at Sotero del Rio Hospital is a regional centre. The obstetric unit has 120 beds, and takes care of 97 per cent of the births (about 10,000 in 1981) in the community. The neonatal unit is attached to the department of paediatrics in the nearby children's hospital (Josepina Martinez de Ferrar Hospital). The neonatal unit has follow-up clinics in the eleven district outpatient departments for mother and child care, which serve our south-eastern area, and the unit also runs a programme of teaching and training for more than 700 doctors and nurses from different parts of the country.

Extent and Importance of the Problem of Low Birthweight (LBW) Deliveries

In south-east Santiago the LBW incidence is approximately 10 per cent and about 75 per cent of neonatal deaths occur in these infants (Table 18.2). The average birthweight in the Sotero del Rio hospital is 3.07 kg, compared with 3.22 kg ($p < 0.001$) in the maternity unit in an area of higher living standards in Santiago.[1]

Table 18.2: Neonatal Mortality by Birthweight, Sotero del Rio Hospital Neonatal Unit, Santiago, South-eastern Area, 1978-81.

Weight (g)	No.	Rate[a] 1978	No.	Rate[a] 1979	No.	Rate[a] 1980	No.	Rate[a] 1981
1,000 or less	36	878	26	702.7	39	795.9	28	736.8
1,000-1,500	30	405	29	408.4	23	338.2	15	241.9
1,501-2,000	22	135.8	24	145.4	10	67.6	8	57.1
2,001-2,500	13	23.2	14	23.9	10	17.1	15	27.7
Sub-total[b]	101	120.6[c]	93	108.5[c]	82	96.6[c]	66	84.6[c]
2,501-3,000	12	5.4	7	3.1	16	6.9	14	6.0
over 3,000	7	1.4	15	2.7	13	2.2	12	1.7
Not restigered	1	–	–	–	–	–	–	–
Total	121	14.8	115	13.3	111	12.1	92	9.1

Notes:
a. Rate per 1,000 live births.
b. Sub-total of low birthweight infants.
c. Rate per 1,000 low birthweight infants.

Mothers of LBW children are usually young primipara or grand multipara more than 35 years of age who have a history of miscarriages. Half of these mothers lack adequate social support; their marriages are often unstable and half of them do not have their own homes, or live in inadequate conditions. The fathers only have basic education, and many are unskilled workers or unemployed. A high percentage of the mothers of LBW children do not attend for antenatal care until after 24 weeks of gestation and 50 per cent of them make less than three antenatal visits. Thirty per cent of them suffer premature rupture of the membranes and the incidence of breech presentation is three or four times greater than normal. These problems increase the risk of perinatal death 30-fold.

In the neonatal period, LBW babies have an increased incidence of asphyxia, hyaline membrane disease (HMD) and infection, and during the first year of life (and in particular the first three months) need frequent re-admissions for respiratory infections and severe diarrhoea with dehydration.

Medical Care of LBW Children in South-east Santiago

Figure 18.2 sets out a flow diagram of the neonatal medical care in our hospital.

Primary Prevention of Premature Birth

Antenatal care is carried out at the eleven district outpatient clinics which deliver a nationally set standard of obstetric care and have their own equipment and staff. The aim is to diagnose and treat quickly and efficiently pathological disorders of pregnancy which can give rise to premature birth. Recently, in an attempt to identify mothers who are at greatest risk of premature delivery we have started to use a system which predicts the theoretical risk of premature birth.[2] This is an adaptation of the systems proposed by Creasey[3] and Papiernik[4].

The factors most frequently linked with the birth of LBW babies are toxaemia, infection, multiple pregnancy, maternal malnutrition with placental pathology, socio-economic problems in the family and inadequate medical care.[5]

Secondary Prevention of Pre-term Birth

Here the object is the early diagnosis of premature labour in order to try to arrest it. In every mother who comes to us with symptoms of

Figure 18.2: Flow Diagram of Intensive Care in Neonatal Unit, Sotero del Rio Hospital, Santiago, Chile.

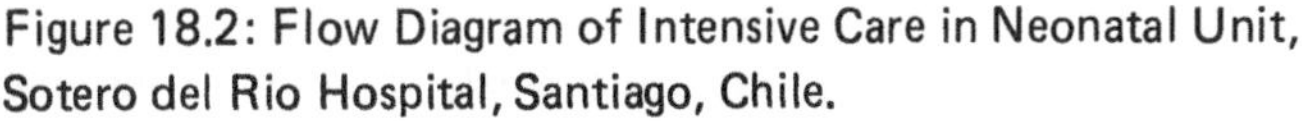

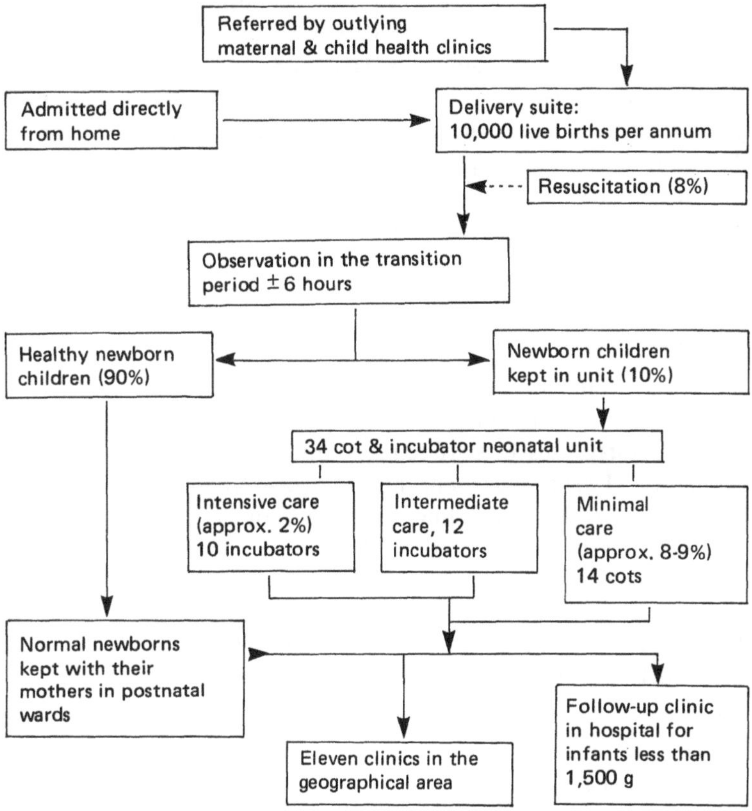

preterm labour we assess gestational age, the stage of uterine contraction and the state of the cervix, to see whether tocolytic agents or betamethasone to induce pulmonary development[6] are indicated. Delivery of babies weighing less than 1.20 kg is usually by Caesarian section in order to avoid the high perinatal risk associated with breech presentation.[7]

Care of the Newborn LBW Child

For the first 6-12 hours, 'at risk' babies are admitted to an observation ward adjacent to the labour ward where experienced nurses and nursing auxiliaries assess the likelihood of infection, monitor temperature control, ventilation and blood glucose and at the same time avoid unnecessary interference which can cause small children to become cold. Here the routine procedures for the identification of the neonate are carried out. The nurses also give BCG, oral polio vaccine, silver nitrate eye drops and intramuscular vitamin K.

Once the temperature is stabilised, the neonate is examined by a paediatrician who takes particular note of weight for dates and neonatal illness. If the infant weighs more than 2.00 kg and is healthy, he is then taken back to his mother in the postnatal section of the hospital, in order to initiate feeding immediately, and avoid a lengthy mother-child separation. All babies who weigh 2.00 kg or less at birth are kept in the hospital neonatal unit whether they are ill or not.

The Neonatal Unit

The NNU has intensive care, intermediate care and convalescence areas, plus sections intended for the admission of parents, a nursing station, a laundry, storage space, staff lounges, offices, a meeting room and a laboratory. Twenty-four hour medical cover is given by residents, teaching supervisors and fellows from the Catholic University of Chile and other parts of the country. The nurse allocation is shown in Table 18.3. The nurses have completed four years of study at the

Table 18.3: Nursing Staff Levels in Neonatal Unit, Sotero del Rio Hospital

Section	Staff Level
Intensive care area	1 nurse per 10 incubators 1 auxiliary per 5 incubators
Intermediate care area	1 nurse per 12 incubators 1 auxiliary per 6 incubators
Convalescence area	1 nurse per 14 incubators 1 auxiliary per 7 incubators

University. The auxiliaries have reached the third year of secondary education and have had a further year of special training.

Intensive Care

The ward is kept at 28°C all the year round. New admissions are placed under radiant heat cradles where their breathing is monitored, as is their heart rate, arterial pressure and temperature. Blood samples are taken together with portable X-ray. Appropriate respiratory support is given for infants with hyaline membrane disease using continuous positive airways pressure and from 1979 intermittent positive pressure ventilation (IPPV) with a Bourns BP200 ventilator. The main indications for admission to this section are given in Table 18.4.

Table 18.4: Conditions Requiring Admission to Neonatal Intensive Care Unit, Sotero del Rio Hospital.

Birthweight less than 1.50 kg
Gestational age less than 32 weeks
Severe neonatal asphyxia
Convulsions
Hypoglycaemia
Need to monitor respiratory rate, temperature or blood pressure
Strict fluid balance
Requiring more than 60% oxygen
Monitoring arterial blood gases
Needing transcutaneous pO_2 measurement
CPAP, IMV, IPPV
Pneumothorax
Intravenous feeding
Pre- and post-operative care

In the laboratory, situated in the unit, a University technician works eight hours per day. The duty houseman covers for the remaining hours. Rapid diagnostic methods are used in this laboratory for blood glucose and urea, bilirubin, hematocrit, urine analysis, gram stain of amniotic fluid and gastric aspirate, biochemical analysis of the liquor amnii, and arterial blood gases.

Convalescence in Progressive Care

Children who receive what we call convalescent care are those who have been hospitalised in intensive care, and also those who receive lesser levels of neonatal care. The basic physical working conditions of this side of the hospital are similar to those described in intensive care but with fewer nurses (Table 18.3). The wards are decorated with pictures designed for infants, and little musical boxes are attached to the cradles and incubators. It is worth noting that nurses rotate regularly through all four parts of the service – the holding station, the intensive care ward, the lying-in wards and the district – so that they are familiar with the work of their colleagues and never get out of practice.

During convalescence special emphasis is placed on promoting lactation and in facilitating the mother-baby relationship. There are no restrictions placed upon the parents visiting their children. Under the supervision of the nurses and auxiliaries they make contact with their baby, caress him freely, talk to him and play with him. The auxiliary in charge of the child establishes a good relationship with the parents, and she is the person who can best assess their adequacy to care for the child in their own home.

Low birthweight babies are discharged home once there is resolution of their basic health problem, provided they weigh more than 2.00 kg and can control their temperature and are feeding well. We also require a favourable assessment of the mother-baby relationship, and the knowledge and attitude of the mother with regard to elementary care of her child.

Feeding the LBW Infant

We use the term 'lactarium' to refer to the organisation which provides colostrum and milk for the early feeding of all our LBW neonates from their own mothers. The lactarium has the following functions:

(1) The education of mothers.
(2) The establishment of early and permanent contact between a mother and her baby.
(3) Use of simple techniques for the manual expression of breast milk.
(4) The collection of milk and its preservation at room temperature for immediate use, or at 4°C for use over a period of time not exceeding 24 hours. We cannot carry out periodic bacteriological control.
(5) The preparation of simple kits for the transportation of mothers' milk drawn off at home, plus written instructions, plastic fridges with ice packs, feeding bottles and materials for cleaning the feeding bottles.

In children weighing less than 1.50 kg at birth, the lactarium has allowed us to begin feeding them within the first 48 hours of life and we reach maximum volumes of 190 cc/kg at 14 days. The babies regain their birthweight on average at 16 days. Babies fed with EBM[8,9] gained weight faster than another comparable group fed with artificial milk (Nan-Nestlé) and their time in hospital was therefore reduced. Energy ingestion was significantly related to the increase in lean mass.[10] Taking more than 180 ml/kg of milk per day was tolerated well without an increased incidence of patent ductus arteriosus.[11]

In our circumstances we are not in favour of milk banks on account of the cost of building them, the difficulties of adequate supervision, and the risks reported by various authors.[12-14] Children who cannot take mothers' milk are fed with formula made up to 86 kcal/100 ml and 1.3 grams protein/ml. Parenteral feeding is normally administered through peripheral veins, and is restricted to pre- and post-operative care and occasional neonates who require prolonged IPPV.

Medical Care of Infants Weighing Greater than 2.00 kg at Birth

All healthy children who weigh more than 2.00 kg stay with their mothers in the hospital for the first three days after birth. Since the child rooms-in with his mother, both lactation and the mother-child relationship are established naturally, and he is often looked after entirely by his own mother. In these parts of the hospital, there is a notorious lack of staff; only one obstetric nurse is provided for every 30 cradles and one auxiliary nurse for every 20-25 cradles. Residents visit twice a day or more. Daily care is carried out by the auxiliary nurse, following precise instructions and standards which are laid down. The nurses supervise the work of the auxiliaries and give personal attention to children whose birthweight was 2.00-2.50 kg; they refer problems to the medical staff.

On discharge only LBW children are examined by a doctor. From the maternity unit newborn babies are referred to the eleven district outpatient clinics in the area. Those that weighed less than 1.50 kg at birth continue to be supervised in the hospital outpatient follow-up clinic.

Care in the Follow-up Clinic

Originally the hospital clinic followed all LBW children. However, for the last three years, follow-up has been restricted to those who weighed less than 1.50 kg at birth – about 90 children per year. Work is carried out in a small hut with a floor area of 80 square metres with a staff of one neonatologist, one nurse and one auxiliary.

In this clinic, medical care is integrated, including the care of the healthy child in accordance with planned schedules of visits, and prevention of various risk factors, as well as coping with intercurrent illness, which is mainly infection and malnutrition. Contributions from neurologists, psychologists, ophthalmologists and audiologists enable neurological problems to be detected and dealt with early. This clinic also takes on the practical teaching of medical and nursing students from the Catholic University of Chile and of other professional people from different parts of the country.

On occasion the nurses from the clinic pay home visits. This backs up the instructions given to the parents on lactation, clothing and basic care of the child. The nurse also makes a direct assessment of the home of the parents, the temperature of the room in which the child sleeps, the degree of possible overcrowding and the experience already acquired by the mother. She makes improvements where possible, gives instruction on matters which require it and plans the dates for future visits to the clinics.

Present Perspectives and Limitations

Figure 18.1 shows that the NNMR in the south-east area of Santiago has fallen in the last few years. The factors which may have contributed to this low NNMR are changes in the pattern of birth, increased urbanisation and the planning of neonatal services. The emphasis placed on the improvement of medical and nursing staff (1974-9), even before the establishment of intensive care (1979), enabled us to reduce the rate of neonatal death to 13.3 per 1,000. The implementation of intensive care techniques is bringing about a reduction in the number of deaths in children with low birthweight, especially among those weighing less than 2.00 kg (Table 18.2), and a change in the death rate from hyaline membrane disease from 59 per cent in 1975 to 36 per cent in 1978.

The average period of lactation in the mothers of children who weigh less than 1.50 kg at birth is now over four months. This means that the number of cases of severe malnutrition in the first year of life has been significantly reduced, as has the number of late child deaths in infants of low birthweight.

Conclusion

The style of neonatal and postnatal care outlined above is the result of eight years of teamwork and of the investment of a great deal of time in the training of staff, despite the limited means at our disposal. We now intend to build into the system a bigger commitment to family and community care. We are improving our teaching methods, doing research, learning and applying suitable technology to the solution of our problem.[2]

I believe that, given our general limitations, nothing is possible without a common effort, and that this kind of participation is the only simple recipe for the success which will enable us to bring together science and the humane wish to serve our children. Their smile is our greatest reward.

References

1. Mardones, F. (1980). Algunos factores condicionantes del bajo peso de nacimiento. *Rev. Med. Chile*, *108*, 839.
2. Torres, J. y col. (1982). Programa de salud perinatal con enfasis en la integración familiar, communitaria y en la formación de recursos humanos. Santiago, Chile, OPS/Kellog.
3. Creasy, R. K., Gummer, B. A., and Liggins, G. C. (1980). A system for predicting spontaneous preterm birth. *Obstet. Gynecol.*, *55*, 692.
4. Papiernik, E. (1969). Le coefficient de risque d'accouchement premature. *La Presse Med.*, *77*, 793.
5. Arteaga, A., Lira, P, and Torres, J. y col. (1978). Efecto de la alimentación durante el embarazo y del estado nutritivo de la gestante sobre el recien nacido. *Rev. Med. Chile*, *106*, 499.
6. Liggins, G. C., and Howie, R. N. (1972). A controlled trial of antepartum glucocorticoid treatment for prevention of the respiratory distress syndrome in premature infants. *Pediatrics*, *50*, 575.
7. Goldenberg, R. L., and Nelson, K. G. (1977). The premature breech. *Am. J. Obstet. Gynecol.*, *127*, 240.
8. Hodgson, M. I., Rathkamp, B., and Torres, J. y col. (1981). Alimentación del recien nacido de muy bajo peso con leche de su propia madre. *Rev. Chil. Nutr.*, *9*, 223.
9. Hodgson, M. I., Rathkamp, B., and Torres, J. y col.(1981). Evaluación de tres formulas lacteas en la alimentación del recien nacido de muy bajo peso de nacimiento. *Rev. Chil. Nutr.*, *9*, 222.
10. Rathkamp, B., Hodgson, M. I., and Torres, J. y col. (1981). Interrelaciones entre ingesta energetica, proteica y progreso ponderal en RN de muy bajo peso de nacimiento. *Rev. Chil. Nutr.*, *9*, 233.
11. Oh, W. Personal communication.
12. Evans, T. J., *et al.* (1978). Effect of storage and heat on antimicrobial proteins in human milk. *Arch. Dis. Child.*, *53*, 239.
13. Liebhaber, M., *et al.* (1977). Alterations of lymphocytes and of antibody content of human milk after processing. *J. Pediat.*, *91*, 897.
14. Siimes, M. A., and Hallman, N. (1979). A perspective in human milk banking. *J. Pediat.*, *94*, 173.

19 SOWETO, SOUTH AFRICA: THE CARE OF NEWBORN INFANTS IN A DEVELOPING COMMUNITY

Samuel Wayburne

Medical and Organisational Problems

Many medical problems in developing countries arise from the high birth rate in populations which are poorly nourished, have limited resources and education, overcrowded living conditions and limited health services coupled with much endemic disease. Infant mortality remains high, contributed to by the excessive number of births, poor maternal care, diarrhoeal disturbances and malnutrition. The improvements in environmental health which could come about in many areas are negated by the effects of the high birth rate, making developing communities even poorer. This is well illustrated by what has happened in the Soweto area of Johannesburg.

Historical Background

Fifty years ago Soweto consisted of a few thousand brick houses on the south-west border of Johannesburg. Soon after the start of the Second World War a huge shanty town mushroomed around the city council development, and tens of thousands of people who had migrated to the Johannesburg area in search of employment lived there in deplorable conditions. By 1939 the population of the Soweto region had reached 40,000, and by 1951 it was 200,000. In his report to the city council of Johannesburg for 1979, the Medical Officer of Health suggests that today's figure is in the region of 1.5 million.

One of the first buildings erected fifty years ago was a local authority clinic. A part-time general practitioner and a number of black nurses conducted curative work, midwifery and some preventive medical services. Any abnormal delivery or medical problems were referred by ambulance to hospitals within the city centre some ten miles distant. In 1938 the City Health Department took over all medical and nursing services and full-time doctors and more nurses were appointed to care for the growing population, while massive housing schemes were under construction.

Baragwanath Hospital now serves the large city of Soweto, but this improvement in hospitalisation, paralleled by better prenatal care and improved living conditions and services for the community, were overwhelmed by the population growth. The hospital opened in mid-1948 in emergency buildings vacated by the British Army. It had no provision for midwifery or 'at risk' newborn infants, but as soon as the hospital opened it was inundated with obstetric emergencies which could not be turned away. This impasse was met by the impromptu conversion of one large open ward into 'delivery' and 'lying-in' areas. The number of patients grew rapidly and in its third year of operation nearly 3,500 deliveries were conducted, using six delivery and twelve lying-in beds. Operative cases were done in the general surgery theatre. Infants in need of special treatment were, like the rest, 'roomed in' at their mothers' bedside, cared for and fed by them and sent home with them after a day or two when usually still in need.

Neonatal Care, 1951-73

In 1951 a large open ward, heated by coal stoves and provided with two hand basins, a small kitchen, a duty room, ablution and toilet facilities, was opened for neonatal special care (Figure 9.1). The 36 × 6 metre area was divided into a babies' section and a mothers' dormitory by moveable screens. Temperature was controlled at 25-27°C by stoking the fires and closing and opening the windows and doors. In this part of southern Africa temperatures range from 30°C in summer to below freezing in winter. Humidification was impractical and was disregarded.[1] There were few nurses, only one of whom had experience of low birthweight infant care, and the doctors fared no better.

Twenty to thirty low birthweight newborns could be admitted to this unit and from the outset mothers were always admitted with their infants and were encouraged to care for them as soon as they were well enough. While the mother was retained in hospital, the rest of her children were usually looked after by the extended family. Good neighbours and friends also helped, but occasionally siblings were lodged in the hospital until family arrangements could be made. Only rarely did a mother have no alternative but to go back to her home, in which case her infant continued under hospital care until well enough to be discharged.

Figure 19.1: The First Premature Baby Ward Opened in 1951, Heated by Coal Stoves and Simply Equipped.

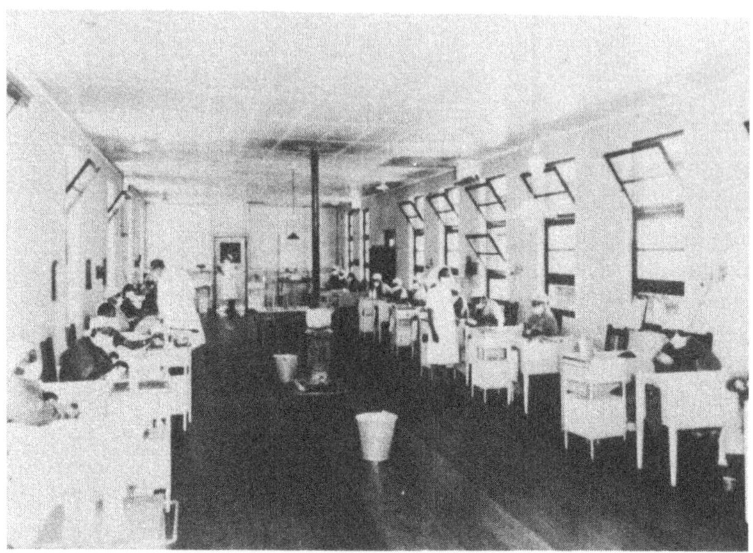

The mothers were taught elementary hygiene and within 2-3 days they were changing, cleaning and feeding their own infants under close supervision, enabling the nurses to do other essentials. Bathing of infants was prohibited in order to prevent hypothermia and cross-infection. Visitors were allowed, but were restricted to the dormitory area or the adjacent lawns. Within several months of opening, the number of cribs had to be increased to 40, and during busy periods as many as 50 infants would be under care, so that conditions became somewhat crowded and the mothers had insufficient room. At times, 40 per cent of the infants were under 1.50 kg and the nurses were hard pressed.

With the continued growth of the midwifery department, so did the neonatal work expand. Results continued to improve as doctors and nurses gained experience and facilities were upgraded. In 1960 we established a second unit almost identical to the first. It held 40 cribs and a mothers' dormitory, and was also heated by coal stoves. Ward lighting was improved and central heating replaced the coal stoves a year or two later (Figure 9.2). However, temperature control still required the opening and closing of windows.

Figure 19.2: First Premature Baby Ward after Upgrading: Central Heating and Oxygen Outlets and Impervious Clean Floor

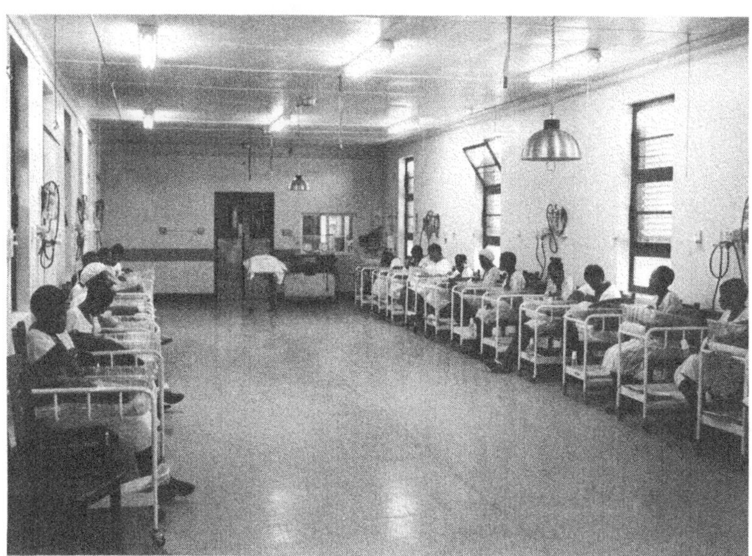

Care on Admission

On admission, all infants under 1.60 kg were well wrapped in cotton wool, including a cotton wool 'bonnet' plus several layers of woollen blankets, leaving only the face exposed (Figure 19.3). Bigger hypothermic infants were similarly treated. They were placed in cribs and electric heating pads set at the lowest temperature were inserted under the uppermost layer of blankets. Rectal temperatures were measured daily with low-reading clinical thermometers and if any abnormality was present this reading was repeated as required to control any necessary treatment. Sometimes 'low-reading' thermometers were inadequate and laboratory instruments were required to measure rectal temperatures which on occasion were 20°C or less.

Well infants over 1.60 kg were wrapped without a primary layer of cotton wool and the head was left exposed. The disadvantage of wrapping infants and keeping them in deep box-like cribs was obvious, but there was no choice at the time and with mothers and supervising nurses constantly present relatively few accidents occurred. In summer, provided they were well wrapped, the warm environment in the infants'

Figure 19.3: Correctly Wrapped Small Premature Infant

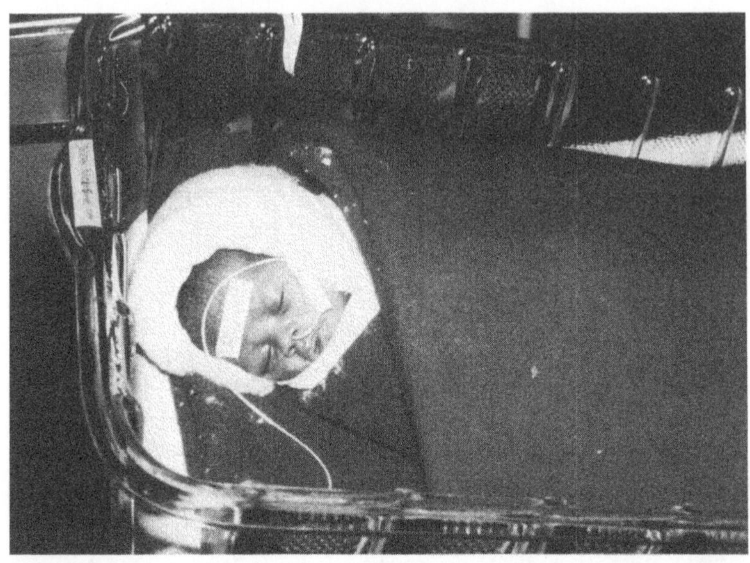

areas permitted the removal of the electric warming pads once the infants' temperature control had stabilised. At this stage temperatures were taken before each feed and most infants of about 1.50 kg or more maintained a normal level after 12-14 days. All infants received an injection of vitamin K on admission and after the first three or four years the dose of the vitamin was reduced from 10 mg to 1 mg or less when its harmful effects became known.

Feeding

At the outset, feeding equipment consisted of rubber-tipped pipettes, narrow-necked standard feeding bottles and nipples, bowls and small containers to hold and keep the feeds warm. As was customary in 1951 in most parts of the world, feeding was delayed for at least 24 hours, after which small feeds of 5 per cent 'dextrin-maltose' solution were given two-hourly for several feeds and followed by undiluted breast milk, increasing the volume daily until 180 ml/kg was given by the age of seven or eight days. The mothers of infants who received supplementary feeds were trained in their preparation and were supplied with the milk powder on discharge from the unit.

When satisfactory nasogastric (NG) tubes became available in about 1960, their use immediately reduced deaths and morbidity from aspiration. All tubes were inserted by nurses and were left in situ for 3-4 days; feeds were then reduced to three-hourly. Before a feed was given, the tube position was tested by means of aspirate on blue litmus paper and adjustments made or a new tube inserted. Mothers coped as well with the tube feeds as with bottles and saved the nursing staff an enormous amount of time (Figure 19.4). Supplements of Vitamin C, D and iron were given throughout this period.

Figure 19.4: Mother Tube Feeding her Infant in an Incubator

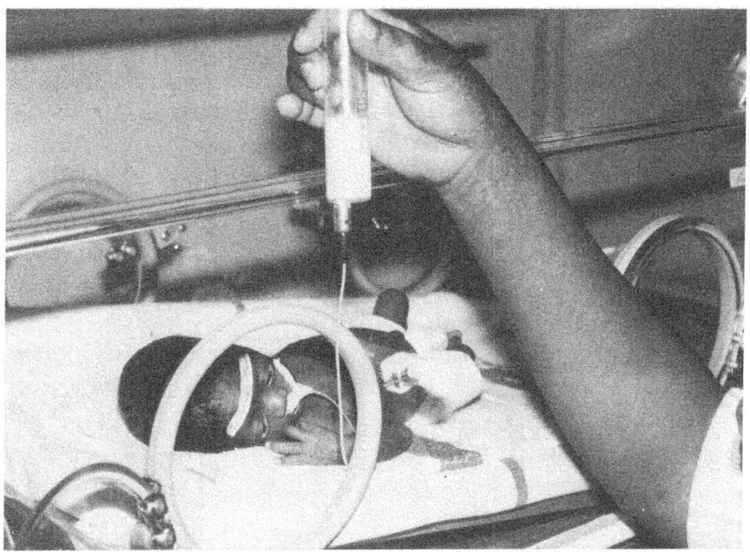

Equipment

The infants' 'beds' consisted of small wooden box-like cribs with an adjustable base which could be raised at one end. They were light enough to be lifted fairly easily. Unfortunately they were about 30 cm deep and infants had to be removed for full examination or resuscitation. These cribs were replaced after nearly 20 years by clear plastic bath-like bassinettes which nestle inside wheeled carriages.

There were no incubators and oxygen was supplied by cylinders and directed over the face of the infant by means of a funnel at a flow rate of 2 l/min. Oxygen analysers and headboxes came into use many years later. Suction apparatus consisted of one electric machine and improvised 'Murphy drip' and oral suction tubes. Disposable intravenous therapy equipment became available after a few years. Two incubators were introduced in 1963 and later more were provided. However, we did not find them necessary as a routine for all small infants and 'normal' neonates above 1.50-1.60 kg.

Most of the mothers proved fully capable of handling their babies in incubators and carrying out all care and feeding. They were taught, encouraged and expected to do so except when the babies were on ventilation or intravenous feeding. Much of the nurses' time was saved through this help provided by mothers.

Initially no laryngoscopes or endotracheal tubes were supplied, making intubation and ventilation impossible, but eventually intubation, CPAP and IPPV became available, which together with the increasing number of incubators constantly improved the outlook for the sickest babies. Exchange transfusions for jaundice were carried out from 1954, and phototherapy was introduced in 1971 (Figure 19.5).

Figure 19.5: Phototherapy in an Outpatient Ward. Infant second from right had an exchange transfusion

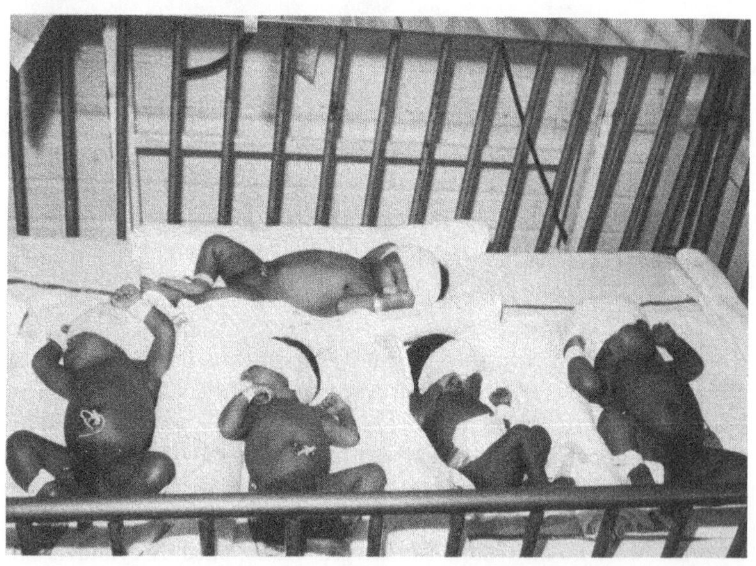

Results

The results of the first 1,000 consecutive admissions to the unit are shown in Table 19.1. Accidental neonatal hypothermia, seen particularly in outborn infants, was a frequent occurrence in winter. This was a major component of the neonatal deaths (Tables 19.2 and 19.3), even with the management outlined above, and the aim was to rewarm them as rapidly and as safely as possible (2°C per hour) with the simultaneous three-hourly nasogastric administration of 25 per cent dextrose solution to prevent the occurrence of hypoglycaemia during rewarming. This was a very important part of the emergency treatment since absorption was excellent at very low temperatures.

Table 19.1: Baragwanath Hospital, Survival Rates of Low Birthweight Infants, 1952/3 (51 per cent were Born outside the Hospital)

Weight (kg)	No. of Infants	Survival %
Below 1.000	47	2.0
1.001-1.500	230	25.0
1.501-2.000	384	62.0
2.001-2.500	339	85.0
Total	1,000	58.0

Table 19.2: Baragwanath Premature Infant Unit Survival, 1965-6.

Group	Number	Percentage
Total Admissions	1,935	
Hypothermia, 33°C and less	372	19.0
Total Survivors	1,385	71.6
Mortality, hypothermias	164	44.0 (as a % of all hypothermias)
Mortality, non-hypothermias	386	24.7 (as a % of all non-hypothermic admissions)

Table 19.3: Baragwanath Premature Infant Unit — Effect of Hypothermia on Survival, 1965-6.

Temp °C on Admission	Subjects	Survivors	Percentage
33-30	252	152	60.3
29-27	89	45	50.5
Below 27[a]	31	11	35.5

Note: a. Lowest recorded temp. 20°

Discharge

On discharge in the early 1950s most of the infants were fully breast fed (77 per cent) or partly breast fed (18 per cent), but in subsequent years, as mothers went back to their employment early, they tended to turn to bottle feeds. It was found to be useful to introduce a system of interrogation by the ward sister and other mothers of those ready for discharge from hospital to ensure that they knew how to care for their infants. A family planning counsellor also made a weekly visit to the unit to discuss informally the problems resulting from having many babies at frequent intervals whom the mothers could not afford to feed, clothe and educate. The counsellor told them how and where to get the help they might need (Figure 19.6).

Neonatal Care 1973-8

A new maternity hospital was opened in 1973 and two special care nurseries attached to lying-in wards were used until the new intensive care and transitional care units (ICU/TCU) were built in 1979 (Figure 19.7) (see below). These nurseries were equipped with a mobile X-ray machine, excellent incubators and monitoring equipment for several infants, ventilators and a special treatment room. Phototherapy equipment on a large scale was incorporated. Mothers continued to be involved initially in the care of their infants in these nurseries.

Neonatal Care 1979 to Present

Baragwanath Hospital and its eight related peripheral clinics now provide full maternity services for 1.5 million people and were responsible for

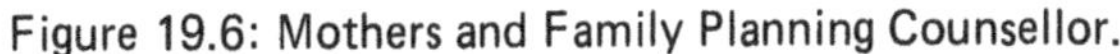
Figure 19.6: Mothers and Family Planning Counsellor.

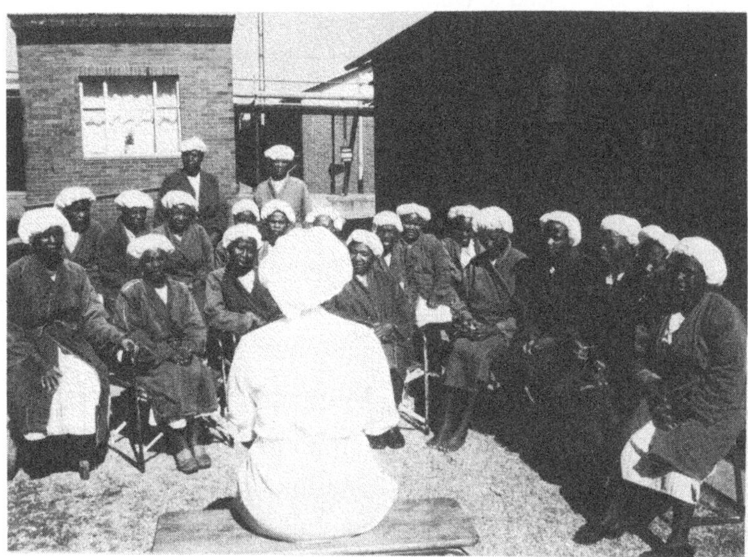

24,000 deliveries in 1980, of which 70 per cent were conducted in the hospital.

Organisation of Neonatal Care

Some 45 per cent of all babies delivered in the hospital are referred to the paediatric staff. Reasons for referral include the following:

(1) Abnormal delivery (currently 16 per cent of patient deliveries are by Caesarean section, of which 86 per cent are emergencies).
(2) All infants below 2.20 kg (below 2.50 kg when referred from outside hospitals).
(3) Prolonged labour, premature rupture of the membranes, clinical evidence of amnionitis, rhesus-negative mothers and those showing positive VDRL tests.
(4) Apgar of 7 or less (assessed by the nursing staff on the labour ward).
(5) Any symptomatic illness or malformation.
(6) Jaundiced infants and apparently well babies of rhesus-negative mothers. Sixty per cent of icteric newborns reveal no underlying cause in spite of full laboratory investigation.

Figure 19.7: Layout of the New Intensive and Transitional Care Unit Which Has been Found to Work Well and Smoothly.

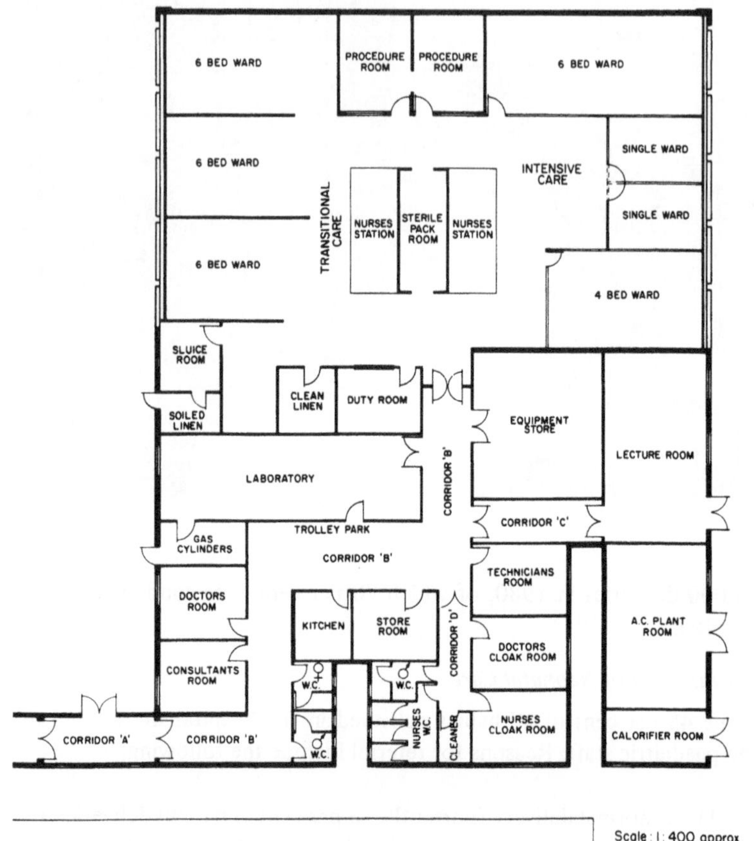

For such infants there are six levels of neonatal care to which they can be sent within the hospital. The initial decision as to where the baby should go rests with a paediatrician on duty in the labour ward, usually a registrar or a senior house officer. One consultant is loosely attached to the labour ward to act as a 'referee' when necessary. Admissions to the ICU are arranged by the labour ward paediatric medical staff liaising directly with the intensive care unit registrar or consultant. Infants less severely ill, but requiring immediate care, are admitted to the TCU. Here they are re-assessed and may be transferred to the ICU if necessary.

Levels of Neonatal Care

(1) Intensive Care Unit (ICU). A twelve-cot fully equipped ICU now exists (Figure 19.7). It is part of a composite ICU/TCU building. It is concerned primarily with the intensive care of infants requiring Intermittent Positive Pressure Ventilation (IPPV) for hyaline membrane disease, meconium aspiration or severe birth asphyxia, plus infants with major neonatal sepsis or undergoing surgery.

(2) Transitional Care Unit (TCU). Eighteen beds are available and equipped (Figure 19.8) to handle care up to and including continuous positive airways pressure (CPAP) and intravenous feeding, and the unit tends to take less severe examples of the conditions admitted to the ICU, plus asymptomatic very low birthweight infants and neurological problems such as convulsions. Both ICU and TCU handle pre- and post-operative surgical emergencies when these are considered to be too ill for the general paediatric surgical ward elsewhere in the hospital.

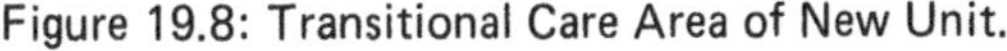
Figure 19.8: Transitional Care Area of New Unit.

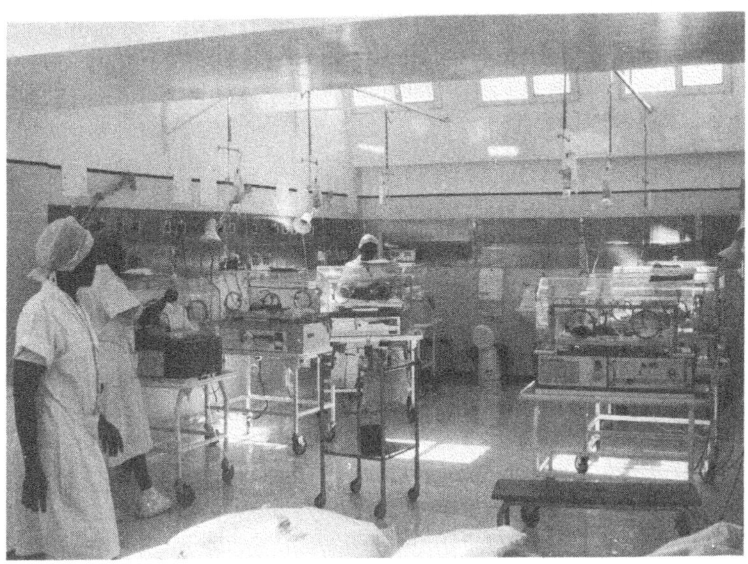

For both these units the mothers are resident in lying-in wards next door and usually stay there until they go with their infants to one of the other levels of care described below. As in the old hospital, other children in the family are looked after by the 'extended' families in Soweto. The mothers are encouraged to spend a lot of time with their infants on the ICU/TCU and help with their care wherever possible, but most procedures, including feeding and changing, are carried out by the nursing staff if the child is critical. The mothers are taught personal hygiene and hand washing and are provided with a complete change of hospital clothing each day. They do not wear extra gowns, masks or overshoes and cross-infection from them is not a problem.

(3) Neonatal 'Special Care'. Fifty cots are available in two nurseries more remotely situated in the maternity hospital, but they may have as many as 80 infants in them at one time. They deal with low birthweight infants who require up to 40 per cent oxygen in incubators or via head-boxes, infants recovering from asphyxia, most metabolic disorders, infections, some congenital anomalies and severely jaundiced babies requiring exchange transfusion, of which about 350 are carried out annually. Outborn infants are freely mixed in with the inborn infants, and no problems with cross-infection arise. Graduates from ICU and TCU are transferred to this area as soon as feasible. The mothers of these infants, trained in hand washing and clothed as above, are resident in adjoining wards but assist much more with their infants' care, including nasogastric tube feeding.

(4) Long-stay Special Care. One ward of 40 beds handles well low birthweight infants of under 1.80 kg who have graduated from the above-mentioned areas, usually when 7-10 days old, having recovered from jaundice, respiratory or other problems. A second ward of 30 beds handles babies over 1.80 kg and those with chronic problems such as neurological deficit, persistent jaundice or infection. This ward also admits jaundiced infants referred from the paediatric OPD and Community Health Clinics for phototherapy or exchange transfusions.

(5) Paediatric Care in Lying-in Wards. There are eight lying-in wards, each with 30 beds. Babies in this category are those seen by paediatric staff daily and who are not considered ill enough to require transfer to specialised paediatric care. Such infants include some requiring phototherapy or observation, those receiving prophylactic antibiotics for premature rupture of membranes and those with minor congenital anomalies and other trivial problems.

(6) Obstetric Care in Lying-in Wards. This concerns normal infants who receive routine care by midwives.

Feeding

In the ICU and, where indicated, in the TCU, intravenous alimentation is administered via a peripheral or central vein using constant infusion pumps. Less commonly infants on ventilators are fed by continuous intra-jejunal or intra-gastric feeds using milk supplied by the mother or milk bank. Feeding of other neonates under 1.50 or 1.60 kg and larger ill babies is done on a three-hourly schedule using expressed breast milk given by nasogastric tube. Breast milk feeds are encouraged at all times and most low birthweight infants are fully breast fed on discharge. If breast milk is insufficient, supplementatry feeds of two-thirds strength cows' milk with added sucrose are given. Most well infants are sent home by the time they reach 2-2.25 kg. Vitamin D and iron are given in the usual way and a supply is given for home use.

Discharge

The discharge routines are similar to those in existence before the new unit was constructed and in general infants have to be feeding well – hopefully on the breast. The mother has to pass her *viva voce* examination from the nursing staff on how to look after her infant and is routinely offered contraceptive advice. Most infants are seen again in a follow-up clinic one month after discharge and further follow-up appointments are arranged as indicated.

Results

The mortality figures during different stages of the unit's development are given in Table 19.4. Detailed figures of causes of death in 1980 appear in Table 19.5 and these reveal that the problem of hyaline membrane disease in low birthweight infants has not been overcome in spite of modern equipment and techniques. Furthermore, asphyxia and its complications, including meconium aspiration, remain a problem at many gestations, but particularly in mature infants.

Summary

The establishment of a special care area in the context of a developing country, short of technical and professional personnel, public funds, infrastructure, communications, etc., requires careful consideration. As

Table 19.4: Baragwanath Hospital, Survival in Low Birthweight Infants Admitted to Special Care.[a]

Birthweight (kg)	1959/60[b] No. Admitted	% Survival	1961/2[b] No. Admitted	% Survival	1980[c] No. Admitted	% Survival
Up to 1.000	116	7	136	14	65	4.5
1.001-1.500	506	51	602	67	276	60
1.501-2.000	510	78	705	91	604	91
2.001-2.500	72	86	77	88	566	94
Totals	1,204	60	1,520	73	1,511	90

Notes:
a. Approximately 45 per cent of infants are small-for-dates.[2]
b. Labour ward deaths excluded.
c. Labour ward deaths included.

shown by experience, it is possible to render a valuable service with modest buildings and basic equipment provided the medical and nursing staff are well motivated, devoted to their duties and reliable. The utilisation of mothers makes a valuable contribution to the successful care of infants, reduces the patient load on the nurses and establishes sound bonding.

Baragwanath Hospital now has a well-equipped and effective perinatal unit which produces improved results and helps to meet the requirements of a developing community with a high birth rate and a large proportion of low birthweight infants (14.5 per cent). The development of the present unit is based upon the experience obtained in the early unsophisticated premature infant unit used with fair success for over 25 years. The main problems which remain are the vast numbers of newborns in need of special care, poor antenatal attendance, low staff/patient ratio and poor socio-economic status of our community. There exists an urgent and compelling need for the training of more medical and nursing staff in the highly technical area of neonatal intensive care. Can there ever be an 'ideal' situation without 'ideal' staff? It is unlikely that any community can afford enough units with enough staff and enough space to meet all requirements, but the aim must be to achieve the highest level of care under prevailing circumstances while improving the community's economic status.

Table 19.5: Neonatal Mortality in Specific Weight Groups – 1980.[a]

	Below 1.00 kg	1.001-1.500	1.501-2.000	2.001-2.500	Above 2.500	Total
Pathology						
Prematurity	26	4	1			31
HMD [b]	32	21	3			56
HMD & complications		43	25			68
Meconium aspiration			1	6	30	37
Asphyxia ± IVH[c]	2	15	8	8	32	65
Other respiratory illness		7	2	2	2	13
Congenital syphilis		4	1	1	3	9
Other infections	1	4	3	4	5	17
Necrotising enterocolitis		8	2	1	1	12
Congenital anomalies tumours		6	4	8	17	35
Miscellaneous			1		4	5
Total	61	112	51	30	94	348
Deaths in each weight group as percentage of total deaths	17.5	32.2	14.6	8.6	27	100
NNM/1,000 L/B	954	399	89	19	6	20.7

Notes:
a. Perinatal mortality, 49.2/1,000 deliveries; neonatal mortality, 20.7/1,000 LB.
b. Hyaline membrane disease.
c. Intraventricular haemorrhage.

Acknowledgements

I wish to thank Professor Harry Stein, Drs K.D. Bolton and Judith M. Rissik for considerable assistance with information and text; Mr R.G. Blair and the Department of Medical Illustration, University of the Witwatersrand, for photographs and figures; Dr B.R. Richard, Medical Officer of Health, for access to population statistics and infant mortality and Dr C. Van Den Heever, Medical Superintendent of Baragwanath Hospital, for access to records and permission to publish.

References

1. Kahn, E., Wayburne, S., and Fouche, M. (1954). The Baragwanath Premature Baby Unit – An analysis of the case records of 1,000 consecutive infants. *S. African Med. J.*, *28*, 453.

2. Stein, H., and Ellis, U. (1974). The low birthweight African baby. *Arch. Dis. Child.*, *49*, 156.

20 STOCKHOLM, SWEDEN: THE SMALL BABY NOT REQUIRING INTENSIVE CARE

Peter de Chateau

Introduction

According to Orme and Boxall[1] transitional care is 'intermediate neonatal care', where babies receive frequent observation and treatment, but not constant surveillance on a minute-to-minute basis 24 hours around the clock. This concept is based on the original idea of the Committee on the Fetus and Newborn of the American Academy of Pediatrics[2]. The Exeter model[1] lays stress on facilities for parents *and* siblings, the encouragement of parent staff co-operation and the joint sharing of responsibility for the newborn, and is provided on specially designated lying-in wards. These same aims underly the organisation of neonatal units in Scandinavia. During the last decade, as the number of intensive care cots has increased, some wards have developed as pure intensive care units while the majority mix intensive and special care. This chapter describes the situation in Sweden where the need for neonatal intensive care cots is relatively low, and describes the attempts made to improve parent-infant relations and parental reactions to the care provided.

The Swedish Health Care System

A low birthrate and the low incidence of prematurity and low birthweight are an important part of the bckground to the Swedish system of perinatal care. In Sweden almost 95 per cent of all medical care, 99 per cent of hospital care and 85 per cent of outpatient and community care is provided through the Community Health Care System. All residents are included in the National Health Care System; even those who visit private practitioners and private specialists get refunds for most of their medical care expenses. Private beds in hospitals are only found in a few hospitals in the largest cities, and no private neonatal care is provided at all. Some of the follow-up of 'at risk' babies with minor problems is done by private paediatricians.

Prenatal Care

The Health Care System reaches about 99 per cent of all pregnant women who make an average of ten visits to a midwife and three to a doctor during pregnancy. Antenatal clinics are located throughout the country, and routine care is given mainly by midwives, who do not, however, deliver the mothers. Each antenatal clinic serves a defined catchment area, so that several clinics together cover the population of pregnant women which uses the facilities of a maternity hospital for delivery and postnatal care. Doctors, general practitioners and obstetricians are consultants and work in the clinics on a part-time basis. In theory at least, midwives and general practitioners handle only normal and uncomplicated pregnancies; all non-optimal cases are referred to an obstetrician. During the last trimester of their pregnancies women usually visit the hospital where they will be delivered to get acquainted with the units and their staff.

Perinatal Care

This is given primarily at the local hospitals and, depending on the presence and degree of complications, also in secondary or tertiary centres. In order to guarantee maximal safety and care for all infants, hospital deliveries are preferred, and only in highly exceptional cases are deliveries elsewhere accepted.[3] According to official government recommendations maternity units should have the following goals:[4]

(1) Close observation of all deliveries and the provision of emotional and psychological support.
(2) Observation of pregnant women to prevent complications for mothers and infants.
(3) Sufficient time and rest for mothers to recover after birth.
(4) Opportunity for mothers to learn about the needs and the care of their newborns.
(5) Surveillance of the babies for optimal adaptation to extrauterine life.
(6) Provision of information regarding establishment of adequate nutrition for new mothers and their offspring.

While these recommendations relating to the medical safety of the mother and her infant are widely observed, the situation for psychosocial aspects of care is more varied. This is despite our belief that delivery is a sensitive period for parents when the foundation for optimal parent-child relationships is laid.

Postnatal Care

This is extremely important in terms of transition from one phase of the mother's life to the next. Great efforts should be made to provide optimal care and support. Social benefits are excellent and varied. One which is almost unique concerns parental leave. All the newly delivered mothers are entitled to almost full pay for nine months' leave after delivery and to another three months with reduced salary. This can be divided between the mother and the father and the one on leave gets about 90 per cent of the normal salary paid through the social security system.[5] Recent statistics show, however, that only a small minority (about 10-15 per cent) of all fathers make use of this possibility and an even smaller proportion of fathers uses the total leave time available. This illustrates very well that social policy cannot provide the means of reaching all desirable goals.

Maternal and Neonatal Care in the Karolinska Hospital

The greater Stockholm area with about one million inhabitants has its perinatal care organised in four main hospitals. The Karolinska hospital is located in the north-western part, and a summary of some perinatal background data in comparison with the whole of Sweden is given in Table 20.1. The frequency of complicated pregnancies, such as diabetes, Rh-immunisation, intrauterine growth retardation and preeclampsia is approximately four times greater than the average for the country. The neonatal ward has a total of 20 beds, eight for intensive and twelve for special care (Figure 20.1). A total of approximately 650 infants per year are admitted, about 125 of whom are admitted from other hospitals in the catchment area. Some 40 infants from hospitals outside this area are referred for intensive care. Annually about 60 infants are treated with assisted ventilation.

The mortality, morbidity and complication rate are comparable with the best to be found in Sweden.[6] For instance, the survival rate for infants with a birthweight of under 1.00 kg is about 65 per cent and of those between 1.00 and 1.499 kg is 88 per cent. The frequency of sequelae like retrolental fibroplasia, bronchopulmonary dysplasia, cerebral palsy and mental retardation is low.[7] The major indications for admission to the neonatal ward are respiratory disease, prematurity, growth retardation, suspected infections and asphyxia, either during or directly after delivery. A great number of infants are admitted for observation or with relatively minor problems. Among these are minor

Table 20.1: Some Perinatal Statistics, Karolinska Hospital (KS), and Comparison with the Whole of Sweden in Percentages of Number of Deliveries (1980).

	KS (n=2,396) %	Sweden (n=94,378) %
Maternal age 35 years or more	12.9	8.5
Breech presentation	1.2	2.5
Vacuum extraction	11.0	6.2
Epidural anaesthesia	20.0	13.2
Birthweight (kg):		
below 1.000	0.3	0.1
1.000-1.499	0.4	0.3
1.500-1.999	1.3	0.8
2.000-2.499	4.0	2.6
All below 2.500	6.0	3.8
Perinatal deaths	0.7	0.8
Neonatal deaths (0-7 d)	0.5	0.4
Apgar less than or equal to at 5 min.	1.1	2.5
Gestational length below 37 wks	4.9	4.8

adaptational difficulties, moderate asphyxia, problems maintaining body temperature, feeding difficulties and hyperbilirubinaemia. In 1981 about 20 per cent of all newborn babies were admitted to the neonatal ward, more than half with minor problems, and stayed 1-2 days. Many of these babies would not have been admitted if it had not been for various staff problems. Among these were the difficulty of providing continuity of staff and staff of sufficient knowledge or confidence during non-office hours. The young doctors on duty alone at night and at the weekend tend, to a greater extent than their more experienced colleagues, to admit babies with minor problems to the neonatal ward and to keep them there for observation, perhaps because signs and symptoms of the newborn are difficult to assess accurately. Midwives, nurses and nurse-aids working in large centres become accustomed to rely rather heavily on medical staff. When slight deviations in the infants' condition from what is considered to be normal are reported, house officers are consulted and the baby is then admitted to the neonatal unit. These circumstances, where staff have few opportunities to develop skills and confidence, create a vicious circle. This trend is reinforced by the fact that more nurses, midwives and nurse-aids are working part-time and are relatively young; they are less experienced

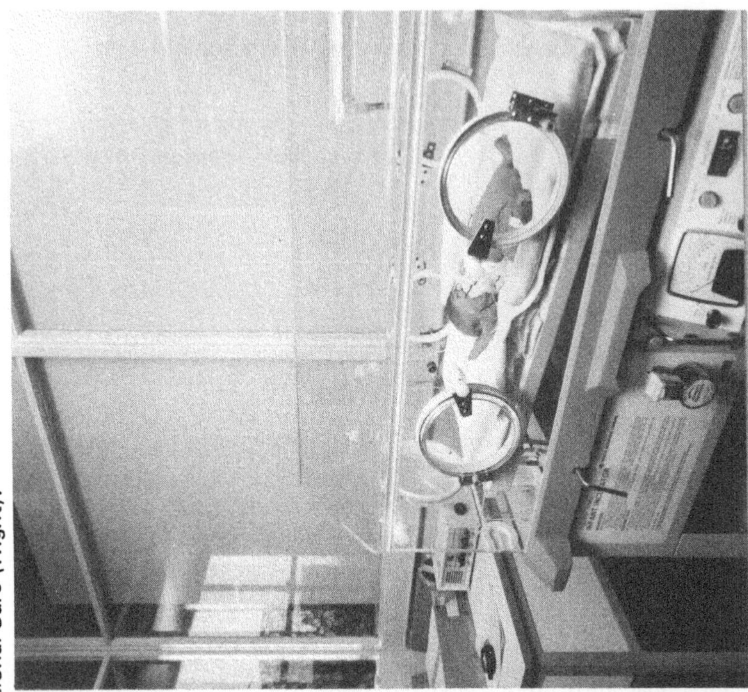

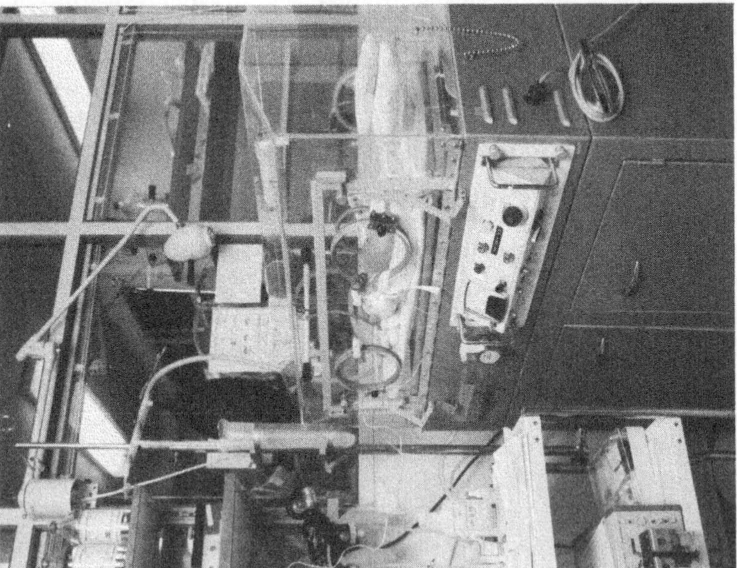

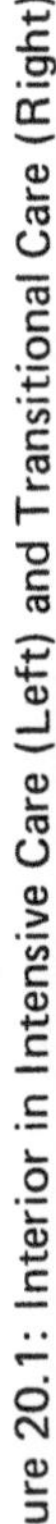

Figure 20.1: Interior in Intensive Care (Left) and Transitional Care (Right).

and, because they are working on a rotating schedule, may lack knowledge concerning the condition of a particular baby.

We are hoping to reduce the transfer of newborns from maternity wards to the postnatal ward by postgraduate training of all staff members and providing facilities on the maternity wards for observation of infants with minor difficulties. There should be rooms on each maternity floor for infant observation with nursery nurses especially trained in the neonatal ward assigned to them. Phototherapy, tube feeding, observation of healthy premature newborns and minor procedures can then be carried out in these rooms. In this way mothers and infants can be kept together, staff will get more experience and responsibility should grow, thus minimising the traumatic effects of separation. We do not yet know to what extent we can institute such a programme and how successful it will be, but it is necessary to break the trend towards more special care and the observation and treatment of infants with very minor problems in special care units.

The development of more technological treatment in neonatal units in the last decade poses dangers and threats to the psychological climate in such units.[8] In an effort to counteract these negative side-effects, more attention has been given to the support of infants, their parents and the staff. A social worker and a psychologist have been working in the neonatal ward at Karolinska for many years. During the last two years a child psychiatrist (half-time) and the hospital minister (part-time) have been introduced.[9] Intensive contact between parents and infants has been encouraged.[10] This is of utmost importance for the mobilisation of fear, anxiety, ambivalence and guilt in parents. During the acute phase of shock[11] a start has to be made with this important and vital work. However, the most difficult period is most probably the subsequent weeks and months, when realisation, reorientation and adjustment have to take place.[9] In our experience the need for support for these parents during this later period is too often forgotten or given a rather low priority. Our new consultants have the time and personal qualifications to carry this load and the work at the unit would be difficult without their presence. They also seem to have more time and skills for the important follow-up work, especially with parents of infants who have died.

Those periods of the day when few parents are present in the neonatal unit are an excellent time to go around and talk to the staff, especially those who watch over the most severely ill infants. At these occasions private discussions with nurses and nurse-aids can take place. Group discussions, originally once a week, have decreased in number as individual consultations have increased, and the relations between staff members and between them, the infants and parents have been clarified. Our new consultants spend on an average 20-25 hours/week at the unit with flexible hours. Individual needs of parents as well as of the staff can therefore be met in a very responsive way. Our intention is that more time can be spent in this way and that the present temporary arrangement will be made permanent. Other research supports this type of care.[12]

Parental Experiences of Special Care

The harmful consequences of neonatal mother-child separation have been reported[12-14] and are reviewed in Chapter 1. If separation can have important effects, we need to know how these can be neutralised. Such research should start with an analysis of factors such as the impact of the severity of the infant's condition, duration of separation, the time of first physical contact between parent and infant, and the mode of delivery. In a small-scale project at the Umea University Hospital, all parents who, during March 1975, gave birth to an infant that was admitted to the neonatal ward immediately after delivery were included. Out of 26 infants, one died the day after birth, another was adopted, and there was one set of twins. Twenty-three parent pairs were then studied.[15]

The most important observation in this small study was that mothers of the infants who were most severely ill felt less important to their infants and had more difficulty in relating to them than mothers with healthier infants. They also took longer to feel that their baby was their own. This can be seen as an expression of anticipatory grief.[5] The mother's fear that the infant will die may also prevent her from accepting her positive feelings towards the infant, in order to avoid some of the pain caused by losing a newborn infant. There was no correlation between the period of time before the mother was first able to touch her infant and her feeling for the baby. Mothers who were delivered by Caesarian section under general anaesthetic had to wait longest to touch their babies, usually more than one day. They, like other mothers, felt that this delay was too long.

There were insufficient data to permit comparison between fathers and mothers. Further analysis of the paternal role is desirable, as the need for contact between father and infant and for support from the father may be especially great when the infant is ill.[16] From our own and Lind's[17] data we believe that fathers should be more involved in hospital care.

The Care of Infants of Diabetic Mothers

For many years there has been general agreement concerning the principles of the treatment of diabetic pregnancies and the perinatal mortality has gradually decreased. Several factors may help to explain these improved results, but probably the most important is the establishment and maintenance of normal maternal blood sugar levels.[18–20] One recommendation concerning the care of these infants in Sweden has been that all newborn babies of diabetic mothers have to be observed, regardless of their symptoms, in a neonatal ward. This policy has automatically resulted in separation of mother and newborn. The potentially deleterious impact of separation has gradually been appreciated and from 1974 onwards all possible emphasis has been made to avoid separation in the neonatal unit at Umea University Hospital.

In 1976 a study was made of the outcome of all diabetic pregnancies treated in the years 1974-6 in comparison with those of 1969-73, when total automatic separation of mothers and babies was the rule. Sixty-five infants were born to 62 diabetic women, 45 during the first period and 20 during the second one. Relationships between important background factors and results are given in Table 20.2. Over the total period 1969-76, the maternal age was found to be positively ($p = 0.01$) correlated with the frequency of severe infant malformation. The mean time of stay in the neonatal ward decreased continuously (Table 20.3), and several children were never admitted to the neonatal ward at all during the latter part of the study. No major differences in medical status or complications were noticed,[20] and the severity of other complications among the infants was not significantly different in the two periods. The rule that all newborn children of diabetic mothers have to be kept on the neonatal ward has consequently been abandoned.

Concluding Remarks

The care of the sick and pre-term infant is an important part of preventive paediatrics, and the education and training of the staff is as basic a part of the paediatrician's duties as the close observation of the newborn and advising and supporting their parents.[21] Extremely prematurely

Table 20.2: Diabetic Mothers and their Babies – the Relations between White-Pedersen Class, Birthweight (kg), Length of Pregnancy (Weeks) and Occurrence of Malformed Infants.

N	White-Pedersen Class	Mean Weight (Range)	Length of Pregn. (Range)	Malformed Infants
14	A	3.4 (2.1-5.0)	37.6 (34-41)	1
18	B	3.8 (1.5-4.6)	36.9 (33-39)	2
14	C	2.9 (2.0-4.0)	37.0 (36-40)	1
16	D	3.1 (1.7-5.0)	36.8 (35-40)	0
3	F	2.8 (2.4-3.7)	36.3 (36-37)	1
65 (total)		3.1 (1.5-5.0)	37.0 (33-41)	5

Table 20.3: Infants of Diabetic Mothers – Length of Postnatal Stay in the Neonatal Ward (Days).[20]

Year	Mean	Stay (Range)	Number of Children	No. of Children Who Were Never Kept in the Neonatal Ward
1969	11.5	(4-22)	7	0
1970	16.3	(5-39)	7	0
1971	18.1	(7-32)	11	0
1972	10.1	(0-33)	13	1
1973	6.1	(2-10)	7	0
1974	6.8	(0-26)	5	1
1975	1.0	(0-2)	3	1
1976	5.6	(0-40)	12	8
Total	10.7		65	11

born and/or severely sick infants and their parents meet in an intensive care unit an environment of stress, separation and special treatment, and often too little time can be devoted to them. Even in special care units, and when babies are waiting to grow so that they can be discharged,[9] an environment of limited human interaction and limited stimulation is often present.

Does separation, on top of the medically and technically complicated care of these babies, cause further harm, especially in the long term? This, apparently simple, question is not very easily answered. An interesting way of conceptualising this problem has been put forward by Bostock and others.[22-23] Basically this suggests a continuity in intra- and extra-uterine gestation. We most certainly have to recognise and understand all aspects of perinatal care procedures in order to make these as safe and humane as possible and attuned to the variety and complexity of goals that have to be realised in this care.[24]

Some measures can be proposed in order to facilitate this goal. Antenatal preparation, education, information, staff involvement and continuity can be promoted. Early post-delivery contact, continuity of personnel, parental information and involvement, education and coaching of the staff as well as the special care for parents of malformed infants and a thorough preparation for discharge, regardless of severity of illness and duration of stay and type of neonatal care, are all means of promoting the best and optimal conditions for the healthy and normal growth and development of the infants who temporarily are put in our care. The environment of pre-term babies has to ensure optimal post-natal adaptation.[25-27]

Acknowledgements

Parts of this review article were aided by the Swedish Medical Research Council (Grant No. 5443), the Krolinska Institute and by Social and Behavioral Science Research Grant No. 11-23 from the Foundation March of Dimes, New York.

References

1. Orme, R.L.'E., and Boxall, J. (1978). The changing pattern of parental involvement in the special care baby unit in Exeter. In *Separation and Special Care Baby Units*, F.S.W. Brimblecome, M.P.M. Richards and N.R.C. Roberton (eds). London, SIMP/Heinemann Medical Books, 64-8.

2. Committee on the Fetus and Newborn (1971). *Standards and Recommendations for Hospital Care of Newborn Infants*, 5th edn. American Academy of Pediatrics.

3. The Swedish National Board of Health and Welfare (1979). *Mödra – och Barnhälso-vård*. Stockholm, Socialstyrelsen.

4. The Swedish National Board of Health and Welfare (1973). *Förlossningvårdens Organisation*. Stockholm, Socialstyrelsen.

5. Winberg, J., and de Chateau, P. (1983). Early social development: studies of infant-mother interaction and relationships. In *Review of Child Development Research, Vol. 6*, W.W. Hartup (ed.). Chicago, University of Chicago Press, in press.

6. Ahlström, H., Lindroth, M., and Svenningsen, N. (1979). Neonatal intensivvård och respiratorbehandling av mycket lågviktiga barn. *Läkartidningen, 76,* 1721.

7. de Chateau, P., *et al.* Unpublished data.

8. Field, T. M., Sostek, A. M., Goldberg, S., and Sherman, H. H. (1979). *Infants Born at Risk*. New York, SP Medical and Scientific Books.

9. Godvik, M., and de Chateau, P. (1982). Barnpsykiatrisk konsultverksamhet vid neonatal – avdelning. *Nord. Med.*, *97*, 78.

10. Klaus, M. H., and Kennell, J. H. (1976). *Mother-infant Bonding*. St Louis, C. V. Mosby Co.

11. Kaplan, D. M., and Mason, E. (1960). Maternal reactions to premature birth viewed as an acute emotional disorder. *Am. J. Orthopsychiatry*, *30*, 539.

12. Barnett, C., Leiderman, P. H., Grobstein, R., and Klaus, M. (1970). Neonatal separation: the maternal side of interactional deprivation. *Pediatrics*, *45*, 197.

13. Kennell, J. H., and Klaus, M. H. (1971). Care of the mother of the high-risk infant. *Clin. Obstet. Gyn.*, *14*, 926.

14. Leiderman, P. H., and Seashore, M. J. (1975). Mother-infant separation: some delayed consequences. In *Parent-Infant Interaction*, Ciba Foundation Symposium, No. 33. Amsterdam, Elsevier, 213.

15. de Chateau, P. (1976). *Neonatal Care Routines*. Medical dissertation, Umea University, No. 20 (new series).

16. Blake, A., Stewart, A., and Turcan, D. (1975). Parents of babies of very low birth weight. In *Parent-Infant Interaction*, Ciba Foundation Symposium, No. 33. Amsterdam, Elsevier, 271.

17. Lind, J. (1973). Die geburt der familie in der frauenklinik. *Med. Klin.*, *68*, 1597.

18. Karlsson, K., and Kjellmer, J. (1972). The outcome of diabetic pregnancies in relation to the mothers' blood sugar level. *Am. J. Obstet. Gynecol.*, *112*, 213.

19. Pedersen, J., Mosted-Pedersen, L., and Andersen, B. (1974). Assessors of fetal and perinatal mortality in diabetic pregnancy. *Diabetes*, *23*, 302.

20. Lithner, F., de Chateau, P., Wickman, M., and Wiklund, D. E. (1977). Treatment of pregnancy diabetics in a scarcely populated region. *Opuscula Med.*, *22*, 119.

21. Brenndorff, von I. (1973). Säuglingspflege. *Med. Klin.*, *68*, 1354.

22. Bostock, J. (1962). Evolutional approach to infant care. *Lancet*, *1*, 1238.

23. Earnshaw, P. A. (1961). The baby's birthright: a plea for a return to exterior gestation and breastfeeding. *Med. J. Austr.*, *48*, 238.

24. Keefer, C. H. (1977). Pollution of the fetus: the delivery experience. Paper presented at the American Psychology Association, San Francisco.

25. Newman, L. (1981). Social and sensory environment of low birth weight infants in a special care nursery. *J. Neur. Ment. Dis.*, *169*, 448.

26. Brody, E. B., and Klein, H. (1980). The intensive care nursery as a small society. *Paediatrician*, *9*, 169.

27. Minde, K., Trehub, S., Cortes, C., *et al.* (1978). Mother-child relationships in the premature nursery: an observational study. *Pediatrics*, *61*, 373.

21 MONTREAL' CANADA: EARLY DISCHARGE OF PRE-TERM NEWBORN INFANTS

Francine Lefebvre and Harry Bard

Ste-Justine's Hospital is a paediatric centre which provides neonatal intensive care as well as care for high-risk obstetric patients. There are 4,000 deliveries per year, 30 per cent of whom are from high-risk mothers. The neonatal intensive care unit admits 1,400 newborns per year, 40 per cent of whom are referred from hospitals elsewhere in the Province of Quebec, which deliver approximately 50,000 babies per annum. The neonatal department is divided into an intensive care unit and normal postnatal wards. The neonatal intensive care unit (NICU) has two sections, an intensive care area which can manage up to 17 newborns, and an intermediate care nursery limited to 40-42 beds.

Pre-term infants admitted to our NICU include those born elsewhere and transferred immediately after delivery as well as those born to high-risk mothers transported to our centre for delivery. When the clinical and social conditions permit, these infants may be transferred back to their local hospital. The majority however are cared for in a postnatal ward within the department until discharge home.

In many hospitals that provide obstetric care in Canada, it is still the custom not to discharge low birthweight infants until they weigh 2.50 kg. However, the importance that has recently been given to the effects of early contact on the establishment of infant-mother bonding[1] has reinforced the belief that early discharge of low birthweight infants could potentiate this process, since a pre-term infant at home will certainly be exposed to more parental contact than in hospital. Discharging the low birthweight infant will decrease his chances of hospital acquired infections – an infrequent but real danger – it will free more beds and nursing time for the more acutely ill, and it will also decrease hospital costs. Furthermore, during the last decade, many studies from industrialised as well as underdeveloped countries have shown that early discharge of low birthweight infants is possible and safe (Table 21.1).[2-10]

Before establishing a similar routine early discharge practice from the NICU in our hospital, a study was carried out to assess its safety. Low birthweight infants (2.00 kg or less at birth), born at Ste-Justine Hospital between October 1979 and June 1980 to mothers living in the

Table 21.1: Summary of the Studies on Early Discharge.

Ref.	Origin	Number of Cases	Mean Discharge Weight (range) (kg)	Results
2	Boston (45% low incomes)	170	2.062 (1.588 – 2.268)	No readmission — no ill effect
3	New York (suitable homes)	57	2.058 (1.720 – 2.280)	Good growth: 89% Lost to follow-up: 7% Bad results: 4% (1 died of sepsis and 1 had a slow growth)
4	Memphis (poverty and inadequate housing)	183	2.076 (2.000 and more)	Comparable weight gain 1 and 4 weeks after discharge In each group, one death and 4-5% readmissions
		198	2.295 (2.268 and more)	
5	Rhodesia (under-developed country)	264	1.838 (1.801 – 1.900)	Readmissions: 9.5% — Mortality: 5.7%
		99	1.959 (1.901 – 2.000)	Readmissions: 1% — Mortality: 1%
		132	2.152 (2.001 – 2.500)	Readmissions: 0.8% — Mortality: 0.8%
6	Denver	44	2.060 (1.600 – 2.800)	No more illnesses than control group of AGA term newborns. One death in study group (? cause)
8	Jamaica	7	1.220 – 1.399	Tube feeding at home Satisfactory evolution: 78%
		25	1.400 – 1.599	Lost to follow-up: 9.6% Readmissions: 12.4% (including one death from
		41	1.600 – 1.816	pertussis in the heavier group)
9	England (adequate homes)	20	1.946 (1.700 – 2.260)	Comparable mean weight at EDC and 3 months No readmissions, no mortality
		20	2.271 (2.200 – 2.250)	

Montreal metropolitan area were studied. Twenty-one infants (born on odd days) were allocated to an early discharge group, and were sent home when they weighed less than 2.20 kg, when the following criteria were met:

(1) They were clinically well and any medical problems were under control.
(2) They had outgrown their birthweight and established satisfactory weight gain.
(3) They had satisfactory temperature control in room air (infants were taken out of the incubator when they weighed 1.80 kg).
(4) They were taking oral feeding by nipple.
(5) On the basis of information obtained from the nurses in the NICU and home visiting nurses, their mother was thought to be capable of caring for them at home.

Seventeen infants (the control group, born on even days) were discharged according to the same criteria, but only when they weighed 2.20-2.40 kg. All infants except one were appropriate in weight for their gestational age. The early discharge and control group were comparable in birthweight (1.66 ± 0.21 kg vs 1.53 ± 0.29 kg), gestational age (32.1 ± 2 vs 31.2 weeks), sex ratio and neonatal illnesses (asphyxia, need for mechanical ventilation, respiratory distress syndrome, apnoea and bradycardia, and need for exchange transfusion). Three sets of twins were included in the early discharge group and one set in the control group. The two groups were similar in respect of mother's age, her marital status, her age (26.1 ± 3.3 years vs 28.3 ± 5.7 years), and her parity (approximately half primiparous, half multiparous).

The early discharge from the nursery was carefully planned for each individual infant. The neonatologists, house staff, nurses, a psychiatrist, psychologist and social worker from the NICU met once a week to discuss problems presented by sick newborns and/or by their families. It gave the members of the group a chance to plan the best approach to the family while the newborn was in hospital, and to elaborate a discharge and follow-up programme. Throughout hospitalisation, but particularly just before discharge, mothers and fathers came into the nursery to handle, bathe, feed and change the diapers of their infants. Breast feeding rooms were available for mothers who had been discharged from hospital. The infants in both groups were followed up in the neonatal clinic. Nurses from the clinic also evaluated the home before and after discharge.

Results

The early discharge group had a mean discharge weight of 2.01 ± 0.08 kg (range 1.89 – 2.19 kg): eleven of the 21 infants were sent home weighing less than 2.00 kg. The control group had a significantly heavier discharge weight, 2.26 ± 0.06 kg (range 2.20 – 2.40 kg, $p < 0.001$). At the expected date of delivery the weight was similar in the two groups (3.09 ± 0.40 kg vs 3.15 ± 0.45 kg; Table 21.2). The two groups had similar lengths, head circumferences and haemoglobin concentrations at the expected date of delivery. Duration of hospitalisation was reduced by a mean of 11.6 days in the early discharge infants ($p < 0.025$, Table 21.2).

Table 21.2: Weight on Discharge and at Expected Date of Delivery and Duration of Hospitalisation for the Two Study Groups.

	Early Discharge Group (n = 21)	Control Group (n = 17)	P
Weight on discharge	2.01 ± 0.08	2.26 ± 0.06	0.001
Weight at EDC[a]	3.09 ± 0.4	3.15 ± 0.45	NS
Days in hospital	26.3 ± 15.2	37.9 ± 14.5	0.025

Note: a. Expected date of confinement.

As judged by visits to the emergency room (four infants in the early discharge group and two control infants), no infant in either group suffered from a serious illness during the interval between discharge and the expected date of delivery. Only one infant – from the early discharge group – was admitted to the hospital for an upper respiratory tract infection. No death occurred in either group. Unfortunately numbers were not large enough to demonstrate a beneficial effect of early discharge on the incidence or duration of breast feeding. However, our data show that when combined with the programme of home visits by nurses and careful follow-up, discharge of infants weighing 2.00 ± 0.1 kg was safe and should be encouraged.

Early Discharge of Infants of Lower Birthweight

In order to determine whether this early discharge policy evaluated during 1979-80 had any impact on the discharge of pre-term infants in other weight categories, the discharge weight and the duration of hospitalisation were compared in inborn infants weighing less than 2.10 kg at birth and discharged home from our hospital in the year prior to (1978), and in the year after (1981) the initial study.

Infants were divided into four groups (Table 21.3): those with a birthweight less than 1.50 kg – group 1; those with a birthweight 1.50-1.79 kg – group 2; those with a birthweight 1.80-1.99 kg – group 3; and those weighing 2.00-2.10 kg – group 4. The mean birthweight and length of gestation were similar in all groups in the two years except for group 2 who, in 1981, had a lower mean gestational age. This study demonstrated that in 1981 there was a decrease in the discharge weight of all groups except those in group 1. However, it was in group 4 weighing 2.00-2.10 kg at birth where the policy of early discharge had the greatest impact. They remained 4.5 days less in hospital in 1981 compared to 1978 (10.7 ± 6.6 $p < 0.025$), and it enabled normal infants of this birthweight delivered in our hospital to be considered for discharge with their mothers.

Table 21.3: Infants of Low Birthweight
Discharge Weight (kg ± 1 SD).

Group	Birthweight (kg)	1978	1981	P
I	below 1.50	2.22 ± 0.1 (n = 32)	2.24 ± 0.34 (n = 75)	NS
II	1.50 – 1.79	2.29 ± 0.15 (n = 42)	2.15 ± 0.18 (n = 57)	0.001
III	1.80 – 1.99	2.27 ± 0.2 (n = 38)	2.12 ± 0.19 (n = 43)	0.001
IV	2.00 – 2.10	2.22 ± 0.15 (n = 33)	2.11 ± 0.15 (n = 27)	0.01

Analysis of the proportion of infants discharged home weighing less than 2.00 kg shows that in 1978 only 4 per cent (4/112) of inborn infants weighing less than 2.00 kg at birth were discharged with their weight still below 2.00 kg, whereas in 1981 23 per cent (41/175) of such infants were discharged weighing 2.00 kg or less ($p < 0.005$, Table 21.4). The lowest discharge weight was 1.84 kg.

In group 2 (birthweight 1.50-1.79 kg) a significantly lower weight was adopted for discharge in 1981 with the result that 19 per cent were discharged home weighing less than 2.00 kg compared to none in 1978. This was despite greater prematurity in the 1981 group (32.6 weeks vs 34 weeks). In the infants weighing 2.00-2.10 kg at birth 44 per cent

Table 21.4: Number of Infants Discharged Home Weighing Less than 2.00 kg.

Group	Birthweight (kg)	1978	1981	P
I	<1.50	2/32 (6%)	18/7 (24%)	<0.05
II	1.50 – 1.79	0/42 (0%)	11/57 (19%)	<0.005
III	1.80 – 1.99	2/38 (5%)	12/43 (28%)	<0.01
IV	All infants 2.00	4/112 (4%)	41/175 (23%)	<0.005

were discharged with their mother in 1981 compared with 27 per cent in 1978. There were no deaths in infants discharged early, but in 1981 one infant (discharge weight 1.93 kg) had to be readmitted four days later with an upper respiratory tract infection causing apnoea for which a short period of assisted ventilation was required.

Conclusion

At Ste-Justine Hospital the policy of early discharge of low birthweight infants has allowed more infants to be discharged home weighing 2.00 kg or less. This has been made possible by using nurses who are assigned to home visits and by close follow-up in the neonatal out-patient clinic. The early discharge policy is certainly a step in the direction of favouring early maternal-infant contact. It encourages early physical contact between parents and their pre-term newborn infants during hospitalisation and should have favourable effects on long-term parental-infant interaction.

References

1. Klaus, M. H., and Kennell, J. H. (1976). *Maternal-infant Bonding*. St Louis, C. V. Mosby Co.

2. Berg, R. B., Salisbury, A. J., and Kahan, R. (1969). 'Early' discharge of low-birthweight infants. *J.A.M.A.*, *210*, 1892.

3. Berg, B., and Salisbury, A. J. (1971). Discharging infants of low birth-weight. *Amer. J. Dis. Child.*, *122*, 414.

4. Bauer, C. H., and Tinklepaugh, W. (1971). Low birth weight babies in the hospital. A survey of recent changes in their care, with special emphasis on early discharge. *Clin. Pediatr.*, *10*, 467.

5. Dillard, R. G., and Korones, S. B. (1973). Lower discharge weight and shortened nursery stay for the low birth weight infants. *N. Eng. J. Med.*, *288*, 131.

6. Singer, B., and Wolfsdorf, J. (1975). Early discharge of infants of low birth weight: a prospective study. *Brit. Med. J.*, *i*, 362-9.

7. Woodall, J. B., Merenstein, G. B., and Merchant, M. (1976). Early discharge of low birth weight (LBW) infants. (Abstract.) *Clinical Research*, *24*, 196A.

8. Singh, M. (1979). Early discharge of low-birth-weight babies. *Trop. Geog. Med.*, *31*, 565.

9. Lowry, M. F., Jones, M. R., and Shanahan, M. D. (1978). Discharge of small babies from hospital. (Letter) *Arch. Dis. Child.*, *53*, 522.

10. Davies, D. P., Haxby, V., Herbert, S., and McNeish, A. S. (1979). When should pre-term babies be sent home from neonatal units? *Lancet*, *i*, 914.

Part Four

THE FUTURE

22 THE FUTURE

J. A. Davis, M. P. M. Richards and N. R. C. Roberton

The contributors to this book have taken a broad look at the evidence concerning the parent-child relationship for those children who begin their lives in a neonatal unit. This evidence supports those who have believed in the importance of providing medical care in such a way that parental relationships are encouraged and given every opportunity to develop and flourish. Quite apart from the difficulties that may arise from the kind of medical care required by a very small or sick infant, the emotional stresses that may accompany the birth of such a baby mean that the parents are often vulnerable, very anxious and lack any confidence in being able to look after their child. Thus, their needs are greater than those of parents of babies whose birth is straightforward. In this book these special needs, and the ways in which they may be met, are illustrated by a number of accounts of the ways in which care is organised in various centres. Each of these centres in their different way places special emphasis on the preservation and fostering of parental relations. Such an emphasis has become much more usual among neonatal paediatricians in recent years and it is now common to find them working in collaboration with other colleagues whose primary concerns are the emotional and social aspects of care. However, such an approach is not universal and we are well aware that the patterns of care described in this book are not typical of all centres.

Problems Which Remain to be Solved

We recognise that several specific difficulties remain to be dealt with before improvements incorporating the practices outlined in this book can take place generally. Some problems will have to be solved by a change of attitude, whereas other problems are only likely to be solved by an improvement in the amount of equipment provided and in the numbers and training of staff. However, little extra building needs to be done, though when neonatal units are replaced they should be much better designed.

The first and perhaps most important difficulty that prevents good psychological as well as good physical care in NNUs is the dualism that lies in the foundation of medical practice. While we all know intellectually that stressed and unhappy patients are less likely to do well, there is still a tendency not only to regard the psychological and physical as separate domains, but to regard the latter as the real business of medicine. According to this view the emotional and social needs of patients are regarded as a kind of icing on the cake: something that is nice to attend to, providing that the important issues have been resolved. We hope that this book will provide no comfort for those who want to cling to this outdated view. It is not possible to provide adequate neonatal care without placing the emotional needs of parents and children at the centre of the scheme of things and seeing them as part and parcel of all that is done.

The second problem which we see arises out of the fact that in population terms the illnesses that a neonatal unit deals with are rare. This means that a large catchment area is needed to provide a reasonable level of activity and thus competence in the specialist unit. Most areas already have, or are moving towards, a system where there is a neonatal unit attached to all the large maternity units and intensive care is available on a regional basis. Logistically, in terms of the availability of experienced staff and special equipment, such a pattern makes sense; but it does make difficulties for parents. Even in densely populated areas, visiting may involve long and expensive journeys[1] and presents particular difficulties to families with older children[2]. There is no simple answer to this problem and solutions are likely to vary with the circumstances, but it is a problem too easily underestimated by those who work within a busy neonatal unit. For those unable, because of geography, family commitments, or poverty to stay in the mother and baby rooms, or to visit their baby as frequently as possible, appropriate financial and home help should be available.

One specific example of the difficulty that faces the neonatologist when patients come from a great distance is that life and death decisions sometimes have to be taken before there is even a chance to meet parents, let alone to have a thorough discussion with them of the issues and feelings involved. The regionalisation of care can mean that a baby arrives at an intensive care unit while the parents are many miles away. The ideal of a situation where a neonatologist can get to know the parents before the delivery and can get some sense of their feelings is seldom obtained. However, considerations of this kind provide support for those who would like to see the neonatal paediatrician much more involved in antenatal and perinatal care. This is now possible in many of the larger appropriately staffed regional units, and is yet another reason for fostering the concept of antenatal transfer of the high-risk pregnant female to the regional *perinatal* centre so that this type of care can be provided before the mother delivers.

A third and very important problem is how to provide appropriate public education. There is scope for being more imaginative in antenatal classes for parents. It is often thought that the mention of anything but the most straightforward deliveries is likely to be counterproductive as it might increase anxiety. However, it is probably true that it is the unknown and unmentioned that provoke most fear, and experience suggests that mention of the more common hazards and the procedures that are used to avert their consequences is appropriate at least for those who have a raised risk of having an abnormal baby. The mere fact that techniques like ventilation or transfer to a regional centre have been briefly mentioned prenatally may allow a much more satisfactory discussion of options of parents whose fetus *in utero* or newborn baby is in jeopardy.

A more complex component of education which would facilitate public and thus parental understanding of neonatal care, and perhaps result in less parental anxiety about their sick neonate, is to create a greater awareness of precisely what neonatal intensive care actually does. The incorrect view that neonatal intensive care merely saves a few babies who would otherwise have died, for a life of profound handicap, and that the agonies of babies who are bound to die are unnecessarily prolonged, needs to be dispelled, as does the equally incorrect, but somewhat paradoxical anxiety, that life support is being withdrawn from many seriously ill, abnormal and deformed babies because the medical profession, but no one else, feels that their future life of handicap would be so unbearable that death is the preferable alternative.

Practising within the constraints arising from these paradoxical anxieties is something that all neonatal paediatricians will have to learn. However their lot can only be made easier by better public understanding of, for example, the chances of neurologically intact outcome for a baby of 27 weeks gestation weighing 800 grams, or for infants surviving perinatal asphyxia or neonatal surgery, or the ultimate quality of life for a child with severe spina bifida.

Handling this public education is difficult. The more sensationalist press has failed in this respect, with dramatic accounts of what are extreme forms of management in extreme cases. Such excesses, by polarising views, can only heighten parental anxiety that *their* child will be treated in some routine, and to them unacceptable, way. But equally, silence on these matters can only encourage suspicion. Perhaps all we can hope for is a gradually increasing awareness of specific problems, backed up by good antenatal teaching, and appropriate, patient, and if necessary repetitive, explanation and discussion when a problem arises for a given family.

Decision making and the holding of responsibility by committees carries grave disadvantages. Nevertheless, discussion with informed and interested lawyers, clergymen and members of other professional and parent groups may be a useful intellectual exercise for all those involved in areas of ethical conflict in neonatal care and will undoubtably help to clarify and bring into sharp focus aspects of their own practice and philosophy which may be woolly and underdeveloped. It is extremely unlikely that a consensus view could be obtained from wide public discussion on, for example, when it is appropriate to discontinue life support in a baby with brain damage but still with electrical EEG activity, operate on children with Down's syndrome or spina bifida, or struggle to sustain life in an infant weighing just over half a kilogram. Furthermore, it is completely impracticable to think that one could apply any such consensus to an individual baby. Each baby has parents from vastly different religious and socio-economic backgrounds, with different ethical values and different concepts of the impact of handicap on their baby and themselves. Coping with each new case which poses these problems is therefore an individual exercise for which only the adequately trained neonatal paediatrician, knowing that he has the support and confidence of his colleagues, will have the breadth of professional knowledge and extent of professional experience to handle.

However, if possible, within the constraints already mentioned, this must always be done with the parents completely and continuously informed. There are some disturbing accounts[3] of how parents can be excluded from decisions about the care of their own infants. Working with parents is a difficult matter, particularly in the context of neonatal care, when complex matters may need to be explained and time may be of the essence. We need to learn much more about how best to carry out these crucial discussions. However, the basic principles are clear; it is parents who will rear their child and it is they who will live with whatever decisions were made neonatally. Experience has already taught us that if there is a sense of exclusion at the beginning, this can become a long-standing anger that can colour all subsequent dealings with a child. If a baby is handicapped, child care can make enormous physical and emotional demands on parents. This will be the fate of a small number of children who pass through NNUs. For these parents in particular, it is the sense of a partnership and a common goal with those involved in providing neonatal care that can make all the difference. The saddest possible situation is where the parents of a handicapped child feel that their child is a failure of the neonatal care system and so is shunned by those who were responsible for the early care.

Planning for the Future

Our guess is that there will be no major breakthroughs in neonatal paediatrics in the near future, though better intrapartum care at short gestation, and techniques for antenatal induction of surfactant or use of artificial surfactant postnatally, are likely to reduce considerably the number of infants severely affected by hyaline membrane disease.[4,5] More and more time is, however, likely to be spent in the care of very low birthweight infants between 500 g (the likely lower limit of viability, imposed by the stage of pulmonary development at this weight) and 800 g birthweight. Already many units are seeing a large number of such infants who have spent months in the unit, requiring artificial ventilation, parenteral nutrition and often complex abdominal and thoracic surgery. For such infants the requirements in terms of parental support and encouragement outlined in this book will be more intense and more prolonged than ever before.

Solutions to the problems of attitude, accessibility, education and ethics of neonatal care, alluded to above, are already appearing and will continue to evolve over the years to come. Human history is, after all, replete with statements about the impossibility of doing things that we have subsequently learnt to do quite easily. However, to facilitate and expedite the solving of these problems we would highlight three areas where we believe there is considerable room for improving attitudes and facilities.

First, we would like to see improvement in the design of neonatal units, though this will have to be a gradual change as old buildings are replaced by new. With the almost unique exception of the unit described by Donald Garrow in Chapter 16, the neonatal units built in Britain and elsewhere have been designed on a rather uniform pattern. In the past the tendency, not surprisingly, has been to view a unit more in the terms of those who work there and less from the perspective of an anxious parent: thus many units have all the internal partitioning glazed, allowing staff maximum visibility but parents no privacy. While it is unlikely that an architect can please everybody all the time, there does seem to be a lot of scope for something rather more imaginative in the design of new units. Hospital design is a very complex matter and to a considerable extent governed by edicts emerging from governments which allow for little latitude in the design of individual units, and may be based on precepts of neonatal unit utilisation and care which are out of date. It should now be crystal clear that there needs to be much greater provision of mother/parent-baby rooms, as well as associated facilities for the parents such as dining rooms, TV lounges and children's playrooms in all neonatal units. There also needs to be a greater flexibility permitted in the design of the units depending on whether they have a large proportion of referral infants, many high-risk cases, or only deal with a tight-knit local community living very close to the maternity hospital.

Secondly we would like to see more staff of all types on the neonatal unit. More properly trained physicians and nurses, who not only have more time to do the basic physical chores of neonatal intensive care, but also are therefore more likely to do them better, will also have sufficient time to spend in supporting, helping and talking to parents, and because they are less stretched and stressed, are less likely to develop the overt problems of 'burnout'.[6] It should be recognised that social workers, psychotherapists and many other types of ancillary professional should be an integral component of the staffing complement of a neonatal intensive care unit, and not a fringe luxury in a few eccentric or privately funded nurseries.

Thirdly, and most important, we would like to emphasise the importance of teaching the attitudes promulgated in this book to all who work in neonatal units. Hopefully new residents will have it drummed into them by senior medical staff, and nurses in training will learn it through the specialised courses for neonatal intensive care which include such topics in their curriculum, but we also hope that ward clerks, social workers, laboratory technicians, radiographers and all the multitude of other staff in neonatal units, will be educated along similar lines – best of all, perhaps, by the example of good practice.

These improvements do, of course, have financial implications which raise perhaps the most fundamental ethical question we have to face, which is the proportion of resources available for medical care that should be devoted to neonatal units. The question is a very complex one involving not only very broad issues about the kind of society which we wish to live in, but also specific and technical questions about what might be achieved by the deployment of new techniques.

It has to be remembered that neonatal intensive care is an *in*expensive specialty to run compared with general adult intensive care, and particularly compared with specialties such as heart and liver transplantion, coronary care and some of the regimes of therapy for malignant disease, all of which have a much less certain justification and are considerably more expensive. Nevertheless, NNUs are but one element of a perinatal health service and we must constantly strive to balance the competing needs in that area. It is only with a wide understanding and confidence in what the neonatologist is trying to do that we can expect the development of the most appropriate facilities for the sick and pre-term baby. We hope that this book will go some way to achieving that end.

References

1. Smith, M. A., and Baum, J. D. (1983). *The Cost of Visiting Babies in Special Care Baby Units. Arch. Dis. Child, 58,* 56.

2. Hawthorne, J. T., Richards, M. P. M., and Callon, M. (1978). A study of parental visiting of babies in a specialised unit. In *Separation and Special Care Baby Units*, F. S. W. Brimblecombe, M. P. M. Richards and N. R. C. Roberton (eds), Clinics in Developmental Medicine, No. 68. London, SIMP/Heinemann Medical Books, pp. 33-54.

3. Stinson, R., and Stinson, P. (1981). On the death of a baby. *Journal of Medical Ethics*, *7*, 5-18.

4. Morley, C. J., Bangham, A. D., Miller, N., and Davis, J. A. (1981). Dry artifical surfactant and its effects on very premature babies. *Lancet*, *i*, 64-8.

5. Lucas, A., and Roberton, N. R. C. (1982). The care of the low birthweight infant. In *Recent Advances in Obstetrics and Gynaecology, No. 14*, J. Bonnar (ed.). Edinburgh, Churchill Livingstone, pp. 115-60.

6. Marshall, R. E., and Kasman, C. (1982). Burnout in the neonatal intensive care unit. *Pediatrics, 65,* 1161.

APPENDIX: A GUIDE FOR PARENTS OF BABIES IN THE SPECIAL CARE BABY UNIT

Joanna T. Hawthorne Amick

What follows is the text of a 20-page booklet made available to parents of babies in the Special Care Baby Unit, Maternity Hospital, Mill Road, Cambridge. Throughout the booklet the baby is referred to as 'he' for convenience.

This booklet has been prepared in order to answer some of the many questions you must have at this moment. Being separated from your baby after birth is upsetting and you probably feel anxious and worried. Even though your baby is having the best possible care, you may wish to know what you can do for him.

Babies have to stay in the Special Care Baby Unit (or SCBU) for many reasons. Your baby may be ill, or he may be a pre-term baby (born before 37 weeks gestation) or he may be of low birthweight (weighing under 2,500 grams (5½ lbs) at birth), or he may have some other problem. Some babies are small (light) for dates which means that they weigh less than is usual for the duration of the pregnancy. You have probably already talked to the doctor about your baby's particular condition and the treatment he will receive. This booklet describes generally some of the reasons a baby might be in the SCBU.

Visiting

The SCBU is open for parents to visit at any time of day or night. You are encouraged to visit frequently in order to get to know your baby and to keep him company. You can also stay as long as you like. Grandparents may also visit as may your other children. It is also possible for you to telephone the SCBU at any time. Information about the babies will be given to the parents only. Each time you visit, you will be asked to wash your hands before you touch your baby. In this way you will not pass any germs on to your baby.

If you have a cold or any signs of infection or illness please do not come into the SCBU without consulting the Sister on duty.

The SCBU often seems very crowded with medical equipment, doctors, nurses, parents and babies. You may feel frightened at first or useless and underfoot, but please remember that you are always welcome to visit your baby and the staff do not feel you are in the way. In fact it helps the nurses to have you visiting and looking after your baby. A doctor, sister, or nurse will always try to answer your questions, though if they are very busy they may not always have a chance to do so straightaway. Don't be afraid of asking them several times for information and explanations. They will always tell you as much as they know.

Sometimes you may come to visit and find that your baby has been moved to another room. This is often necessary depending on the type of care he requires. If you ring the bell before you come into the SCBU, one of the nurses will show you where your baby is.

When you are staying in the postnatal ward, it will be easy for you to visit at any time. Some mothers find it upsetting to be in the postnatal ward without their baby. Always remember that you can spend as long as you like with him in the SCBU. If you have had a Caesarian section you may not be able to see your baby right away. He may be brought to see you depending on his condition, or you will be wheeled in a chair to see him if necessary. It will be possible for you to have a Polaroid photograph of your baby if you cannot visit him right away or if he has been transferred from another hospital without you.

It may be possible for you to stay in the postnatal ward for the length of time your baby is in the SCBU, depending on the availability of beds. In this way, you can get to know your baby better before you leave hospital and have to visit from home. If you would like to lengthen your stay, discuss this with the Sister and your obstetrician (the hospital doctor who looks after you during your pregnancy).

Although some parents say that they find it upsetting to visit at first, especially if their baby is ill or small, when they look back at this time they are glad they saw their baby from the beginning. It is natural to feel anxious or upset. Parents sometimes feel that they don't want to get too close to their baby in case anything happens to him. However, psychologists have shown that parents feel much better if they get to know their baby as soon as possible so that they can see what he is really like rather than imagining the worst from a distance. You are encouraged to visit often, to touch, cuddle and talk to your baby as well as to participate in his care as much as possible. The most important thing to remember now is that you, the parents, are the people your baby needs most.

Visiting from Home

Often the distance between your home and the hospital, the care of your other children, or a transport problem can make visiting difficult. If you would like some financial help with transport costs, ask the Sister on duty who will inform the social worker. You may have been away from your other children for some time already and they may not understand why you keep leaving them. A clear and simple explanation about their new brother or sister will help, along with a photograph of the baby if possible. Perhaps you can keep a growth chart at home so they can watch the baby gaining weight.

The Special Care Baby Unit

The Unit was purpose-built in 1969. It has room for 24 babies. The unit is divided into six separate rooms. One or two are used as intensive care rooms where the baby will be if he is ill enough to require special treatment. When he is better, he will be moved to one of the other rooms. If your baby has an infection, he will be cared for in a room by himself. In order to keep the babies warm, the temperature in the SCBU must be high. You are advised to wear light clothes in order to be comfortable while visiting.

Mother-and-baby Room

Near the SCBU there is a bedroom for mothers with a kitchen and bathroom for their use. It is possible for you to come and stay here to be near your baby. You may be asked to stay here with him for about two days before he is discharged home, especially if he has had to stay in the SCBU for some time. This gives you a chance to get to know your baby better before you take him home. Most mothers are delighted to be able to be alone with their babies at last, and also to know that they can ask the staff if they have any questions. This also gives you a chance to look after him on your own, feed him and bath him. The staff will explain the dosages of any medicine or vitamins which your baby will need to take when he goes home.

If it is extremely difficult for you to come to stay with your baby overnight because of your other children, you are encouraged to come to spend the day in the mother-and-baby room. If you would like to come at any other time while your baby is in the Unit, please ask the Sister on duty.

When you are in the mother-and-baby room you will eat your meals with the other mothers on postnatal ward 7B. When you come to stay, it is suggested that you might like to bring your own radio, a book, or something else to do.

What You May See

In the intensive care rooms, you will see machines used to help the babies who have breathing difficulties. The most common cause for this is respiratory distress syndrome (RDS), a condition of some newborn babies in which they have difficulty in keeping their lungs inflated. If your baby has this condition and requires extra oxygen to breathe, a large plexiglass hood (or head box) will be placed over his head to increase the oxygen content in the air he breathes.

There are other machines called ventilators which help to expand the baby's lungs when he cannot do it himself. If your baby requires ventilation, he will have a tube down his throat or nose, leading to his lungs. In order for the tube to stay firmly in place it is usually strapped over the baby's head with bandages. He may also be wearing little gloves, so that he cannot pull out any of the tubes, and a hat and bootees to keep him warm.

When your baby is admitted, he will probably be put in an incubator. The main purpose of the incubator is to keep him warm; this is very important if he is ill or small or was cold at delivery. Small babies tend to lose heat rapidly and need help to keep themselves warm. An incubator is the best place in which to do this. It also makes it easier for the staff to observe him, and for this reason he is usually left undressed.

Your baby may have small paper discs taped to his chest, arms or legs with wires leading to a monitor. The monitors record his heart beat, respiration and blood pressure. You will probably hear the ticking sound made by these monitors. The monitors are also equipped with alarms that sound if your baby's condition changes. He will be taken off the monitor as soon as he is better. He may also spend some time on an apnoea mattress which monitors his breathing.

Intravenous Medicine or Feeding

If your baby needs to be given medicine or food intravenously (directly into the blood) he may receive it either through an umbilical catheter (thin tube passed into his umbilical artery or vein) or through a scalp vein. Scalp veins are more accessible in small babies and the needle is easier to keep in place. The needle is small and does not hurt your baby once it has been inserted. In order to find a vein into which the needle can be inserted, it may be necessary to shave some of your baby's hair. This will grow back, but it may take several weeks to do so. The needle may be held in place by some plaster of Paris which will be washed off when the needle is taken out.

Phototherapy

If your baby has jaundice (yellowness of the skin due to the accumulation of a pigment in the body), he will be put under the fluorescent lights which will eliminate his jaundice. This treatment is called phototherapy.

One-third of all newborn babies get mild jaundice between 2-6 days of age. It is not an illness as in other types of jaundice in adults. If your baby needs treatment, he may be under the light for several days until the jaundice clears. When he is under the light he must wear a mask to shield his eyes from it since it is very bright. If you are bottle or breast feeding your baby he may be removed from under the light at feeding times, and his mask can be taken off while you feed him.

Low birthweight babies who are ill are more prone to this condition.

Occasionally, if the jaundice persists, your baby may need an exchange blood transfusion to wash away the pigment-filled blood.

Special Tests

If your baby is ill, and particularly if he is in the intensive care rooms, he will need several types of blood tests done. The blood is usually obtained from a catheter (thin tube) that is inserted into his umbilical artery or vein. Blood may otherwise be obtained from a heel prick or from an arm vein as in an adult. All these tests guide the doctors and nurses in deciding what treatment your baby needs. If he is having trouble with his breathing a blood-gas test will tell how effectively he is breathing, and the amount of oxygen the baby is breathing can be adjusted if necessary and other medicines given if indicated. A great deal can be told about a newborn baby's condition by various tests done on the blood.

Other tests on your baby may include X-rays, electrocardiograms (ECG or heart tracings) and blood pressure measurements. The staff will be pleased to explain these tests to you.

If your baby requires an operation, he will be sent to Addenbrooke's Hospital in Cambridge or possibly a hospital in London, depending on his condition. He will be transported in an ambulance in a special portable incubator to keep him warm. The doctor or nurse with your baby will have all the necessary equipment required to look after him during the journey. It may be possible for you to go with your baby. The Sister on duty can tell you.

Your Feelings

The doctor will have already informed you about your baby's problems. As much information as possible will be given to you.

Although it is natural for you to search for the causes of low birthweight, premature delivery or illness in your baby, it is hard to pinpoint one cause in an individual case. This is a matter you should discuss with the obstetrician and paediatrician. Perhaps the course of your pregnancy was perfectly normal. Some mothers feel that it is something they did that caused their babies' problem, but there is no reason to blame yourselves.

It is quite natural to feel worried and upset when your baby is in the SCBU. When he is small and ill you may worry about his chances of survival. Later on when he is holding his own, you may still have worries and doubts about whether he will continue to improve and whether or not he will develop normally. Because you're anxious and perhaps shocked you may find it difficult to believe your baby is really alright when the staff tell you this. It is a normal reaction to need constant reassurance.

Most parents find it difficult to feel that they really do have a baby when he has to stay in the SCBU. They often feel he is a little stranger.

These feelings may last for a long time. The best way to get to know him is to visit as much as possible, stay as long as you can and do as much as you can for him.

Looking After Your Baby

You can help to feed your baby from the very beginning, either by tube bottle or the breast. There are other things you can do as well. If he is in an incubator you can hold his hand and stroke him, change his nappies through the port-holes and hold him out of the incubator for a short time as soon as his condition permits. When he is in a cot, you can change his gown and nappies, and his cot sheet and blankets. You will also be able to bath your baby or give him a wash with Hibitane cream.

Your baby wants to get to know you and likes to be held and talked to by his mother and father like any newborn baby. He will soon learn the sound of your voices and may turn his head towards you. When he is awake, he may like to look at your face and may notice light, bright colours and patterns. If you would like to bring in a new, clean toy for your baby, arrange this with the Sister on duty.

If your baby is very small, it may seem frightening to handle him at first. However, he will not break and you'll find that you will get used to his size quite quickly.

Staff Looking After Your Baby

Your baby is cared for by a staff of experienced doctors, sisters and nurses. In the intensive care area one nurse is assigned to care for one or two babies, and in the other areas, one nurse is assigned to care for three or four babies.

The Senior Nursing Officer in charge of the SCBU is Miss Whitby. There are five Sisters. Other staff in the SCBU are: Staff Midwives, Staff Nurses, Nursery Nurses, Student Nurses and Nursing Auxiliaries. There are also trained nurses taking a special Neonatal Nursing Course in the SCBU.

A Senior Paediatrician (children's doctor) is in the Unit most of the time, who specialises in the care of the newborn and is concerned with the day-to-day running of the Unit. In addition there are three full-time doctors (house officers) who work in the Unit for six months at a time. The Paediatric Registrars from Addenbrooke's Hospital (New Site) are also involved in the care of the infants in the SCBU. Some medical students who are learning more about neonatology (the care of infants during the first 28 days of life), may also be working in the SCBU.

There is a social worker in the hospital, who is available to help with difficulties you may have in the way of money, accommodation, travelling expenses and also problems with personal relationships in the family. She is also there to advise you on services that are available outside, which you may need either now or at a later stage. If you would like to see her, you can ring her at the hospital number in the mornings, or ask the Sister on duty. The health visitor attached to the SCBU will inform you local health visitor about your baby's condition. There is a special liaison between the hospital health visitor and your own health visitor. They are responsible for helping with the care of you and your baby once he goes home. Your health visitor may also visit you for a chat while your baby is still in the SCBU and you are at home. Your GP will be sent a letter about your baby when he is discharged.

If you would like to have your baby christened, there is a hospital chaplain available for you to talk to and the Sister on duty will help you with the necessary arrangements.

Tube Feeding

If your baby is ill or small, his sucking reflex will be too weak for him to be fed by a bottle or the breast, so he will be fed through a small tube passed through his nose and into his stomach. This tube will be kept in place by adhesive tape on his face. If your baby is pre-term, he will usually be able to start sucking at 35 weeks from his conception. Other babies can start sucking when their condition permits. If he is very small or ill his feeds will be given hourly or two-hourly initially and then will be gradually decreased to three or four-hourly as his condition improves. He may then be taken out of his incubator and fed by bottle or the breast.

You will be told when your baby can have his first breast or bottle feed. At first, he will receive one bottle or breast feed a day, then gradually increase until he can have alternate tube and bottle (or breast) feeds. When he can have all bottle (or breast) feeds, the tube will be removed.

Breast Feeding

Even though your baby may be ill, small or pre-term, you may still be able to breast-feed him once he is better and his weight has increased. Until that time, you can express your milk for him.

Breast milk is the best milk for your baby, especially when he is ill or small, and so you are encouraged to express your milk, especially the high protein milk of the first week. The staff of the SCBU and post-natal ward will show you how to express the milk from your breasts so that it can be given to your baby. In addition, by regularly expressing your breasts you will stimulate your lactation in the same way as a baby suckling. In this way, your lactation can be established and maintained until your baby is big enough and fit enough to go to the breast.

It is important to remember that if you want to keep your milk flowing, you must always empty both your breasts every four hours (or five or six times daily). The SCBU staff will give you bottles in which to store your milk. You can keep the bottles in your refrigerator at home for up to 48 hours only, or in your deep-freeze for a longer period until you can bring it in for your baby. The staff will make sure that your baby receives your milk.

Even if your baby has to stay in the SCBU after you are discharged from hospital, you can express your milk at home with a hand-pump which you get on prescription from the chemist, or a mechanical pump which you may be able to hire. The Sister on duty can give you details on how to hire a mechanical breast pump. There are mechanical pumps on the SCBU and Ward 7B which you can use while you are in hospital or when you come to visit. It is important to learn the correct method of using these pumps in order to make expressing easier for you.

It can be difficult to keep your milk flowing, especially if your baby has to be in the SCBU for a long time. Worry or anxiety or living far away from the Unit, so that you are unable to visit frequently, also may have the effect of decreasing your milk flow. It can be just as tiring to express your milk for your baby as it can be to breast-feed him. Expressing also takes time and perseverance. However, feeding your baby yourself is a positive thing you can do for him at the moment. When your baby is well enough, you will be able to come in to breast-feed him several times a day in his room in the SCBU. If you would prefer some privacy, you may be able to breast-feed in a room on your own. You may prefer to come to the mother and baby room before your baby's discharge in order to establish breast feeding.

If you have a lot of milk, you might like to donate any extra to the milk bank which stores breast milk in the SCBU. Mothers from the community also send in any extra milk they may produce. Even a small amount of breast milk can feed a tiny baby for several days.

Bottle Feeding

The bottle milk which is used in the SCBU is close to the composition of human milk. As soon as your baby is well enough to feed from a bottle, you can feed him yourself. When you are visiting from home, you can telephone the SCBU to see what time your baby's feeds will be that day.

Weight

It is quite normal for your baby to lose weight during the first week of life. Babies who are ill or small may continue to lose weight for longer. It may take two weeks or more before your baby gradually starts to put on weight again. Don't be disappointed if one day he loses weight or stays the same because the next day he might gain. These variations are quite normal. Once your baby has started gaining weight and is feeding well, he will gain about 200 grams (6½-7 oz.) per week. When your baby weighs about 1500 grams (3 lb. 5 oz.) he will be transferred from his incubator to a cot if his condition permits. When your baby weighs about 2,000 grams (4lb. 7 oz.), he will be able to go home if there are no other problems and he is feeding well.

The babies are weighed every day, and their length, head circumference and chest circumference are measured every week. There is a conversion chart for kilos into pounds and metres into inches at the back of this booklet.

What Your Baby Looks Like

By the sixteenth week of pregnancy, the fetus is fully formed, so if your baby is born early, he will be small but perfectly developed.

If your baby is pre-term, his head may look too big for his body. This is only a stage in his development and will be perfectly normal when he reaches term. His chest may look small to you and his abdomen large but this too will change with age. Your baby's legs and arms may look skinny and his skin may look folded and is covered with a light covering of hair. He will fill out as he grows older – his skin allows him room to grow! The hair will gradually disappear. Your baby will also sleep quite a lot until he is older or feeling better. All newborn babies sleep for 20 hours a day or more.

A tiny pre-term baby may seem to you to move in a strange way. This is because his ability to control his movements is not fully developed owing to his immaturity. When he reaches his expected date of delivery he will move just like any other newborn baby. Small babies can be very strong so there is no need to fear that you may hurt him by handling him.

Babies Transferred from Other Hospitals

Your baby may have been sent to this SCBU from another hospital because this Unit is the one in the region specially equipped to look after small and ill babies. Every effort will be made to transfer you to the postnatal ward here to be near your baby if you so wish. If you cannot come with your baby you can telephone the SCBU about his progress and come to visit him as soon as you are able. When your baby is better, he may be transferred to a hospital near where you live. The staff will usually send you a Polaroid photograph of your baby if you cannot be near him.

Discharge

It can seem a long time before you are finally able to take your baby home. You may have been feeling tense, edgy and irritable at home or at work and you may have found it difficult to concentrate or to settle into your normal routines. It helps to talk your feelings over with others. When the staff finally tell you that he is ready to go home, you may feel nervous or unsure even though it is an exciting moment. Parents are so often anxious about taking home a baby who was ill or small at birth. This is quite a normal feeling. Getting to know your baby while he is in the Unit will help you.

Your baby will be discharged from the SCBU when he weighs about 2,000 grams, provided he is medically well and feeding normally. When he is discharged you can treat him like any other baby. You can take him out in his pram, as long as he is warmly clothed and wrapped. Here are some answers to the most usual questions from parents:

Q. How long can you leave the baby before waking him for a feed, especially at night?

A. Feed the baby as late as possible and leave through the night if he will sleep. Do not leave more than five hours during the day time.

Q. How careful should the mother be in protecting the baby from infectious diseases, e.g. common cold in the family?

A. The baby need not be protected from its own immediate family, mother, father, brothers and sisters (as this would be virtually impossible) but avoid other people and other children, especially those with colds, from kissing, etc., the baby.

Q. When should the baby be vaccinated?

A. Discuss this with your doctor or health visitor. The times are different in different parts of East Anglia. The usual times in Cambridgeshire are:

(1) 3-4 months old – diphtheria and tetanus, polio, and whooping cough
(2) 6-8 weeks later – repeated
(3) 4-6 months later – repeated

Q. How will the premature baby grow during the first year?

A. Babies who are just premature will gain weight normally. Babies who are small for dates will usually stay comparatively small for their age.

Q. With the greater risk of anaemia in the premature baby, should he be weaned earlier, or continue with vitamins and iron supplements in his feed?

A. He should not be weaned earlier, but be given iron and vitamin supplements as prescribed by the doctor.

Q. How long should you keep the baby's room at a temperature of 70°F?

A. The baby will very quickly adapt to your own home temperature and provided he is well wrapped or the room is warm, you need not worry after the first 3-4 weeks.

Q. When can you take the baby out?

A. As soon as he goes home.

Q. What size hole should the feeding bottle teat have for a premature baby?

A. Large-holed teat at first; then medium.

Q. How far in advance can I make up the feeds?

A. Feeds can be made and kept for 24 hours in the fridge, but no longer.

Q. Can I use a hot water bottle to keep the baby warm?
A. Hot water bottles are dangerous and you should not use them at all for your baby.

It is important to prevent your baby getting too fat. The best way is:

- not to make bottle feeds 'stronger' by adding extra scoops of powder,
- not to add more than the recommended amount of sugar to the baby's bottle, and don't give sweetened drinks,
- not to add cereals or rusks to the baby's bottle,
- not to introduce solid foods too early; keep your baby on milk only for at least 10-12 weeks, preferably until he is three months old (from his expected date of delivery and not from his actual birth-date).

Follow-up

Your health visitor will come to visit you when your baby goes home. She is a trained nurse and often a midwife who has had further training and experience in caring for babies as they grow up. She will give you advice on feeding, and on any other matters that may be worrying you. She will also give you the address of your nearest child health clinic where you can go to weigh your baby or ask questions. If you need any further help you should consult your GP or you may ring the SCBU at any time.

There is a Baby Clinic held at Mill Road every Tuesday afternoon. You may be asked to bring your baby back to one of these Clinics or to the SCBU for a check-up. The doctors like to follow up some babies for 1-2 years depending on their problems at birth.

Just as full-term babies develop at different rates, so do pre-term babies who were very ill at birth also develop at different rates at first. Babies reach their own developmental milestones such as smiling, sitting without support, standing and walking at a set time from conception. If your baby was born two months early, he will appear to be two months late in reaching his milestones. By the time he is two years old, these differences will be very small, so this initial difference is nothing to worry about.

At Home with Your Baby

It can be tiring to have a new baby in the house, so try to get enough rest and let the housework wait. You will find it almost a full-time job looking after the baby. Small babies sometimes need feeding more often and take longer over their feeds than larger babies. Just enjoy your baby, follow his needs and you will both be content.

If you would like to talk to other parents who have had a baby in the Special Care Baby Unit in the past, or meet others whose baby is in at the same time as yours, please tell the Sister on duty. If you don't mind talking to other parents, perhaps you would like to leave your name and address with the Sister.

We hope this booklet has answered some of the many questions you may have at the moment. The doctors and nurses want you to feel that you can share in the care of your baby while he is in the SCBU. Any observations you make of your baby are important to the staff. They also welcome any ideas you have which can make this period easier for you and your baby.

Chart for Conversion of Grams into Pounds and Ounces
(100 grams = 3½ ounces)

grams	lbs	ounces	grams	lbs	ounces
700	1	8	2,000	4	6½
740	1	9½	2,040	4	8
800	1	11½	2,100	4	10
840	1	13	2,140	4	11½
900	1	15½	2,200	4	13½
940	2	1	2,240	4	15
1,000	2	3	2,300	5	1
1,040	2	4½	2,340	5	3
1,100	2	7	2,400	5	4½
1,140	2	8	2,440	5	6
1,200	2	10½	2,500	5	8
1,240	2	11½	2,540	5	9½
1,300	2	14	2,600	5	11½
1,340	2	15	2,640	5	13
1,400	3	1½	2,700	5	15
1,440	3	3½	2,740	6	0½
1,500	3	5	2,800	6	3
1,540	3	6	2,840	6	4
1,600	3	8½	2,900	6	6½
1,640	3	10	2,940	6	7½
1,700	3	12	3,000	6	10
1,740	3	13½	3,040	6	11
1,800	3	15½	3,100	6	13½
1,840	4	1	3,140	6	14½
1,900	4	3	3,200	7	1
1,940	4	4½	3,240	7	2½

Approximate Conversion Chart for Centimetres to Inches

Centimetres	Inches
1.0	0.4
2.5	1.0
5.0	2.0
10.0	4.0
13.0	5.0
15.0	6.0
18.0	7.0
20.0	8.0
23.0	9.0
25.0	10.0
30.0	12.0
35.0	14.0
40.0	16.0
45.0	18.0
51.0	20.0
55.0	22.0
60.0	24.0
65.0	26.0

Glossary

Apnoea	Periods of cessation of breathing.
Aspiration	Entrance of fluids or secretions (meconium, mucus, stomach juices) into windpipe and lungs.
Bilirubin	A pigment produced in the breakdown of red blood cells, causing jaundice.
Blood gas	Laboratory test to determine the amount of oxygen and carbon dioxide in the blood. It reflects lung function and to some degree heart function.
Bradycardia	Slowing of the heartbeat.
Continuous positive airways pressure	A way of giving oxygen under pressure to a baby when he has RDS. It gets more oxygen into the baby's blood than when he breathes on his own.
Cyanosis	Condition in which the skin, lips and nailbeds are bluish in colour from lack of adequate oxygen in the blood.
Dextrostix	A reagent strip which gives a colour change proportional to the level of glucose in the baby's blood.
Endotracheal tube	A tube inserted into the windpipe (trachea) to maintain an open airway and to assist ventilation or breathing.

Gestational age	Age of the unborn baby in weeks from the time of conception.
Grunting	Deep, short noises heard when a baby is having difficulty breathing.
Heat shield	Plexiglass half-cylinder placed over a small baby to concentrate heat around his body.
Headbox	Plexiglass box placed over a baby's head to deliver oxygen.
Incubator	Enclosed plexiglass cot which provides the baby with proper warmth and humidity.
Intravenous (IV)	Tube inserted directly into a vein. Used to deliver nourishment from various solutions or to administer medication.
Jaundice	Yellowish colour of the skin caused by an excess of bilirubin in the blood.
Kilogram (kg)	A unit of weight: 1 kilogram = 2.2 pounds 2½ kilograms = 5½ pounds.
Lumbar puncture	Inserting a needle through the baby's back into the fluid around the spinal cord to check for the presence of infection.
Meconium	Dark greenish waste product that accumulates during fetal life and is expelled as the first bowel movement (stool).

Oxygen (O_2) — Colourless, odourless gas found in the air and drawn into the lungs by the process of respiration. Room air, or the amount of oxygen in the normal atmosphere, is 21 per cent. Various equipment can be used to supplement room air up to 100 per cent oxygen.

Phototherapy — Treatment for jaundice by fluorescent lights placed over the incubator or cot. An eye mask is used to shield the baby's eyes from the light.

Pneumothorax — Trapped air leaking outside the lung and accumulating under the chest wall. This air takes up space and can cause the lung to collapse. It can be drained with a chest catheter so the lung can re-expand.

RDS — Respiratory Distress Syndrome or Hyaline Membrane Disease: a disease of premature babies due to immaturity of their lungs.

Retraction — Pulling in of the chest wall during inspiration.

SUBJECT INDEX

AUTHOR INDEX